vironments

erceptions
and Objective Measures

Obesogenic Environments

Complexities, Perceptions and Objective Measures

Edited by

Amelia A. Lake
BSc(Hons), RD, RPHNutr, PhD

Tim G. Townshend
BA(Hons), MA

Seraphim Alvanides
MA, PhD, FRGS

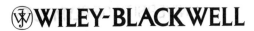

WILEY-BLACKWELL

A John Wiley & Sons, Ltd., Publication

This edition first published 2010
© 2010 Blackwell Publishing Ltd

Blackwell Publishing was acquired by John Wiley & Sons in February 2007. Blackwell's publishing programme has been merged with Wiley's global Scientific, Technical, and Medical business to form Wiley-Blackwell.

Registered office: John Wiley & Sons Ltd, The Atrium, Southern Gate, Chichester, West Sussex, PO19 8SQ, United Kingdom

Editorial offices: 9600 Garsington Road, Oxford, OX4 2DQ, United Kingdom
            2121 State Avenue, Ames, Iowa 50014-8300, USA

For details of our global editorial offices, for customer services and for information about how to apply for permission to reuse the copyright material in this book please see our website at www.wiley.com/wiley-blackwell.

The right of the author to be identified as the author of this work has been asserted in accordance with the Copyright, Designs and Patents Act 1988.

Wiley also publishes its books in a variety of electronic formats. Some content that appears in print may not be available in electronic books.

Designations used by companies to distinguish their products are often claimed as trademarks. All brand names and product names used in this book are trade names, service marks, trademarks or registered trademarks of their respective owners. The publisher is not associated with any product or vendor mentioned in this book. This publication is designed to provide accurate and authoritative information in regard to the subject matter covered. It is sold on the understanding that the publisher is not engaged in rendering professional services. If professional advice or other expert assistance is required, the services of a competent professional should be sought.

Library of Congress Cataloging-in-Publication Data
Obesogenic environments : complexities, perceptions, and objective measures / edited by Amelia A. Lake, Tim G. Townshend, Seraphim Alvanides.
    p. ; cm.
  Includes bibliographical references and index.
  ISBN 978-1-4051-8263-8 (pbk. : alk. paper) 1. Obesity – Epidemiology. 2. Obesity – Prevention.
I. Lake, Amelia A. II. Townshend, Tim G. III. Alvanides, Seraphim.
  [DNLM: 1. Obesity – epidemiology. 2. Diet. 3. Environment. 4. Feeding Behavior – psychology.
5. Health Promotion – methods. 6. Obesity – etiology. WD 210 O129 2010]
  RC628.O333 2010
  614.5′9398 – dc22

                                                                                2010001847

A catalogue record for this book is available from the British Library.

Typeset in 10/12 Sabon by Laserwords Private Limited, Chennai, India
Printed in Singapore by Ho Printing Singapore Pte Ltd

1   2010

Contents

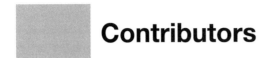

Contributors

Editors

Lake, Amelia A.
Senior Lecturer in Food and Nutrition, Applied Biosciences, School of Applied Sciences, Northumbria University, UK.

Dr Amelia A. Lake trained as a dietitian and worked in the NHS before taking up a research post with Newcastle University where she completed a Ph.D. and held a National Institute for Health Research Postdoctoral Fellowship on the theme of Obesogenic Environments. Amelia is currently a Senior Lecturer in Food and Nutrition at Northumbria University and her research interests include the obesogenic environment, food environments and food choice.

Townshend, Tim G.
Director of Planning and Urban Design and Senior Lecturer in Urban Design, School of Architecture, Planning and Landscape, Newcastle University, UK.

Tim Townshend is a Senior Lecturer, Director of Planning and Urban Design and a member of the Global Urban Research Unit (GURU) at the School of Architecture, Planning and Landscape, Newcastle University. He was recruited to academia from practice in 1993 and since then he has developed a national and international profile in a wide range of areas in urban design research, most recently exploring the links between urban form and obesity.

Alvanides, Seraphim
Social Geographer, School of Geography, Politics & Sociology, Newcastle University, UK.

Dr Seraphim Alvanides is an academic geographer with postgraduate studies in computational geography and consultancy experience in geographical project management. His current research is concerned with the evaluation of obesogenic environments and environmental supportiveness for physical activity within an environmental justice framework.

Contributing authors

Ball, Kylie
Associate Professor, Centre for Physical Activity and Nutrition Research, Deakin University, Melbourne, Australia.

Brown, Caroline
Research Associate, School of the Built Environment, Heriot-Watt University, Edinburgh, UK.

Brug, Johnannes
Director of the EMGO Institute for Health and Care Research, Chair of Division VI and the Department of Epidemiology & Biostatistics, and Professor of Epidemiology at the VU University Medical Center, Amsterdam, the Netherlands.

Cooper, Ashley
Reader in Exercise and Health Science, Department of Exercise, Nutrition and Health Science, Bristol University, UK.

Crawford, David
Alfred Deakin Professor and Director of the Centre for Physical Activity and Nutrition Research, Centre for Physical Activity and Nutrition Research, Deakin University, Melbourne, Australia.

Day, Peter
Researcher and GIS Analyst, GeoHealth Laboratory, Department of Geography, University of Canterbury, New Zealand.

Edwards, Kimberley L.
Lecturer in Epidemiology, Division of Epidemiology, Leeds Institute of Genetics, Health and Therapeutics, University of Leeds, UK.

Ells, Louisa
Obesity and Physical Activity Lead, North East Public Health Observatory, Wolfson Research Institute, University of Durham, Queen's Campus University Boulevard, Stockton on Tees, UK.

Giles-Corti, Billie
Winthrop Professor and Director, Centre for the Built Environment and Health, School of Population Health, The University of Western Australia, Crawley, Western Australia.

Grow, H. Mollie Greves
Assistant Professor of Paediatrics, Seattle Children's Hospital Research Institute and the University of Washington, USA.

Jackson-Leach, Rachel
Senior Policy Officer, International Association for the Study of Obesity, London, UK.

James, W. Phillip T.
President of the International Association for the Study of Obesity, Hon Prof. London School of Hygiene and Tropical Medicine, London, UK.

Jones, Andy
Reader, Centre for Diet and Activity Research (CEDAR), School of Environmental Sciences, University of East Anglia, Norwich, UK.

Mackett, Roger L.
Professor of Transport Studies, Centre for Transport Studies, University College London, UK.

Midgley, Jane L.
Lecturer in Planning, School of Architecture, Planning and Landscape, Newcastle University, UK.

Page, Angie
Senior Lecturer, Department of Exercise, Nutrition and Health Science, Bristol University, UK.

Panter, Jenna
Research Associate, Centre for Diet and Activity Research (CEDAR), School of Environmental Sciences, University of East Anglia, Norwich, UK.

Pearce, Jamie
Reader in Human Geography, Institute of Geography, School of GeoSciences, University of Edinburgh, Edinburgh, UK.

Rigby, Neville
Former Director of Policy and Public Affairs International Obesity TaskForce, London, UK.

Robertson-Wilson, Jennifer
Assistant Professor, Department of Kinesiology and Physical Education, Wilfrid Laurier University, Ontario, Canada.

Saelens, Brian E.
Associate Professor of Pediatrics and Psychiatry & Behavioral Sciences, Seattle Children's Hospital Research Institute and the University of Washington, USA.

Salmon, Jo
Associate Professor, Centre for Physical Activity and Nutrition Research, Deakin University, Melbourne, Australia.

Timperio, Anna
Senior Lecturer, Centre for Physical Activity and Nutrition Research, Deakin University, Melbourne, Australia.

Van Lenthe, Frank J.
Assistant Professor, Social Epidemiology, Department of Public Health, Erasmus Medical Centre Rotterdam, the Netherlands.

About the Editors

Dr Amelia A. Lake is a dietitian and public health nutritionist and works as a Senior Lecturer in Food and Nutrition at Northumbria University. Amelia's current work is to explore the obesogenic environment. She has particular interest in the food environment, the environments of young people and the workplace environment. Her research involves transdisciplinary collaborations to examine how the environment interacts with individual's behaviours. Amelia received her first degree from Glasgow Caledonian University and worked in the Health Service before taking up a research post with Newcastle University, where she completed a Ph.D. Amelia is a committee member of the Association for the Study of Obesity, a council member for the Nutrition Society and also member of the British Dietetic Association. Along with Tim Townshend, Amelia is a co-founder of the North East Obesogenic Environment Network (NEOeN; www.neoen.org.uk). Amelia is currently a Beacon for Public Engagement Fellow (www.ncl.ac.uk/beacon) apart-from being a regular contributor to her profession's publications. Amelia has extensive experience of working with non-specialist audiences as well as academics and has produced various training programmes and related material.

Tim G. Townshend is Senior Lecturer in urban design and a member of the Global Urban Research Unit (GURU) at Newcastle University; he has been Director of Planning and Urban Design since August 2008. Tim was recruited to academia from practice in 1993; since then he has developed a national/international profile in urban design research. He has published on a range of topics addressing the impact of the design of the built environment in relation to contemporary social concerns – in particular, fear of crime, sustainable neighbourhoods and, most recently, obesity. Tim is further interested in issues of transdiciplinarity and the role of transdisciplinary working in tackling complex issues. He has exemplary links into practice. His work attempts to maximise its impact and as such is always policy relevant. He has been a consultee on a series of planning policy documents and sits on a number of external committees and panels. Along with Amelia Lake, Tim is a co-founding member of the North East Obesogenic Environment Network (NEOeN) www.neoen.org.uk.

Dr Seraphim Alvanides is a social geographer with the Research Cluster Society, Space and Practice in Geography at Newcastle University. Seraphim has extensive experience of geographical information technologies from his engagement with practice and academic research. His current research interests involve the measurement and evaluation of obesogenic environments, focusing on physical activity within an environmental justice framework. Following his undergraduate studies, Seraphim was employed as a geographical project manager and consultant in the private sector. Subsequently, he returned to academia to complete an MA (with distinction) in Geographical Information Systems and a Ph.D. in Human Geography (University of Leeds, UK). He has since published on methodological aspects of geographical information science and its application in understanding the obesogenic environment. Seraphim is a Fellow of the Royal Geographical Society (with IBG) and a committee member of Geography of Health Research Group. He is committed to public engagement and outreach through consultancy projects with local authorities and voluntary organisations, as well as delivery of training programmes and events.

This book is dedicated to transdisciplinary working and international co-operation.

Acknowledgements

The editors would like to acknowledge the contribution of the chapter authors in developing this transdisciplinary volume. The international experts who have contributed to this volume are representative of a broad range of disciplines and illustrate the range of disciplines required to tackle the global issue of overweight and obesity.

In addition, the editors would like to acknowledge Carolyn Fahey who designed the front cover, the UK Government's Foresight Programme (Foresight Government Office for Science, Department of Innovation Universities and Skills, Crown Copyright URN 07/1179) for permission to use the Foresight Obesity Systems Map in Chapter 2 of this book and the World Health Organisation for permission to use Table 7 from p. 63 of the WHO 916 Report in Chapter 1 of this book. Every attempt has been made to contact copyright holders of materials used in this book.

1 An International Perspective on Obesity and Obesogenic Environments

W. Philip T. James,
Rachel Jackson-Leach
and Neville Rigby

1.1 Introduction: the emergence of obesity

The obesity epidemic started becoming a serious public health issue in most western societies only in the early 1980s.[1] The problem emerged later in lower income countries as they went through the extraordinary economic and societal changes accompanying what is known as the 'nutritional transition'. Nevertheless, in countries emerging from extreme circumstances, for example, in post-war Germany or in the richer classes of poor countries, for example, Brazil, women characteristically put on weight first; then the business man's 'paunch' became an index of success. The same persists in African countries where prevailing malnutrition is accentuated by the new fear of 'slim disease' – a consequence of HIV infection. Recent studies[2,3] show that in affluent societies obesity emerged in children in the early 1980s and since then has become an intense societal concern because no longer could one ignore the fact that environmental pressures must be a major factor in determining this extraordinary development.

Obesity was first highlighted as a major global concern by World Health Organisation (WHO) in 1997, preliminary work having been undertaken by the newly formed International Obesity Task Force (IOTF). In its report the full range of complications from excess weight gain were set out.[4] The WHO acceptance of 'normal' weights for a population was based on the body mass index (BMI) method for relating weight to height, that is, weight (kg)/[height (m)]^2. So people of normal shape and composition but of varying heights had the same BMI, with 'healthy' values being taken as between 18.5 and 25, for both men and women of all ages. These values were based on early US insurance figures.[1] However, the ready acceptance of the importance of obesity came with the WHO millennium analyses of the major risk factors underlying the burden of premature death and disability from all the major diseases throughout the world.[5] The IOTF's contribution[6] showed that the optimum average BMI for a population was only about 21 because the risk of diabetes, high blood pressure and coronary heart disease increased throughout the so called 'normal' range. Thus, the risk of diabetes was 5–6 times greater at a BMI of just under 25 than at BMIs of 21. Obese people – that is, with BMIs ≥ 30 – had more extreme risks.

1.2   The magnitude of the problem

The risks of weight gain include the development of diabetes, heart disease, strokes, high blood pressure, cancers of the breast (post-menopause), colon and rectum, kidney and gallbladder, together with physical handicaps, for example, arthritis. These effects made excess weight, that is, BMIs ≥ 21, rank as the sixth greatest global risk factor for all illnesses accounting for sickness and early death throughout the world! Since then, further analyses in 2006 by WHO, the World Bank and the Centers for Disease Control and Prevention in the United States showed that excess weight is now the third highest risk factor in the affluent world and is within the top 10 risk factors in the regions of the world with the poorest people.[7]

New IOTF analyses in 2008 showed that there were over 525 million obese adults, with over 1 billion already being overweight (BMIs 25–29.9). This problem is affecting ever younger adults; now in every region of the world, women aged 45–60 years have the maximum rates of overweight and obesity. In the Middle East over 80% of women are affected (of whom >40% are obese), these values exceeding the North American, Latin American, European and Oceania prevalences of >25–35% obesity, with a total prevalence for overweight and obesity of 50–70%. Only Africa and Asia have lower prevalences and even here the middle-aged have obesity rates of 8–15% with totals of 30–40% for BMIs ≥ 25. Men in general have lower values, with North American men showing the greatest prevalence of obesity. In most countries, 50–70% of middle-aged men have BMIs ≥ 25, with obesity rates of >30% in North America, and 15–20% in Latin America, Europe, Middle East and Oceania. Only Asia and Africa have significantly lower rates.

Within more affluent societies there is a strong relationship between the socio-economic circumstances of a group of children and adults and their susceptibility to gain weight. This also relates to their educational status, with the more affluent and educated groups having much lower obesity rates and a longer life expectancy.

1.3   The basis for the current underestimated burden of obesity

Childhood obesity rates now seem to be accelerating. Four years ago IOTF estimated that 10% of children in the world were overweight or obese[8] when the internationally accepted IOTF criteria of overweight were used.[9] Yet Figure 1.1 reveals that on average over 15% of the world's children are now affected; over one-third of North American (including Cuban) children are overweight or obese. Only Africa has an overall prevalence of <10%. The rates are going up remarkably rapidly and now there is clear evidence in affluent societies that even modestly overweight children have a greater lifelong risk of early death and cardiovascular disease, i.e. with high blood pressure, heart disease and strokes.[10] Thus, the current burden of ill-health from excess weight gain is an underestimate because the earlier an adult becomes overweight, the greater their future handicap. Current estimates of the burden of overweight and obesity have not included the future impact of such high proportions of overweight children now entering adult life.

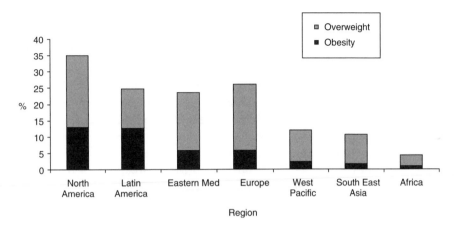

Figure 1.1 Overweight and obesity in children around the globe (based on IOTF cut off points).

The other underestimate of the impact of obesity relates to the fact that Asian communities are far more prone to developing type 2 diabetes and cardiovascular disease than Caucasian adults in western environments.[11] This is ascribed to genetic differences, but this is probably incorrect because the body's susceptibility to adult disease is often programmed by the health and nutritional status of the mother during pregnancy and the child's growth and well-being in the first 2 years of post-natal life. Thus, European and North American children who are born small and/or grow slowly in the first 2 years of life are much more susceptible to developing selective abdominal obesity with its higher risks of diabetes, cardiovascular disease and some cancers, particularly if they put on excess weight after 2 years of age. This is also evident in India, China and several other developing countries. In India it is being linked to vitamin B_{12} deficiency and abnormalities of the body's handling of folic acid metabolism probably exacerbated by low intakes of animal foods.[12] Asian adults, at any BMI above 23 (now considered the upper 'acceptable' BMI limit for Asians), have a 2–5 fold increased risk of diabetes and high blood pressure. Mexicans are also more susceptible to diabetes and hypertension than US non-Hispanic Whites and acquire the problems rapidly as they gain weight in early adult life.[13] So throughout the world the previously termed 'maturity-onset' diabetes is now being seen in early adult life and even in children, particularly in the poorer countries.

These data suggest that the majority of the world's populations may well be more prone to the consequences of excess weight gain than we originally thought. Therefore, given the prevalences of childhood overweight and obesity in the poorer parts of the world (Figure 1.1) we are now confronting a huge global medical problem. Medical costs are rising rapidly; financial analysts show that the medical costs of treatment have increased by 2% per annum above the economic growth of both affluent and poor countries for many decades and about 50% of the increasing medical costs in the United States relate to increasing rates of overweight and obesity. Many lower income countries, previously geared to coping with childhood malnutrition, are already overwhelmed with the problems of the adult chronic diseases. Already over 4 times as many adults die from cardiovascular disease in lower income countries as in Europe, North America, Australasia and Japan. World Bank also shows the irretrievable debts incurred by 40% of Indians' attempt to cover their medical care costs, and in China the latest parliamentary session recognised the medical plight of the hundreds of millions of poor Chinese rural dwellers as critical. Thus, whether we are dealing with rich or poor countries, the future medical costs are unsustainable. So the challenge is how to convert the political processes which focus on single, short-term solutions to recognise and respond to the need to prevent these problems.

1.4   Individual susceptibility to weight gain and the persistence of obesity

An individual's susceptibility to put on excess weight is very dependent on his or her genetic make-up. The effect is powerful and explains 50–75% of the difference in the range of weights within any one group living in a particular environment. Thus, in any socio-economic class or educational level those who develop obesity first are the genetically prone to weight gain. Their environmental circumstances or resulting behavioural patterns are still important but it is unwise to blame individuals within a society for their poor health. They can improve their prospects by changing their diet and physical activity patterns, but this is much more difficult for people who are susceptible to weight gain. Also, once adults have gained weight, it is now clear that the brain adapts – perhaps physically in terms of neural pathways – to resist subsequent slimming. This seems to be a strong contributor to the persistence of the epidemic despite the public pressure to lose weight and the billions of dollars spent on weight loss remedies. It is also true that the prevailing environmental pressures are intense; so to overcome these pressures, a family must create its own 'microenvironment' to cope. This is a task few can accomplish and there is much inappropriate prejudice relating to both obese children and adults' excess weight when the most appropriate response is to consider their environmental circumstances and their particular need for help.

1.5   The environmental basis for the obesity epidemic

The fundamental environmental basis for the obesity epidemic was recently highlighted by the UK government analysis known as the Foresight report.[14] Some implications of this report are summarised in Box 1.1. The emphasis on the normal biological response in terms of weight gain is important because it emphasises the environmental basis for the current epidemic. Therefore, one has to consider both the changes in the energy demand for physical work etc. as well as factors affecting food intake. The latest WHO summary of the factors affecting weight gain is given in Table 1.1. The fall in the demand for physical exertion seems to have come several

---

Box 1.1   Understanding the obesity epidemic and the need for prevention now

1   Obesity is a normal 'passive' biological response to our changed physical and food environment.

2   Some children or adults are more susceptible for genetic, social and economic reasons.

3   Overwhelming environmental impact reflects outcome of normal industrial development.

4   Obesity reflects failure of the free market.

5   Obesity is similar to climate change:

- Outcome of numerous societal and industrial developments/forces
- Action now essential – exceptionally difficult to reverse adult obesity
- No single remedy will suffice
- Coordinated central and local government, industrial, societal and individual changes necessary
- Major environmental changes needed – not just individual advice to eat less and walk more
- Immediate action necessary despite many logical remedies remaining unproven

---

Table 1.1   The contributors to the development of obesity as set out by WHO and categorised by the level of evidence for each contributor.

Evidence	Decreases risk	No relationship	Increases risk
Convincing	Regular physical activity. High dietary non-starch polysaccharides (NSP) (fibre) intake		High intake of energy-dense nutrient-poor foods. Sedentary lifestyles
Probable	Home and school environments that support healthy food choices for children.[a] Breastfeeding		Heavy marketing of energy-dense foods[a] and fast food outlets. Adverse social and economic conditions (in developed countries, especially for women) High intake of sugars – sweetened soft drinks and fruit juices
Possible	Low glycaemic index foods	Protein content of the diet	Large portion sizes High proportion of food prepared outside the home (western countries) 'Rigid restraint/periodic disinhibition' eating patterns
Insufficient	Increasing eating frequency		Alcohol

[a]Associated evidence and expert opinion.
Source: Table taken from Diet, Nutrition and the Prevention of Chronic Diseases, WHO 2003, TRS 916. Geneva

decades ago in affluent countries with the progressive mechanisation of society, which has reduced the need for physical work. Globally, one of the important factors has been urbanisation with the consequent reduction in the need for the strenuous physical work normally required of peasant farmers. Thus, we calculated that Chinese men and women, formerly living a hard farming life, on transfer to an urban setting but still involved in long hours of building activity or other forms of manual labour, reduced their energy needs by 300–400 kcal/day. This automatically means that this is the reduction in food intake needed by the brain's automatic regulatory system to prevent weight gain.[15] The differences between cycling to work, taking public transport or becoming sufficiently affluent to have one's own car are also important. Transferring from bicycles – the normal mode of Chinese transport 10 years ago – to public transport saves a further 150 kcal/day or so; having a car reduces the energy demand by about another 100 kcal/day. Thus, the total impact of increasing mechanisation, the constraints of city living and the pressure to sit watching television means that food intakes may need to fall by 400–800 kcal/day for a Chinese adult to compensate for the changes in their working and living conditions: it is a world away from the physical demands of their traditional agricultural subsistence way of life. Indeed, they readily opt for these changes perhaps because the evolutionary demand for intense and/or prolonged physical activity meant that the human race evolved to recognise the value of minimising the demands for physical work.

These dramatic changes with urbanisation and technological developments involve both irreversible processes and some options, for example, in the design of the urban physical and social environment. These options can either limit or promote routine and spontaneous physical activity and are primarily determined by central and local governments. These decision makers are, however, influenced by massive industrial pressures attempting to persuade us to use personal motorised transport, personal entertainment and gadgets which minimise the need for any physical activity in the home, in transport or at work. Table 1.2 summarises some of the optional changes in the physical environment which condition everyday physical activity. These changes are heavily influenced by industrial interests and have been very poorly analysed compared with those environmental factors affecting food intake.[16]

Food intakes should have fallen substantially throughout the world on the basis of the decades' long progressive fall in the demand for physical work, but for centuries societies everywhere have been concerned with food deprivation. Thus, in several countries intakes have risen and in others they have not fallen enough to match reducing energy needs. The cultural emphasis on food governs adults' responses to its value and their own perceived need for food as well as their approach to feeding their children. Furthermore, we have evolutionary mechanisms with specific taste buds linked to brain pleasure centres which respond positively to salt, meat, sweetness and fats in the form of essential fatty acids. Now these food components are abundantly available in the industrialised food chain which now forms the most powerful marketing consortium in the world. The global food chain is, therefore, completely inappropriate for a world which is now predominantly

Table 1.2   Inevitable and optional changes in physical activity.

Inevitable

- Rural to urban transition from agricultural work reducing demand for work
- Labour changes from manual to service occupations limiting activity
- Mechanisation/computerisation of standard work; also home duties, for example, cooking, washing, cleaning minimising physical exertion

Optional

- Urban building policies: high intensity or US style sprawl has huge impact on dominance of cars and pedestrian activity
- Road and community design affect safe and ready access for play/walking
- Office and supermarket location policies determine transport needs
- Car/traffic policies based on preference for cyclists/pedestrians?
- Policies on free spaces for children's play; lighting for safety, e.g. for older people
- Park/leisure/sports facilities/school physical activity lessons
- Reducing the retail food environment index, i.e. the density of fast food outlets in urban environments
- Ease of transport of perishable foods into towns/cities

sedentary. In a free-market-based world the agricultural, food and marketing sectors continue to maximise their profits, with food outlets and supermarkets filling their shelves with items selected by taste panels. The vast arrays of products are also marketed intensively on the basis of price and they are made available everywhere. 'Branding' is also promoted with all the subtlety that psychologists and others can devise. These developments have led to an overwhelming 'obesogenic' environment which particularly affects the more vulnerable sectors of society and is transforming the food systems of lower income countries. These pressures operate throughout society with additional lobbying of prime ministers and ministers to ensure that no coherent response is prepared which could threaten the booming food chain profits. These forces are more difficult to combat than the pressures of the tobacco industry.

The British government's Foresight report set out the immense challenges which require immediate action but far more political resolve is needed than is currently evident. One ray of hope, however, relates to urban planning and the promotion of physical activity as set out in this book. Urban design not only relates to factors influencing physical activity but also to those affecting food intake. Thus, the retail food environmental index relates to the density of fast food restaurants and convenience stores. This density has been found to relate to the prevalence of obesity and diabetes,[17] and new plans in China are to have a MacDonald's restaurant in every new petrol station built!

The current emphasis on climate change provides a synergy with the need to transform our physical environment so that we promote spontaneous rather than sports-related or deliberate physical activity. The challenge then is for urban designers to include the health benefits of more physical activity in their assessments of competing schemes and to present them as a bonus accruing from the many strategies being developed to tackle climate change. Both changes in food intake and physical activity are needed, but if we could, by changes in urban design, induce an increase in *spontaneous* activity of 200 kcal/day (equivalent to an extra hour on one's feet moving/walking/day) and if this affected the whole of society these measures would make the required additional fall of perhaps 300 kcal/day in total food intake by limiting fat/sugar energy rich snacks and reducing the energy density of normal foods to achieve energy balance at lower body weights much more readily achievable.[15]

References

1. Black, D. (1983) Obesity – a report of the Royal College of Physicians. *Journal of the Royal College of Physicians of London.* 17(1):3–58.
2. Norton, K., Dollman, J., Martin, M., Harten, N. (2006) Descriptive epidemiology of childhood overweight and obesity in Australia:1901–2003. *International Journal of Pediatric Obesity.* 1(4):232–238.
3. Wang, Y. Lobstein, T. (2006) Worldwide trends in childhood overweight and obesity. *International Journal of Pediatric Obesity.* 1(1):11–25.
4. World Health Organization. (2000) *Obesity: Preventing and Managing the Global Epidemic.* World Health Organisation Technical Report Series No. 894. WHO, Geneva.
5. Ezzati, M., Lopez, A.D., Rodgers, A., Vander Hoorn, S., Murray, C.J. Comparative Risk Assessment Collaborating Group. (2002) Selected major risk factors and global and regional burden of disease. *Lancet.* 360(9343):1347–1360.
6. James, W.P.T., Jackson-Leach, R., Ni Mhurchu, C., Kalmara, E., Shayeghi, M., Rigby, N.J., Nishida, C., Rodgers, A. Overweight and obesity (high body mass index). In: *Comparative Quantification of Health Risks. Global and Regional Burden of Disease Attributable to Selected Major Risk Factors.* (Eds. Ezzati, M., Lopez, A.D., Rodgers, A., Murray, C.J.L.) Chapter 8, Volume 1. World Health Organization, Geneva, 2004 pp. 497–596.
7. Lopez, A.D., Mathers, C.D., Ezzati, M., Jamison, D.T., Murray, C.J.L., eds. *Global Burden of Disease and Risk Factors.* New York, NY, Oxford University Press, 2006.
8. Lobstein, T., Baur, L., Uauy, R. (2004) Obesity in children and young people: a crisis in public health. *Obesity Reviews.* 5(s1):4–85.
9. Cole, T.J., Bellizzi, M.C., Flegal, K.M., Dietz, W.H. (2000) Establishing a standard definition for child overweight and obesity worldwide: international survey. *British Medical Journal.* 320:1240–1243.
10. Baker, J.L., Olsen, L.W., Sørensen, T.I. (2007) Childhood body-mass index and the risk of coronary heart disease in adulthood. *New England Journal of Medicine.* 357(23):2329–2337.
11. Huxley, R.T., James, W.P.T., Barzi, F., Patel, J.V., Lear, S.A., Suriyawongpaisal, P., Janus, E., Caterson, I., Zimmet, P., Prabhakaran, D., Reddy, S., Woodward, M. on behalf of the Obesity in Asia Collaboration. (2008) Ethnic comparisons of the cross-sectional relationships between measures of body size with diabetes and hypertension. *Obesity Reviews.* 9(Suppl. 1):53–61.
12. James, W.P.T. (2008) The epidemiology of obesity: the size of the problem. *Journal of Internal Medicine.* 263(4):336–352.
13. Sanchez-Castillo, C.P., Velasquez-Monroy, O., Lara-Esqueda, A., Berber, A., Sepulveda, J., Tapia-Conyer, R., James, W.P.T. (2005) Diabetes and hypertension increases in a society with abdominal obesity: results of the Mexican National Health Survey 2000. *Public Health Nutrition.* 8(1):53–60.
14. Foresight (2007). *Tackling Obesities: Future Choices – Project Report.* 2nd Edition, London, Government Office for Science. http://www.foresight.gov.uk.

15. James, W.P.T. (2008) The fundamental drivers of the obesity epidemic. *Obesity Reviews.* 9(Suppl. 1):6–13.
16. James, W.P.T., Rigby, N. The challenge of the chronic diseases epidemic for science and society. In: *Essentials in Human Nutrition.* (Eds. Mann, J.I., Truswell, A.S.) 3rd Edition. Oxford, Oxford University Press, 2007 pp. 249–259.
17. California Center for Public Health Advocacy. (2008) *Designed for Disease: The Link between Local Food Environments and Obesity and Diabetes.* California Center for Public Health Advocacy, Policy Link, and the UCLA Center for Health Policy Research. http://www.publichealthadvocacy.org/designedfordisease.html.

2 Towards Transdisciplinary Approaches to Tackle Obesity

*Tim G. Townshend, Louisa Ells,
Seraphim Alvanides and Amelia A. Lake*

2.1 The focus on interdisciplinary research

It has been argued that the traditional academic disciplines set around specific knowledge areas – the sciences, arts and humanities – have thrived on specialisation and differentiation, each establishing isolated academic cultures with their own language[1,2] and ethos,[3,4] regardless of whether this reflected the real world.[5] In the more recent past, however, there has been increased emphasis on academic research that addresses real-life issues[6–8] and research that is carried out in the context of application.[9,10] A key dynamic is that 'real life' issues often do not fit neatly into disciplinary boundaries. Further, as observed by Khan and Prager,[11] the idea of the solitary academic toiling away in search of solutions to problems was a myth which served as a barrier to preventing a collective response from academia to the problems of mankind. Increasingly, academic foundations and policymakers have accepted the need for interdisciplinary working, reflecting a reality that over the next decades many of the major challenges in research will cross over the boundaries of disciplines that have their roots in previous centuries.[12,13]

The challenge of obesity is a clear case in point, for until recently, it was framed as a medical problem and understandably so, since obesity is linked to so many medical conditions. More recently, however, there is growing recognition that the medical profession alone are unable to successfully arrest the rise in obesity rates and that a more holistic approach is required. This is not to suggest, however, that taking an interdisciplinary approach to health problems is new. A vote in 2007 in the *British Medical Journal* on the most important medical advance since the journal was published in 1840 was awarded to the 'sanitary revolution',[14] recognising that, in the 19th century, epidemics of contagious diseases, such as cholera and typhus, were treated with a combination of newly emerging medical knowledge and treatments, engineering improvements to water supply and sanitation and urban planning regulations. This approach was typified by the comprehensive health acts and bills passed on either side of the Atlantic in the second half of that century.

In the 20th century, as highlighted by Ceccarelli, there have been a number of key texts that were of 'broad interdisciplinary persuasion' (p. 2)[15] and she argues that these are, in fact, part of a long tradition of texts, some of which have been accepted and others, which have caused huge controversy. Yet, today there seem to be more inhibitors to interdisciplinary working that must be addressed than have traditionally been the case. The general organisation of Universities into discipline-specific departments and research institutes is demonstrative proof of the longevity of academic adherence to disciplinary boundaries and certainties. Universities themselves often specialise in particular disciplines and sub-disciplines; funding bodies like narrowly focused research proposals and specialisation wins academic advancement and accolades. Such issues as outlined below may provide major hurdles to interdisciplinary advancement.

2.2   Defining modes of interdisciplinarity

What exactly is meant by interdisciplinary research? There are a number of terms, interdisciplinary, multidisciplinary, pluri-disciplinary, cross-disciplinary and transdisciplinary,[16] which, erroneously, are often used interchangeably. Analyses of interdisciplinarity, for example, suggest three levels or stages of working.[17,18] Firstly, multidisciplinary research suggests that researchers work on a common problem, but in discrete environs, the results of their work are brought together, but with little actual engagement between the various individuals concerned. Interdisciplinary working, on the other hand, suggests common epistemological approaches linking different discipline areas employed by a team of experts, as Pellar puts it 'in an organized program to attack a challenging problem' (p. 502)[19]; this mode of working does not, however, involve the re-evaluation of research practice within the individual disciplines, or the adoption of methods and techniques from one discipline to another.

Beyond these modes, 'radical interdisciplinarity'[17] or transdisciplinary[16,18] working involves the sustained interrogation of the different research approaches from the disciplines involved, to question the assumptions and cultures of the various disciplines and to generate new collective ways of working. It, therefore, develops a common conceptual framework that bridges the relevant disciplines and serves as a basis for generating new research approaches defined directly by the research questions in hand. An aspect of transdisciplinarity, therefore, is that the focus of academic endeavour is outside traditional disciplinary boundaries. In effect, there is something of a continuum with multidisciplinary working at one end and fully integrated transdisciplinary research at the other.

The key advantage of transdisciplinary working is that by bringing different disciplines together it has the potential for fostering innovation, to create novel interventions, policies and practice; this is highly pertinent in the fight against obesity where traditional approaches have largely failed. An advantage of bringing the social sciences into the traditional medical arena should be that the social scientist is able to stand as a proxy for society and as such help the medical sciences become as responsive to societal needs as possible. Though one must be wary of this argument, since it might be claimed it positions the social sciences in overly idealistic light. In the recent past, geographers, for example, have been criticised for being uncritical of the corporatisation of their discipline.[20] Interdisciplinary working highlights such issues and therefore is challenging to those involved.

2.3 The complexity of obesity

As reviewed in Chapter 1, obesity has only been recognised as a serious problem since the 1980s. In the interim period, however, it has developed into a major global pandemic, interlinked with the greatest challenge facing mankind, climate change. At one level, the issue of energy balance appears deceptively simple – to encourage people to increase their physical exercise (energy expenditure) and to modify their diet to reduce their energy intake. At the individual-level, however, the propensity of people to become overweight, or obese, varies between subsets within the overall population and, indeed, at different stages in any individual's life cycle.[21] Thus obesity is a complex interplay between individual biology, eating behaviour and physical exercise. It has been suggested that 'human biology has become out of step with the structure of society' (p. 791).[22] The underlying biological tendency for humans to acquire and store energy, and the desensitisation of our appetite control system (at the core of the obesity systems map[21]) within the context of an obesogenic environment, means individuals exert less control and choice over their lifestyle patterns, which impacts on their weight.[23]

Moreover, as pointed out by the UK Foresight report, this is set against a 'social, cultural and environmental landscape' (p. 79)[21] and raises complex social and economic issues, encompassing food manufacturing, production and retailing, healthcare and education, and includes the way we plan and develop our towns and cities – subjects which have been addressed throughout the chapters of this book. In addition, key influences, particularly the thrust of years of public policy and competition and market forces, have worked together since the end of World War II to encourage greater food availability and the accommodation of the private car. These two aspects, taken as norms of life in the developed world (and increasingly in the developing world), now run counter to the need to reduce food intake and encourage exercise.

In their development of a framework for interdisciplinary research on environment, design and obesity, Wells *et al.*[23] suggested that clothing, food, technology (labour-saving devices), buildings and neighbourhood design, in addition to the natural environment, are all implicated in the obesity equation. The UK Foresight report suggests seven key subsystems that should be considered in the obesity epidemic:

- Physiology – biological variables related to obesity, such as genetic predisposition
- Individual physical activity – for example, the levels of activity involved in one's employment, or home life
- Physical activity environment – opportunities for physical exercise, the nature of the living environment, and so on
- Food consumption – the amounts and types of food consumed

- Food production – drivers of the food industry, such as efficiency, growth and profit
- Individual psychology – stress levels, degree of social interaction
- Social psychology – influence at societal level, for example, education, media

Interrelated issues emerge from this list of sub-themes. Firstly, it is clear that much of this is outside the traditional medical and life sciences arena, where most obesity-related research has been located. Secondly, the sheer number of traditional disciplines that are involved in studying and understanding the relationships within and between the subsystems is extremely large, and those disciplines operate at different levels and through different legal structures. Further, by looking at the interfaces between just two or perhaps three sub-theme areas might appear to break the complexity into manageable tasks. However, because the system is so highly interconnected (Figure 2.1) – 108 variables and 304 causal links involved in the 'obesity system' – tackling any particular interface, or causal link, carries its own risks.

This obesity systems map suggests that the consequence of intervention at any one interface may actually be discharged away from the original focus; or may even be compensated for by unintended changes elsewhere in the system. For example, a campaign to encourage children to walk to and from school may expose them to the temptation of more sweet shops and fast food outlets, potentially producing a null

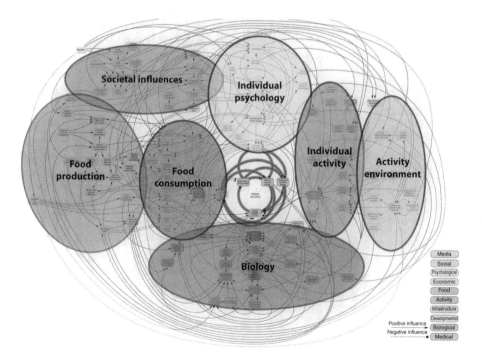

Figure 2.1 Foresight obesity systems map showing thematic clusters. With permission from the Government Office for Science, London.

effect. In adolescents, the attempted suppression of risky behaviour, for example, through a media campaign aimed at highlighting obesity risk to their age group, may actually lead them to engage in other health risk behaviours (the theory of reactance) such as drug taking, smoking or eating disorders.[24] This may, in part, explain why interventions to tackle obesity have thus far had limited success.

2.4   The challenge of interdisciplinary understanding

The Foresight obesity systems map provides us with insight into the complexity of, and interrelationships between, various determinants of obesity. Moreover, research on obesity from the medical, life and social sciences has explained a great deal about many of these complex determinants; however, most work to date has not been 'well integrated across the disciplines' (p. 43).[21] How best might this be achieved and what barriers to effective working might be met? Since the amount of interdisciplinary work that has been carried out in the study of obesity is limited, the following sections look more broadly at debates on interdisciplinary research, as well as the editors' own experience in attempting to answer these key questions.

2.4.1   Lessons from the field of sustainability

The field of sustainability provides some interesting insights in relation to interdisciplinary working. Issues around sustainable urbanism were recognised as requiring input from the natural, engineering and social sciences from the 1980s onwards. A review of three research programmes funded by UK Research Councils and specifically tasked with developing new forms of interdisciplinary working, however, found significant challenges.[17] Firstly, the authors suggested that in the studies they had reviewed, the social and cultural dimensions (and differences) of knowledge and its location within specific epistemic cultures had not been addressed sufficiently. In particular, they suggested that the funding bodies themselves were incapable of 'breaking down the distinctions that gave their own identity meaning' (p. 1025).[17] This is extremely important since if interdisciplinary projects on obesity are to be appropriately funded, then funding bodies may have to radically address their research funding processes and the criteria on which they give awards (see Section 2.4.3). Moreover, since transdisciplinary projects will almost certainly need more lead-in time in order for academics from different disciplines to fully understand each other's perspectives, they may appear relatively expensive and contain large amount of unproductive time. These, in particular, challenge normal institutional working practices where expectations of what constitutes a 'worthwhile' project to fund, based on value for money, precedents and track record are often deeply engrained.

The problems of disciplinary cultures and norms will also be a challenge for those working in an interdisciplinary team. Evans and Marvin suggest that being part of a particular discipline is 'not just a matter of mastering a technical discourse, it is also a matter of being a particular kind of person' (p. 1018)[17]; though, to some extent, there are, in reality, universally upheld values and beliefs within broad disciplines (such as geography) might seem open to question. Moreover, different outlooks by individual researchers may not necessarily be drawn along discipline boundaries. It may be, therefore, that difference in culture and values are highlighted by interdisciplinary working and might be used as an excuse for creating barriers to effective working.

2.4.2 Language as a barrier

On a relatively pragmatic note, the co-editors note that language may be a key barrier to effective working, particularly in the early stages of a research project when disciplinary differences are unknown and unexpected. The difficulties of language in interdisciplinary projects have also been highlighted elsewhere.[1,2] However, language may prove problematic in more than one way, for example, when trying to address issues that lie outside the usual boundaries of their discipline, an academic team with the best intentions may develop their own vocabulary for phenomena that are already prescribed by specific terminology by others. In setting out to map health problems investigated for possible links with the built environment, Rao et al.[25] use the term 'appearance'; this is not, however, a term that has a particular meaning in the built environment disciplines. Examining the sense in which 'appearance' is being used, the term 'quality of the public realm' would actually be applied by those disciplines.

A further difficulty is where terms or expressions have different meanings between disciplines. In Chapter 4 Jones and Panter review the concept of 'accessibility' from the perspective of the field of health service delivery planning. They note that accessibility implies that people with the same type and degree of health need to have an equal chance of receiving appropriate and equal quality treatment. In the field of urban design, however, 'accessibility' has a totally different connotation. Here the term is used as a tripartite notion of visual, physical and symbolic (psychological) qualities of public space,[26] that is, would someone understand how to get to a public space, could they physically traverse the environment to enter it and would they feel comfortable and safe in doing so? There are, in fact, many terms like 'access', 'environment' and 'surveillance' which are in common everyday use in both the health and built environment professions, but which carry quite different disciplinary 'baggage' with them.

2.4.3 Academic positioning

A problem faced by any individual working in a team outside his or her own academic discipline, however, is that of academic positioning. Those journals, which are often most highly regarded in almost any discipline, are usually discipline specific, making it difficult to publish interdisciplinary work in them. In the social sciences, moreover, there is strong emphasis on demonstrating one's ability to be an independent researcher with sole-authored articles in top journals being highly prized. This model is different in the field of medicine where team publications are more usual. Even so, top accolades, the Nobel Prize being the most obvious example, are about the individual rather than the team.

Academics and academic departments are increasingly judged by the quantity/quality of publications produced, for example, the UK Research Assessment Exercise (RAE) 2008[27] and the upcoming Research Excellence Framework (REF).[28] In the United Kingdom, for example, the medical sciences use impact factor and citation metrics as part of this judgement, the social sciences have, thus far, not followed this method; though whether this will be imposed by the REF is still being debated. Where articles of multidisciplinary teams get published, this can, therefore, create problems for individual team members.

Related to this, there is the somewhat delicate issue of epistemic superiority that might traditionally have been assumed by some quantitative researchers over 'softer' qualitative research. Medical research has tended to base much of its findings on strictly controlled and regulated clinical trials, with bodies such as the United Kingdom's National Institute for Health and Clinical Excellence (NICE) having strict criteria as to what they will accept as 'evidence'. In relation to their physical activity and environment guidance, however, NICE allowed a much wider interpretation of evidence, suggesting greater recognition in the value of a range of work. For their part, social-science researchers need to acknowledge the value in contributing to evidence-based policy, as much as to the development of academic theory.

2.4.4 Summary of barriers

These (potential) barriers, however real or imaginary, need to be addressed rather than be ignored, and several approaches might be adopted. Longer start-up phases for interdisciplinary projects (though this obviously involves cost and a basically unproductive period in the life of a research project), sensitive management of teams which respect traditional working practices while allowing them to be challenged, flexibility on the part of team members and a willingness to understand others' perspectives are all key to overcoming this challenge. Such issues also apply to working across academic and policy/practice boundaries.

2.5 Interdisciplinary policy and practice

The Foresight report[21] not only stressed the multifaceted nature of obesity but also the importance of tackling this right from the individual to the policy level. In England, the Government has pledged to tackle obesity through a cross-Government strategy: 'Healthy Weight, Healthy Lives',[29] which supports the creation of a healthy society: from early years to school and food, sport and physical activity to planning, transport and health services. The aim of this strategy is 'to be the first major nation to reverse the rising tide of obesity and overweight in the population by ensuring that everyone is able to achieve and maintain a healthy weight' (p. 5).[29] This strategy has been further supported by *Healthy Weight, Healthy Lives: One Year On*[30] and the physical activity strategy: 'Be Active, Be Healthy: a Plan for Getting the Nation Moving'.[31]

One of the key features of Healthy Weight, Healthy Lives: One Year On[30] focuses on creating an environment that promotes healthy weight, as a result of the Foresight acknowledgement of the need to address wider social and economic issues in order to achieve this aim. This focus is divided into four key visions: (i) children, healthy growth and healthy weight, (ii) promoting healthier food choices, (iii) building physical activity into our lives and (iv) creating incentive for better health. These visions are supported by the Change4Life campaign, which is a society-wide movement that aims to prevent overweight and obesity by encouraging the population to 'eat better and move more'.[32] As part of the Change4Life movement, nine 'Healthy Towns' (Tewkesbury, Halifax, Thetford, Tower Hamlets, Manchester, Middlesbrough, Dudley, Sheffield and Portsmouth) have also been selected for a trial of new holistic approaches to promoting physical activity and healthy eating within their community and town infrastructures.

A key focus of the physical activity plan 'Be Active, Be Healthy' is creating an active environment. This centres around evidence from the NICE physical activity and environment[33] guidance, to inform the creation of safe play spaces, enhancements to planning policy around open spaces, sport and recreation, alongside the Sport England Active Design report[34]; this is in addition to encouraging activity within the natural environment.

The initiation of policies and guidance to combat the obesogenic environment will help the fight against obesity; however, to be successful and sustainable these must be (i) initiated by interdisciplinary teams to ensure a combined approach with a consistency in messages and (ii) thoroughly evaluated to ensure policy and practice evolve in a positive feedback loop. Given the current weaknesses in the evidence base around the effective prevention of obesity, the National Obesity Observatory issued a standard evaluation framework for all weight management interventions[35] to ensure a consistent standardised best practice approach to evaluation.

The challenge for policy is to find a way to address these issues from an interdisciplinary perspective, and if this is not established, then policymakers risk being bombarded with different perspectives from different academic disciplines. These perspectives will use different theories and different models and policymakers will face an impossible challenge to bring these together into a coherent policy approach.

2.6 Discussion

The complexity of obesity is overviewed in this chapter and discussed in detail in this book. The Foresight obesity systems map graphically highlights the vast array of variables and causal links that have been investigated in relation to obesity and even this may be something of a simplification. Furthermore, this systems map shows that many of these links cross over traditional disciplinary boundaries.

In this volume, we bring together writers from backgrounds in policy, nutrition and dietetics, epidemiology, environmental sciences, medical sciences, town planning/urban design, geography and physical activity. The editors have worked on a number of interdisciplinary projects and are fully convinced of the need to challenge our own established disciplinary perspectives. Furthermore, while true transdisciplinarity remains a goal rather than an achieved state of our work, we would argue that the very complexity of obesity demands that a move towards transdisciplinary research is in fact inevitable.

References

1. Schoenberger, E. (2001) Interdisciplinarity and social power. *Progress in Human Geographies.* 25:365–382.
2. Bracken, L., Oughton, E. (2006) What do you mean? The importance of language in developing interdisciplinary research. *Transactions of the Institute of British Geographers.* 31:371–382.
3. Giacomini, M. (2004) Interdisciplinarity in health services research: dreams nightmares, maladies and remedies. *Journal of Health Services Research and Policy.* 9(3): 177–183.
4. Nowotny, H. (2003) The potential of transdisciplinarity, http://www.interdisciplines.org/interdisciplinarity/papers/5, accessed 01.08.09.
5. NcNeely, I.F., Wolverton, L. *Reinventing Knowledge: from Alexandria to the Internet.* London, WW Norton, 2008.
6. Latour, B. *The Politics of Nature: How to Bring the Sciences in Democracy.* Cambridge, MA, Harvard University Press, 2004.
7. Nowotny, H., Scott, P., Gibbons, M. *Rethinking Science: Knowledge and the Public in an Age of Uncertainty.* Cambridge, MA, Polity, 2001.
8. Martin, R. (2001) Geography and public policy: the case of the missing agenda. *Progress in Human Geography.* 25:189–210.
9. Ward, K. (2005) Geography and public policy: a recent history of policy relevance. *Progress in Human Geography.* 29:310–319.
10. Ward, K. (2006) Geography and public policy: towards public geographies. *Progress in Human Geography.* 30:495–503.
11. Khan, R.L., Prager, D.L. (1994) Interdisciplinary collaboration are a scientific and social imperative. *Scientist.* July 11:12.
12. European Science Foundation. *Strategic Plan 2006–10.* Strasbourg, France, European Science Foundation, 2005.
13. H.M. Treasury. *Science and Innovation Framework 2004–14.* London, H.M. Treasury, 2004.
14. Ferriman, A. (2007) BMJ readers choose the "sanitary revolution" as the greatest medical advance since 1840. *BMJ.* 334:111.
15. Ceccarelli, L. *Shaping Science with Rhetoric: The cases of Dobzhansky Schrödinger, and Wilson.* Chicago, IL, Chicago University Press, 2001.
16. Nowotny, H. (2009) The potential of transdisciplinarity. Available from http://www.interdisciplines.org/interdisciplinarity/papers/5, [cited 2009 01.08.09].
17. Evans, R., Marvin, S. (2006) Researching the sustainable city: three modes of interdisciplinarity. *Environment and Planning A.* 38:1009–1028.
18. Barry, A., Born, G., Weszkalnys, G. (2008) Logics of interdisciplinarity. *Economy and Society.* 37:20–49.
19. Pellar, T.C. *Bridging Discipline in the Brain, Behavioural and Clinical Sciences.* Washington, DC, National Academies Press, 2000.
20. Lindley, T. 2009 Academic capitalism and professional reproduction at the conference. *ACME.* Available from http://www.acme-journal.org/vol8/Lindley09.pdf, [cited 2009 01.08.09].
21. Foresight. *Tackling Obesities: Future Choices – Project Report.* London, Government Office for Science, 2007.

22. King, D.A., Thomas, S.M. (2007) Big lessons for a healthy future. *Nature*. 449(7164): 791–792.
23. Wells, N.M., Ashdown, S.P., Davies, E.H.S., Cowett, F.D., Yang, Y. (2007) Environment, design, and obesity: opportunities for interdisciplinary collaborative research. *Environment and Behavior*. 39(1):6–33.
24. Dooley, J.A., Deshpande, S., Adair, C.E. (2009) Comparing adolescent-focussed prevention and reduction messages. *Journal of Business Research*. doi 10. 1016/j.busres.2009.02.011.
25. Rao, M., Prasad, S., Ashead, F., Hasitha, T. (2007), The Built Environment and Health. *The Lancet*. 370(9593):1111–1113. Web Extra Material, accessed 01.08.09.
26. Carr, S., Francis, M., Rivlin, L.G., Stone, A.M. *Public Space*. Cambridge, Cambridge University Press, 1992.
27. UK Research Assessment Exercise (2008) http://www.rae.ac.uk/, [cited 2009 01/08/09].
28. UK Research Excellence Framework (2009) http://www.hefce.ac.uk/research/ref/, [cited 2009 01/09/09].
29. Department of Health. *Healthy Weight, Healthy Lives: A cross-government research and surveillance plan for England*. London, Department of Health, 2008.
30. Cross-Government Obesity Unit, Department of Health and Department of Children, Schools and Families. *Healthy Weight, Healthy Lives: One Year On*. London, Department of Health, 2009.
31. Department of Health. *Be Active, Be Healthy: A Plan for Getting the Nation Moving*. London, Department of Health, 2009.
32. http://www.nhs.uk/change4life (2009), accessed 01.08.09.
33. NICE. *NICE Public Health Guidance 8: Promoting and Creating Built or Natural Environments that Encourage and Support Physical Activity*. London, National Institute for Health and Clinical Excellence, 2008.
34. Sport England. *Active Design Promoting Opportunities for Sport and Physical Activity Through Good Design*. London, Sport England, 2008.
35. www.noo.org.uk/sef (2009), accessed 01.08.09.

3 Walkability, Neighbourhood Design and Obesity

*Jennifer Robertson-Wilson
and Billie Giles-Corti*

3.1 Introduction

As discussed in Chapter 1,[1] the high rate of obesity among youth and adults worldwide is of increasing concern. The obesity epidemic is discussed in terms of energy balance.[2-4] In subscribing to social ecological models,[5-7] researchers now recognise that to address issues of obesity, diet (energy in) and physical activity (energy out), there is a need to look beyond simply focusing on individual factors to consider broader factors (e.g. social, physical, policy and economic environments) with a view to developing targeted environmental and policy interventions.[5,8]

In this chapter, we examine evidence on the relationship between obesity and neighbourhood design with a particular focus on neighbourhood walkability. For a discussion of various aspects of the broader economic and physical (or built) environment related to obesity in adults and youth, we direct the reader to several recent reviews.[9-14] A brief overview of walkability and key terms is followed by a presentation of the literature relating obesity to walkability and related indicators. The last section of the chapter discusses key issues related to study measurement, design and conceptualisation, which require attention to advance this body of research.

3.2 What is walkability?

Creating pedestrian-, cycling- and transit-friendly environments is now recognised as being important for both the environment[15] and for health.[16,17] Motor vehicle travel is encouraged in low density auto-dependent urban development that separates land uses; and excessive motor vehicle travel is detrimental to human health.[15] Examples of several studies also show that time spent driving increases the odds of being obese[18,19] while time spent walking decreases the risk of obesity.[18,20]

There is now a growing body of cross-sectional evidence summarised in an ever-growing number of reviews in adults,[21-27] and, to a lesser extent in children,[28-30] that walking, particularly walking for transport, is associated with living in compact neighbourhoods with well-connected street networks, mixed use planning, public open space, footpaths and access to high-quality public transport. Neighbourhoods with these characteristics are said to be more *walkable*. To better help understand the impact of the built environment on walking, Frank et al.[31] break the built environment into three components: the transportation system, land use patterns and urban design characteristics. The transportation system is defined as the 'network of physical infrastructure within a region, such as its street network, its transit system and separated systems for non-motorised users such as jogging and biking paths' (p. 100).[31] The ease with which one can reach destinations within one's neighbourhood or region is based on the transportation system.[31] The presence of destinations is determined by land use patterns.

Land use patterns relate to the 'spatial arrangement of structures on the landscape' (p. 100).[31] It determines the proximity between residential, retail, commercial, industrial and service (schools, libraries, etc.) destinations and the types of transportation required to reach these destinations.[31] Land use mix refers to 'the degree to which different types of users (residential, commercial, retail) are located within close proximity to one another' (p. 102).[31] The level of land use mix or structural density is governed by the level of population density. Higher levels of population density are associated with more intensified land use, which increases proximity to a variety of destinations and 'reduce[s] trip lengths, thereby increasing travel options (walking, bicycling and transit) as well as obviating the need to own a vehicle' (p. 101).[31]

Another factor that influences the proximity of destinations is the connectivity of the street network that links destinations. Street networks that are highly connected provide a relatively direct route between destinations and many alternative routes to reach a specific destination.[31] Moreover, for such street networks, there is little difference between the distance between an origin and destination using the street network and the straight-line distance (or 'the crow fly distance', p. 100).[31] This is contrary in suburbs with disconnected street networks as is found in areas with many cul-de-sacs. In these suburbs, the straight-line distance between an origin and destinations is often considerably shorter than the distance using the street network.[31]

Finally, urban design features refer to often micro-level infrastructure that makes a neighbourhood feel safe and attractive.[31] These include the presence of sidewalks, the presence of trees and benches, whether or not a street has good surveillance, and traffic lane characteristics.[31,32] Micro-scale urban design features contribute to creating convivial neighbourhoods and, over and above destination accessibility and proximity, may determine whether or not residents choose to walk or cycle to local destinations.[31]

Together these factors influence an area's walkability. Walkable environments have proximate destinations, traversable landscapes that are safe and leafy and have pedestrian amenities present (e.g. sidewalks, street trees).[33] On the basis of this[33] and other definitions,[31] walkability can be therefore defined as the extent to which walking is supported in an area through the provision of pedestrian-friendly macro- and micro-level infrastructure including the above-noted well-connected street network with a variety of land uses and higher densities. The opposite of walkability is urban sprawl which, Frumkin et al. (p. 1)[17] define using the Smart Growth

Vermont[34] definition of 'dispersed, automobile-dependent development outside of compact urban and village centres, along highways, and in rural countryside'.

3.3   Measuring walkability

Various methods are used to measure overall walkability and its components.[18,35] However, examples of studies assessing walkability generally include measures of

- *street connectivity*: measured by indices such as intersection density per road miles[36] or per defined area,[18,20,37–40] block length,[39,40] link-node ratio or pedestrian route directness[39];
- *mixed land use*: measured by the consistency or diversity of different land uses in a defined area[18,20,41] including ratios of retail or commercial floor area,[20,41] and ratios of non-residential to total buildings[37] or commercial to residential building land use per defined area[38];
- residential[20,41,42] or population *density*.[37,43,44]

A major problem in comparing studies is that walkability, like many other physical environment features, is often measured at different geographic scales.[10,13,45,46] For walkability studies specifically, these have included examples such as buffers around a participant's home of 0.1, 0.5 and/or 1 km[18,20,41,47] or 0.25, 0.5 or 1 mile[48] or larger areas such as one's census tract,[38] county[42,49] or metropolitan area of residence.[50–52] At the aggregate level of scale, examples exist of walkability or related indicators being evaluated at the county level[53] and state level.[54,55] Clearly, the lack of standardisation of measures and scale is problematic as it often produces conflicting or mixed findings and limits comparison across studies.[10,13,25,46] Lack of specificity between environmental and behavioural measures is also likely to attenuate the associations between variables.[46,56]

3.4   Linking neighbourhood design aspects of walkability to obesity

To help shift the agenda, the main question explored here is whether neighbourhood walkability is associated with levels of obesity. In this section, we review the evidence examining the association between obesity indicators of walkability as a specific feature of neighbourhood design. The main neighbourhood design features of interest include walkability (including indicators of density, land use and connectivity), urban sprawl and other features such as geographic location and sidewalk presence.

3.4.1   Walkability and obesity

The association between walkability and obesity is one of the few neighbourhood design features to have been studied across different age groups. Four studies examined walkability and weight status among adults and an inverse relationship was consistently reported across all studies.[20,36,41,57] Only one published study to date appears to have examined weight status and walkability among young children.[58] This study used a commonly adopted walkability index and found an inverse relationship between walkability and weight status for preschool-aged girls (but not boys), even when using different weight status cut-off points were explored.[58]

Nevertheless, the impact of walkability appears to vary according to subgroup. For example, null findings were reported in a study of older adults (over 65 years of age),[47] and two studies with adolescents.[48,59] Whether these findings reflect a differential in the impact of the built environment on different age groups is not clear as the studies varied in measures used and study designs. For example, as noted by the authors, it is possible that study variations may be due to the measure of years spent in one's home or variations in the walkability index used[47] or sample size.[47,48]

Although there appears to be consistent evidence in adults that neighbourhood walkability is associated with weight status, as previously stated, additional evidence is required that enables comparison within and between countries and of the impact of walkability on different population groups.[10,13] This research is important given that the neighbourhood design factors that create walkable neighbourhoods provide the blueprint for neighbourhoods that last for decades, if not centuries. Thus, ensuring that the right design and the needs of different sub-populations is considered is critical.

3.5   Breaking down walkability

As noted earlier, measures of neighbourhood walkability incorporate a number of sub-components: residential or population density; mixed use planning and connectivity. It is possible that these indicators act synergistically to influence levels of obesity; however, it is also possible that one or other of these components drives the relationship. A number of studies have attempted to unpack the walkability index to examine the association between various components of the index and weight status, suggesting that some indicators may be more important than others.

3.5.1   Density

The evidence for the relationship between density and weight status is mixed, regardless of the level of analysis. At an ecological (aggregate) level, modest evidence supports a negative association between county-level density[53] and state-level density[54,55] and obesity. However, at the individual level, using neighbourhood or census tract residential or dwelling density, the relationship is mixed depending upon the population under study and the measure of weight status adopted.

For example, five studies found no association between weight status and density in adult populations[37,43] or children and adolescent populations,[58-60] while a number of other studies found negative associations for specific sub-populations depending upon how the weight status was measured. Specifically, in bivariate and/or multivariate analyses, density indicators were negatively associated with body mass index (BMI) in whites but not other subgroups,[18] as was overweight among males,[61] overweight/obesity among women and girls,[62] and overweight (but not BMI or obesity) among men (95% CI: $0.993-1.00$, $p = 0.051$).[63] Conversely, two studies found positive associations for women in the sample: one between obesity (not overweight) and density for non-degree holding white women only[61] and the other among obese women (although not for indicators of overweight or BMI).[63] An inverse association between waist-to-hip ratio (not BMI) and postcode area density was reported in a UK sample.[44]

More recently, another variation in studies relates to statistical techniques being adopted. Results are also mixed across studies employing multilevel modelling techniques, reporting either no association[52] or a positive association[64] between density and BMI, while other studies report a negative association between density and weight status.[38,51] However, the studies vary considerably in terms of whether they measure dwelling[52] or population density[38,51,64] and in terms of study design and location. For example, one study involved a longitudinal cohort study of Filipino women and found that 'women living in areas with higher population density had larger increases in BMI over time' (p. 618).[64] However, in developing countries, other factors may be at play. For example, in developing countries, density 'may be an indicator of economic development and wealth...women living in places with less economic development had smaller changes in weight over time. Areas with lower population density may have developed more slowly. Fast food options and transportation in these areas might be limited so that people walk more and eat healthier food than people in more developed areas' (p. 621).[64]

As with walkability, the evidence on weight status and density highlights the need for more consideration to be given to how weight status is measured and for studies of sub-populations across different countries in order to examine how the relationship varies across age, ethnicity, gender and other demographic factors. The impact of density on weight status in developing countries, for example, may vary due to factors related to socio-economic status and changes in means of transportation.[65] This warrants prospective investigation particularly as many developing countries are rapidly changing in a globalised economy and are beginning to enjoy the benefits of economic development and wealth creation.

Another consideration for studies that involve density is the type of housing people inhabit in densely populated areas. For example, a Cyprian study found that adults living in apartments were less likely to be classified as overweight/obese, but girls living in apartments were more likely to be overweight than their counterparts living in homes with a yard.[62] The authors suggest that it could be that while adults benefit from apartment living because there are proximate destinations to walk to, the same environment curtails children's play and activity.[62]

3.5.2   Land use mix

Land use mix provides destinations to walk to and also appears to be inversely associated with weight status among adults[18,38,66] and older adults.[67] However, as with density, the relationship appears to vary by subgroup. For example, in one study correlational differences across ethnicity were observed,[18] while another study found an inverse relationship between land use mix and obesity for degree-holding men but not among other subgroups.[61] Further, land use mix was not associated with weight status among preschool children[58] or youth aged 11–15.[59]

Only one published study involving a largely female Hispanic population[37] found a positive association between land use mix and weight status. The authors attribute this inconsistency to both the variables adjusted for in the model and the land use assessment adopted.[37] Together, these results suggest that the diversity of land uses may not influence all groups equally with respect to weight status.

3.5.3   Street connectivity

The level of street connectivity influences the ease with which residents can walk to access location destinations. Like other components of the walkability index, the relationship between intersection density or street connectivity and weight status is mixed. Irrespective of how connectivity and weight status (BMI, overweight or obesity classification) is measured, several studies report an inverse relationship between connectivity and weight status at both the individual level[18,58,61,63] and the ecological (neighbourhood) level ($p = 0.05$).[68]

However, variation and inconsistencies are again found by subgroup and according to the specific weight status outcome adopted. For instance, while two studies found an inverse association in men, the finding by Frank et al.[61] holds for obesity and not overweight status among degree-holding men, while that by Smith et al.[63] holds for overweight and obesity status but not BMI, suggesting that the relationship is not linear. Smith et al.[63] further report an inverse relationship for overweight women (95% CI = 0.985–1.000, $p < 0.05$). Similarly, another study found that the weight status of preschool girls, but not boys, was inversely related to intersection density.[58] Conversely, a positive relationship between connectivity and weight status emerged among certain subgroups of adults.[61] Yet, a number of studies have reported null effects,[37,38,59,60] particularly after adjustment for potential confounders.[51]

3.6   Urban sprawl, geographic location and obesity

Urban sprawl is another composite neighbourhood design measure used to examine the relationship with obesity. As noted above, urban sprawl denotes an urban form that is car friendly rather than pedestrian friendly, is spread out rather than closely connected and is often further characterised by low-density neighbourhoods with disconnected street networks and poor access to shops and services.[17]

The evidence on the association between weight status and urban sprawl is mixed depending upon the statistical analytical methods adopted and the level at which 'sprawl' is assessed. One ecological study of US states explored changes in rates of obesity as impacted by changes in sprawl as assessed by land development changes.[55] Weight status was positively associated with increased land development. This positive association is consistent with other studies using multilevel modelling techniques examining the link between weight status and *county-level sprawl*.[42,49,50,69] However, perhaps not surprisingly, at the larger *metropolitan level*, the evidence on the impact of sprawl is mixed, with several authors reporting a positive association[52,70] while others do not.[42,50]

Broadly, rural or suburban environments may also be considered as an indicator of neighbourhood sprawl. Poortinga[71] found that the prevalence of obesity was higher among English adults in a suburban (vs. urban) environment. Geographic location was also significant in another study, but only for adult women in a bivariate analysis.[62]

Issues in developing countries may also vary. For example, in a Chinese study, youth living in either urban or suburban compared with rural environments were more likely to be classified as overweight or obese.[72] The authors suggest that access to both food outlets and transportation in urban/suburban environments may in part account for these findings.[72] However, in addition, it is plausible that in developing countries in particular, work- and travel-related energy expenditure is substantially higher than in urban and suburban areas in those countries, which may also help explain the results. Further studies in developing countries are warranted, particularly given that many of these countries are currently experiencing rapid change with shifts in the way they are built, the transportation options available and rapid urbanisation. Taken together, these studies suggest that increasing levels of sprawl is associated with increasing levels of obesity. However, future studies should consider the level at which sprawl is assessed as this appears to influence this relationship.[13]

3.7   Other design features and obesity

Several other neighbourhood design features have also been examined in relation to obesity and warrant discussion. For example, area of residence and housing features may impact weight status. Among Australian adults, living on a highway (as opposed to a cul-de-sac) was associated with higher levels of overweight (but not obesity).[73] Further, some evidence of density of bus and subway stops being linked to weight status is now emerging.[38]

Two studies[60,63] examined the association between age of home or neighbourhood as a proxy for neighbourhood walkability in that older areas tend to have a grid pattern street design rather than 'the discontinuous cul-de-sac or loop pattern' (p. 1)[33] found in newer neighbourhoods.[33,60] The studies found that youths living in older homes were less likely to be overweight[60] as were adults, irrespective of whether weight status was measured by BMI, overweight or obesity.[63]

Finally, both objective and subjective indicators of sidewalk availability or condition have been shown to be related to weight status, although once again the evidence is mixed. A number of studies have found that weight status is reduced in areas where sidewalks or trails are present or are in good condition.[73–76] Nevertheless, this is counterbalanced by a number of other studies of perceptions of the presence of sidewalks reporting null findings.[69,77,78] As with other neighbourhood design indicators, the evidence appears to vary according to the level of adjustment[74,76] whether the outcome measured was overweight, obesity or BMI,[73,76] and the population studied.[75]

3.8   Neighbourhood design as a moderator

In addition to the direct effects of walkability and related neighbourhood design indicators on weight status, several studies have found a moderating effect of walkability indices on weight status. In one study, 'in Higher Population Density Townships, increased amounts of vegetation surrounding a child's residence were associated with less risk of overweight' (p. 321).[79] In examining the effect of county sprawl on weight status, another study found that while sprawl was positively related to BMI, this relationship was impacted by the number of perceived barriers an individual reported.[69] Specifically, the more personal barriers identified, the stronger the BMI–sprawl relationship.[69]

Finally, in a study that adjusted for neighbourhood selection factors,[41] an inverse relationship between obesity and having the highest neighbourhood walkability was found when neighbourhood selection was adjusted for, even though this factor was not directly associated with obesity itself. However, in another sample in the study that adjusted for neighbourhood preference, obesity was associated with neighbourhood preference, but not walkability.[41] This suggests that additional research is needed to elucidate whether the effects of neighbourhood design features on weight status is direct or is mediated or moderated by other factors,[10,14] with one focus being the impact of self-selection factors.[41]

3.9   Summary of findings and future directions in research on the impact of neighbourhood design and/ or walkability and obesity?

As evidenced by this and other recent reviews,[10,11,13] there is growing interest in the relationship between the built environment and obesity. Neighbourhood design provides a blueprint that influences generations of local residents. Hence if a passive intervention such as improving the way communities are built has an impact on weight status – even if small – it provides an important population-wide intervention worthy of future consideration.

The evidence suggests that indeed there is a relationship between weight status and neighbourhood walkability and other related neighbourhood design features. In general, the literature suggests that more walkable areas with higher density, land use mix and connectivity are associated with a reduced risk of overweight and obesity, whilst urban sprawl and newer urban environments with few destinations and mixed use areas increase the risk of overweight and obesity. That being said, the evidence in some areas is 'mixed' because the impact of the built environment appears to vary by population, unit of analysis and different methods for measuring weight status.

Given the embryonic nature of this field, some of the initial challenges to this research (e.g. putting the obesity–environment link on the research agenda; measurement of neighbourhood design features) have been an impediment to producing consistent evidence, and undoubtedly, measurement of outcome and exposure measures will continue to evolve and improve. However, to advance this field of research and take it to its next level, researchers need to give due consideration to several of the challenges and limitations in conducting obesity–walkability research that the majority of authors of the studies reviewed here commonly cite, specifically, issues of study design, neighbourhood scale definition and measurement, as well as the differential impacts of built environment on subgroups. It will be difficult to advance our knowledge of the relationship between obesity and neighbourhood design unless these factors are considered when designing future studies. Each issue is addressed below.

3.9.1   Study design

One of the main goals of walkability and related built environment research is to inform the development of policies and programs to curb obesity. Policymakers, government officials, urban and transportation city planners, public health practitioners, researchers and community members alike are now asking questions such as 'How should a community design new neighbourhoods in a way that might reduce obesity?', 'Are sidewalks needed in neighbourhoods and is this sufficient to reduce the risk of obesity or overweight?' or 'What specific neighbourhood design features should be included in community growth plans and how will obesity and overweight be impacted?'

In a recent paper,[80] the authors review calls for improved public health intervention evidence and turn their attention to the challenges of 'collecting robust evidence on outcomes' (p. 752).[80] As noted in other reviews,[10,11,13] almost all studies reviewed here exclusively employed cross-sectional designs (with certain exceptions[49,55,64] based on longitudinal or cross-sectional change data). Further, of the studies reviewed here, the majority of authors employing cross-sectional designs cite this as limitation of their research. Overall, the use of cross-sectional designs is consistently recognised as a research limitation because causal inferences cannot be drawn.[10,14] Thus, study design has implications for the high-quality evidence base for policy and neighbourhood and future studies need to consider establishing cohort studies or natural experiments that will enable longitudinal evidence to be accumulated.[80,81]

As Handy et al.[82] point out, cross-sectional designs demonstrate associations between outcome variables like physical activity and walkability, but the 'chicken and egg' question remains; rather than obesity (or physical activity or diet) being influenced by neighbourhood features, people with a certain weight status (or physical activity or dietary pattern) may decide to live in a certain neighbourhood because it supports their preferred lifestyle.[10,41,82] Thus, in cross-sectional studies, it is equally plausible that self-selection is the reason for any impact of neighbourhood features on obesity or other related outcomes.[10,41,82,83] From a public health perspective this is important because if people choose neighbourhoods that are consistent with their behaviour, then interventions designed to enhance neighbourhood designs may have little impact on obesity or physical activity outcomes and our efforts are best targeted towards individual behaviour change. Although the study by Frank et al.[41] attempted to account for self-selection by assessing neighbourhood preferences and attitudes, the authors concede that the study was limited because self-selection was assessed in a cross-sectional study design and the other factors that may impact an individual's preferences need to be assessed in future studies.[41]

The challenges of using randomisation in public health research, particularly for environmental or policy changes, have been discussed elsewhere.[80,81] As these authors have pointed out,[10,80,81] generally it is not possible to randomise individuals in environment or policy change interventions, for example, to walkable or less walkable communities to examine obesity trends over time. Thus, natural experiments (or longitudinal, quasi-experimental designs) have been advocated as a viable alternative for environment-based research in the areas of obesity, physical activity and diet.[10,14,45,80,81,84]

Although not without limitations and challenges, evaluating natural experiments will advance our knowledge in this area and provide evidence that goes beyond purely cross-sectional evidence.[80,81] In a natural experiment, 'some environmental or policy change allows for data collection prior to and following a change' (p. 23),[14] but this change is not typically manipulated by the researcher.[80] Ramanathan et al.[81] identified several recent or ongoing natural experiments, including the Residential Environments Project (RESIDE) conducted in Perth, Australia.[83] In the RESIDE project, the walking, cycling, public transport use, sense of community and weight status of participants is being tracked over time before and after they move into new homes built in neighbourhoods, some of which were designed according to a state government subdivision design code aimed at creating more pedestrian-friendly neighbourhoods.[83] This study will enable the effect on residents of government policy designed to create 'liveable' neighbourhoods to be assessed and will provide some insights into the influence of the built environment on a range of resident outcomes including their health and travel behaviours, as well as their preferences and attitudes and social health outcomes.[83]

To further advance the field, researchers will need to collaborate with key partners and officials from a variety of fields at a variety of levels.[5,84] In bringing researchers and practitioners together in a concept mapping exercise, Brownson et al.[84] identified several priority environment and policy topics relevant to both physical activity researchers and practitioners. In addition to mutual agenda setting and planning, strong pre-established partnerships may enable researchers to be aware of the activities of those responsible for the planning and implementation of (say) a new sidewalk policy or municipal neighbourhood design guideline. This relates to the idea noted in the concept mapping study of 'the creation of research teams that could be ready to conduct studies or evaluations should the opportunity become available (e.g. natural experiments)' (p. 497).[84] This speaks of the idea that researchers need to not only be aware of opportunities but also have the skills to do so, and stand in readiness to respond quickly in order to capitalise on opportunities that present themselves. However, even in cases where the researchers are not aware of such opportunities in advance, evaluation may still be possible using for instance existing databases, and this is worthy of consideration.[81] Finally, access to funding opportunities is also essential to evaluate natural experiments.[81] Funding agencies such as *Active Living Research*[85] and as Ramanathan *et al.*[81] note the *Canadian Institute of Health Research*[86] have provided some recent opportunities.

In order to capitalise on opportunities such as natural experiments, mechanisms that facilitate funding bodies to be responsive to the funding requirements of natural experiments rather than having to wait for the 6–18 month peer-review process, which is often too slow and may result in the collection of valuable baseline data being missed, are required.

3.9.2 Neighbourhood definition

In addition to study design, a key issue limiting the consistency of findings is the scale at which neighbourhood walkability is being measured.[10,11,13,45,46,87] As previously mentioned, a variety of 'neighbourhood' definitions, typically based on researcher-defined distance from home (e.g. 1 km, person-specific 'neighbourhoods') or existing boundaries (e.g. census tracts), have been used to assess neighbourhood design features.[10,11,13,45,46,87] At present, no optimal scale has been identified.[13,46] This is highly problematical for several reasons. Firstly, different scales may differentially influence the impact of walkability (or related indicators) on outcomes like physical activity and obesity.[10,13,46] For example, as illustrated here and consistent with the observation by Papas *et al.*,[13] the impact of urban sprawl on obesity differs by the spatial scale adopted, undoubtedly due to the variation within any spatial area.

In addition, the neighbourhood scale relevant to study the neighbourhood design–obesity relationship may vary according to the population being studied.[45,46] In line with the rationale to explain the differential effects of apartment living on adults versus children,[62] one example may be that walkability within a shorter buffer around the home or for smaller block size groups may be more appropriate for children or older adults who may be restricted in how far they may or are allowed to travel, when compared with able-bodied adults.

For researchers interested in differences between objective and perceived neighbourhood design indicators in relation to obesity, inconsistencies between researcher ('objective') and resident ('perceived') neighbourhood definitions are also a problem.[45,46] Several review authors have suggested that both perceived neighbourhood and objective neighbourhood data should be captured[11,13] and recent studies[74] have attempted to clarify the contribution of the two types of data on obesity.[10]

Finally, a major issue in the literature to date is that using different neighbourhood scale indicators across studies impedes the generalisability of findings.[10,46] To remedy these issues, some authors recommend that researchers 'investigate the implications of using different sized-buffer zones for different environmental exposures, behaviours and across different target groups' (para 24),[45] advice that is reiterated by others.[13] Thus, researchers may benefit from reviewing the work of Berke et al.[47] who assessed BMI and walkability at different-sized area buffers.

3.9.3 Measurement

If what is measured and how it is measured is not sound or sufficient, the conclusions drawn will be biased. First, the 'soundness' or validity of outcome measures needs to be considered. In previous reviews,[10,11] the reliance of self-reported height and weight across studies examining neighbourhood design and obesity has been questioned. Bias is introduced as self-reported BMI is often lower than measured assessments as study participants often underestimate weight and overestimate height.[88–91] Future studies could examine the difference in self-reported versus measured BMI in studies of walkability and neighbourhood design to assess whether in environmental studies, the use of self-reported measures reduces associations found. Further, the impact of walkability and neighbourhood design on other weight-related indicators,[11] such as waist circumference or waist-to-hip ratio (as used by Stafford et al.[44]), could also be examined. Moreover, while Spence et al.[58] did not find any differences in the neighbourhood design–obesity relationship when using two different obesity cut-offs for preschool children, a similar approach could be for other studies to ensure that differential cut-offs do not introduce additional bias in the outcome measure.

The second measurement issue is the 'soundness' or validity of measures of neighbourhood design and walkability. Again, Ball et al. succinctly note that 'there appears a tendency for studies to be guided more by the data that are available than by careful a priori theoretical selection and conceptualisation of key environmental exposures' (para 10).[45] The use of existing data often means accepting a predetermined neighbourhood scale.[13] Thus, Booth et al.[11] contrast the merits of direct (e.g. environmental audits), intermediate (e.g. phone books, perceived indicators) and indirect (e.g. Census, GIS) measures of the neighbourhood design environment. Although such data are available and may be expedient as some suggest,[45] the validity of data from the latter two sources is questioned on the basis of the extent to which the collected intermediate data is accurate and the elapsed time between data collection and changes to the real world with indirect assessments.[11] Even in recognising the time and cost-intensive nature of primary data collection, they recommend using direct measurements such as audits to ensure quality data.[11] In a recent 2006 supplement of the *Journal of Physical*

Activity and Health, several audit tools related to neighbourhood design and the broader built environment are presented.[92–94] However, before direct measurement is recommended as the 'standard', validation studies are required of existing data sources to assist in assessing its quality and levels of measurement error.

The third measurement issue relates to the need for a better conceptual and theoretical understanding of the underpinnings of the relationship between obesity and the built environment.[45] Based on social–ecological models,[5–7] ecological models consider multiple levels of influence on the basis that research and future interventions must look beyond the individual. Similarly, others[45,46] use physical activity behaviours to advocate examining the relative influences of not only physical environment factors, but also social and individual factors. In their recent review, Black and Macinko remark that 'few of the studies reviewed have tested a comprehensive model of the determinants of obesity at the neighbourhood level' (p. 14).[10] They provide a framework that includes physical activity and dietary behaviour, individual factors (e.g. demographics, attitudes), environment (e.g. physical features, social support) and broader factors (e.g. policy, history), and how these factors may interact to influence obesity, as a way to stimulate research and hypothesis testing.

To take this point further, Wells *et al.*[14] consider the role of mediators and moderators of obesity-related behaviours of physical activity and diet and built environment features. However, mediators and moderators may also be examined with obesity as an outcome. Building upon Black and Macinko's[10] framework, researchers may wish to consider testing the relative influence of physical activity and diet in terms of accounting for the obesity–neighbourhood design relationship. Several studies reviewed explicitly explored how adjustment for each type of obesity-related behaviour impacted the obesity–environment relationship, yet many studies reviewed did not test for the range of relevant obesity-related risk factor behaviours. For instance, one study[42] found that sprawl influences obesity directly and indirectly through physical activity while in another study, accounting for obesity-related behaviours strengthened the link between weight status and sprawl, which, in one model, had previously been insignificant.[49] However, other research found no mediating effect of physical activity for obesity and neighbourhood design variables of interest.[37,44,71]

As for moderators, the impact of the neighbourhood design features of obesity-related behaviours (and, as we note here, for obesity itself) may be relevant only for some populations[14] as seen in some of the studies reviewed in this chapter.[18,58,61,63] For example, the extent to which the neighbourhood design–obesity relationship varies by age[13] is worthy of future consideration, as are the moderating influences of population density in developing countries[64] and variations that might result according to other design features[79] or personal factors.[69] Examining these conceptual and theoretical pathways and taking into account context-specific environment and behaviour-specific measures (e.g. specific types of physical activity and dietary indices)[45,46] may assist in fine-tuning relationships and thus, advancing our understanding of neighbourhood design influences on obesity.

3.10   Summary

The study of the impact of neighbourhood walkability on obesity and overweight is a new field of endeavour and is gaining traction. To date, there is promising evidence that the way we build cities may influence weight status partly because urban design impacts whether or not residents are easily able to walk, cycle or use public transit, and how much time they spend driving. Reported automobile use or time spent driving has been shown to be associated with weight status[18,19,43] as have county-based indices of commute time and vehicle miles travelled.[53] As the evidence base unfolds and the mediating and moderating influences of urban design are considered, future studies will strengthen the evidence base by paying greater attention to study design (and the need for more longitudinal and natural experiment evidence in order to address the issue of causality) and measurement of both weight status and the built environment (in particular the issue of geographical scale), examining differences that might be evident across different sub-populations across the life-course and paying better attention to the conceptualisation and theoretical underpinnings of studies and the hypothesised relationship. Without addressing these issues, the evidence base will continue to present a confusing picture, which will impede policymakers taking action and will provide a convenient excuse for inaction due to 'insufficient' or 'inconsistent' evidence. Given the challenge of the task ahead, there is clearly an urgent need for advice about best buys with the greater leverage if we are to better address the obesity issue.

The health sector may only encourage environmental change rather than facilitate or implement change. Thus, it is important for researchers to form partnerships with policymakers and practitioners to ensure that they pursue research that will directly inform policy and practice, and in so doing, help to facilitate and galvanise action. In this regard, funding bodies have a role to play by actively encouraging these partnerships through funding requirements for active and demonstrated partnerships.

References

1. James, W.P.T., Leach, R., Rigby, N. Introduction: an international perspective on obesity and obesogenic environments. In: *Obesogenic Environments: Complexities, Perceptions and Objective Measures*. (Eds. Townshend, T., Alvanides, S., Lake, A.) Wiley-Blackwell, United Kingdom, 2009.
2. Hill, J.O. (2006) Understanding and addressing the epidemic of obesity: an energy balance perspective. *Endocrine Reviews*. 27:750–761.
3. Hill, J.O., Melanson, E.L. (1999) Overview of the determinants of overweight and obesity: current evidence and research issues. *Medicine and Science in Sports and Exercise*. 31(Suppl. 11):S515–S521.
4. Hill, J.O., Peters, J.C. (1998) Environmental contributions to the obesity epidemic. *Science*. 280:1371–1374.
5. Sallis, J.F., Cervero, R.B., Ascher, W., Henderson, K.A., Kraft, M.K., Kerr, J. (2006) An ecological approach to creating active living communities. *Annual Review of Public Health*. 27:297–322.

6. Sallis, J.F., Owen, N. Determinants of physical activity. In: *Physical Activity and Behavioral Medicine*. Sage, Thousand Oaks, CA, 1999 pp. 110–133.
7. Sallis, J.F., Owen, N. Ecological models of health behaviour. In: *Health Behavior and Health Education: Theory, Research and Practice*. (Eds. Glanz, K., Lewis, F.M., Rimer, B.K.) 3rd Edition, Jossey-Bass, San Francisco, CA, 2002 pp. 462–484.
8. Swinburn, B., Egger, G., Razza, F. (1999) Dissecting obesogenic environments: the development and application of a framework for identifying and prioritizing environmental interventions for obesity. *Preventive Medicine*. 29:563–570.
9. Anderson, P.M., Butcher, K.F. (2006) Childhood obesity: trends and potential causes. *Future Child*. 16:19–45.
10. Black, J.L., Macinko, J. (2008) Neighbourhoods and obesity. *Nutrition Reviews*. 66:2–20.
11. Booth, K.M., Pinkston, M.M., Poston, W.S.C. (2005) Obesity and the built environment. *Journal of the American Dietetic Association*. 105(5, Suppl. 1):S110–S117.
12. Brisbon, N., Plumb, J., Brawer, R., Paxman, D. (2005) The asthma and obesity epidemics: the role played by the built environment. A public health perspective. *Journal of Allergy and Clinical Immunology*. 115:1024–1028.
13. Papas, M.A., Alberg, A.J., Ewing, R., Helzlsouer, K.J., Gary, T.L., Klassen, A.C. (2007) The built environment and obesity. *Epidemiologic Reviews*. 29:129–143.
14. Wells, N.M., Ashdown, S.P., Davies, E.H.S., Cowett, F.D., Yang, Y. (2007) Environment, design, and obesity. *Environment and Behaviour*. 39:6–33.
15. Woodcock, J., Banister, D., Edwards, P., Prentice, A.M., Roberts, I. (2007) Energy and transport. *Lancet*. 370:1078–1088.
16. Frank, L.D., Engleke, P. *How Land Use and Transportation Systems Impact Public Health: A Literature Review of the Relationship between Physical Activity and Built Form*. Atlanta, GA, Centers for Disease Control and Prevention, 2000. Available at: http://www.cdc.gov/nccdphp/dnpa/pdf/aces-workingpaper1.pdf.
17. Frumkin, H., Frank, L., Jackson, R. *Urban Sprawl and Public Health: Designing, Planning, and Building for Healthy Communities*. Washington, DC, Island Press, 2004.
18. Frank, L.D., Andresen, M.A., Schmid, T.L. (2004) Obesity relationships with community design, physical activity, and time spent in cars. *American Journal of Preventive Medicine*. 27:87–96.
19. Wen, L.M., Orr, N., Millett, C., Rissel, C. (2006) Driving to work and overweight and obesity: findings from the 2003 New South Wales Health Survey, Australia. *International Journal of Obesity (London)*. 30:782–786.
20. Frank, K.L., Sallis, J.F., Conway, T.L., Chapman, J.E., Saelens, B.E., Bachman, W. (2006) Many pathways from land use to health associations between neighbourhood walkability and active transportation, body mass index, and air quality. *Journal of the American Planning Association*. 72:75–87.
21. Badland, H., Schofield, G. (2005) Transport, urban design, and physical activity: an evidence-based update. *Transportation Research Part D – Transport and Environment*. 10: 177–196.
22. Humpel, N., Owen, N., Leslie, E. (2002) Environmental factors associated with adults' participation in physical activity: a review. *American Journal of Preventive Medicine*. 22:188–199.
23. McCormack, G., Giles-Corti, B., Lange, A., Smith, T.K., Martin, K., Pikora, T.J. (2004) An update of recent evidence of the relationship between objective and self-report measures of the physical environment and physical activity behaviours. *Journal of Science and Medicine in Sport*. 7(Suppl. 1):81–92.
24. Owen, N., Humpel, N., Leslie, E., Bauman, A.E., Sallis, J.F. (2004) Understanding environmental influences on walking: review and research agenda. *American Journal of Preventive Medicine*. 27:67–76.
25. Saelens, B.E., Sallis, J.F., Frank, L.D. (2003) Environmental correlates of walking and cycling: findings from the transportation, urban design, and planning literatures. *Annals of Behavioral Medicine*. 25:80–91.

26. Transportation Research Board. 2005 *Does the Built Environment Influence Physical Activity? Examining the Evidence*. Washington, DC, TRB. Available at: http://onlinepubs. trb.org/Onlinepubs/sr/sr282.pdf.
27. Wendel-Vos, W., Droomers, M., Kremers, S., Brug, J., van Lenthe, F. (2007) Potential environmental determinants of physical activity in adults: a systematic review. *Obesity Reviews*. 8:425–440.
28. Davison, K.K., Lawson, C.T. (2006) Do attributes in the physical environment influence children's physical activity? A review of the literature. *International Journal of Behavioral Nutrition and Physical Activity*. 3:3–19.
29. Ferreira, I., van der Horst, K., Wendel-Vos, W., Kremers, S., van Lenthe, F.J., Brug, J. (2006) Environmental correlates of physical activity in youth: a review and update. *Obesity Reviews*. 8:129–154.
30. Salmon, J., Booth, M.L., Phongsavan, P., Murphy, N., Timperio, A. (2007) Promoting physical activity participation among children and adolescents. *Epidemiologic Reviews*. 29:144–159.
31. Frank, L.D., Engelke, P.O., Schmid, T.L. *Health and Community Design: The Impact of the Built Environment on Physical Activity*. Washington, DC, Island Press, 2003.
32. Pikora, T.J., Giles-Corti, B., Knuiman, M.W., Bull, F.C., Jamrozik, K., Donovan, R.J. (2006) Neighborhood environmental factors correlated with walking near home: using SPACES. *Medicine and Science in Sports and Exercise*. 38:708–714.
33. Forsyth, A., Southworth, M. (2008) Guest editorial: cities afoot: pedestrians, walkability and urban design. *Journal of Urban Design*. 13:1–3.
34. Smart Growth Vermont. (2008) What is sprawl. Available at: http://www. smartgrowthvermont.org/learn/sprawl/?no_cache=1&sword_list%5B0%5D=sprawl.
35. Leslie, E., Saelens, B., Frank, L.D., Owen, N., Bauman, A., Coffee, N., Hugo, G. (2005) Residents' perceptions of walkability attributes in objectively different neighbourhoods: a pilot study. *Health and Place*. 11:227–236.
36. Doyle, S., Kelly-Schwartz, A., Schlossberg, M., Stockard, J. (2006) Active community environments and health. *Journal of the American Planning Association*. 72:19–31.
37. Rutt, C.D., Coleman, K.J. (2005) Examining the relationships among built environment, physical activity, and body mass index in El Paso, TX. *Preventive Medicine*. 40:831–841.
38. Rundle, A., Diez Roux, A.V., Freeman, L.M., Miller, D., Neckerman, K.M., Weiss, C.C. (2007) The urban built environment and obesity in New York City: a multilevel analysis. *American Journal of Health Promotion*. 21(Suppl. 4):S326–S334.
39. Dill, J. (2004) Measuring network connectivity for bicycling and walking. *Joint Congress of ACSP-AESPO*. Leuven, Belgium. Available at: http://www.enhancements.org/download/ trb/trb2004/TRB2004-001550.pdf.
40. Handy, S.L., Boarnet, M.G., Ewing, R., Killingsworth, R.E. (2002) How the built environment affects physical activity: views from urban planning. *American Journal of Preventive Medicine*. 23:64–73.
41. Frank, L.D., Saelens, B.E., Powell, K.E., Chapman, J.E. (2007) Stepping towards causation: do built environments or neighbourhood and travel preferences explain physical activity, driving, and obesity? *Social Science and Medicine*. 65:1898–1914.
42. Ewing, R., Schmid, T., Killingsworth, R., Zlot, A., Raudenbush, S. (2003) Relationship between urban sprawl and physical activity, obesity, and morbidity. *American Journal of Health Promotion*. 18:47–57.
43. Pendola, R., Gen, S. (2007) BMI, auto use, and the urban environment in San Francisco. *Health and Place*. 13:551–556.
44. Stafford, M., Cummins, S., Ellaway, A., Sacker, A., Wiggins, R.D., Macintyre, S. (2007) Pathways to obesity: identifying local, modifiable determinants of physical activity and diet. *Social Science and Medicine*. 65:1882–1897.
45. Ball, K., Timperio, A.F., Crawford, D.A. (2006) Understanding environmental influences on nutrition and physical activity behaviours: where should we look and what should we count? *International Journal of Behavioural Nutrition and Physical Activity*. 3:33.
46. Giles-Corti, B., Timperio, A., Bull, F., Pikora, T. (2005) Understanding physical environmental correlate: increased specificity for ecological models. *Exercise and Sport Sciences Reviews*. 33:175–181.

47. Berke, E.M., Koepsell, T.D., Moudon, A.V., Hoskins, R.E., Larson, E.B. (2007) Association of the built environment with physical activity and obesity in older persons. *American Journal of Public Health*. 97:486–492.
48. Kligerman, M., Sallis, J.F., Ryan, S., Frank, L.D., Nader, P.R. (2007) Association of neighbourhood design and recreation environment variables with physical activity and body mass index in adolescents. *American Journal of Health Promotion*. 21:274–277.
49. Ewing, R., Brownson, R.C., Berrigan, D. (2006) Relationship between urban sprawl and weight of United States youth. *American Journal of Preventive Medicine*. 31:464–474.
50. Kelly-Schwartz, A.C., Stockard, J., Doyle, S., Schlossberg, M. (2004) Is sprawl unhealthy? A multilevel analysis of the relationship of metropolitan sprawl to the health of individuals. *Journal of Planning Education and Research*. 24:184–196.
51. Lopez, R. (2007) Neighbourhood risk factors for obesity. *Obesity*. 15:2111–2119.
52. Ross, N.A., Tremblay, S., Khan, S., Crouse, D., Tremblay, M., Berthelot, J.M. (2007) Body mass index in urban Canada: neighborhood and metropolitan area effects. *American Journal of Public Health*. 97:500–508.
53. Lopez-Zutina, J., Lee, H., Friisa, R. (2006) The link between obesity and the built environment: evidence from an ecological analysis of obesity and vehicle miles of travel in California. *Health and Place*. 12:656–664.
54. Maddock, J. (2004) The relationship between obesity and prevalence of fast food restaurants: state-level analysis. *American Journal of Health Promotion*. 19:137–143.
55. Vangergrift, D., Yoked, T. (2004) Obesity rates, income, and suburban sprawl: an analysis of US States. *Health and Place*. 10:221–229.
56. Owen, N., Cerin, E., Leslie, E., duToit, L., Coffee, N., Frank, L.D. (2007) Neigbourhood walkability and the walking behavior of Australian adults. *American Journal of Preventive Medicine*. 33:387–395.
57. Saelens, B.E., Sallis, J.F., Black, J.B., Chen, D. (2003) Neighborhood-based differences in physical activity: an environment scale evaluation. *American Journal of Public Health*. 93:1552–1558.
58. Spence, J.C., Cutumisu, N., Edwards, J., Evans, J. (2008) Influence of neighbourhood design and access to facilities on overweight among preschool children. *International Journal of Pediatric Obesity*. 3:109–116.
59. Norman, G.J., Nutter, S.K., Ryan, S., Sallis, J.F., Calfas, K.J., Patrick, K. (2006) Community design and access to recreational facilites as correlates of adolescent physical activity and body mass index. *Journal of Physical Activity and Health*. 3(Suppl. 1):S118–S128.
60. Grafova, I.B. (2008) Overweight children: assessing the contribution of the built environment. *Preventive Medicine*. 47:304–308.
61. Frank, L.D., Kerr, J., Sallis, J.F., Miles, R., Chapman, J. (2008) A hierarchy of sociodemographic and environmental correlates of walking and obesity. *Preventive Medicine*. 47:172–178.
62. Lazarou, C., Panagiotakos, D.B., Panayiotou, G., Matalas, A.L. (2008) Overweight and obesity in preadolescent children and their parents in Cyprus: prevalence and associated socio-demographic factors – the CYKIDS study. *Obesity Reviews*. 9:185–193.
63. Smith, K.R., Brown, B.B., Yamada, I., Kowaleski-Jones, L., Zick, C.D., Fan, J.X. (2008) Walkability and body mass index: density, design, and new diversity measures. *American Journal of Preventive Medicine*. 35:237–244.
64. Colchero, M.A., Bishai, D. (2008) Effect of neighborhood exposures on changes in weight among women in Cebu, Philippines (1983–2002). *American Journal of Epidemiology*. 167:615–623.
65. Popkin, B.M., Paeratakul, S., Zhai, F., Ge, K. (1995) Dietary and environmental correlates of obesity in a population study in China. *Obesity Research*. 3(Suppl. 2):S135–S143.
66. Mobley, L.R., Root, E.D., Finkelstein, E.A., Khavjou, O., Farris, R.P. (2006) Environment, obesity, and cardiovascular disease risk in low-income women. *American Journal of Preventive Medicine*. 30:327–332.
67. Li, F.Z., Harmer, P.A., Cardinal, B.J., Bosworth, M., Acock, A., Johnson-Shelton, D. Moore, J.M. (2008) Built environment, adiposity, and physical activity in adults aged 50–75. *American Journal of Preventive Medicine*. 35:38–46.

68. Heinrich, K.M., Lee, R.E., Regan, G.R., *et al.* (2008) How does the built environment relate to body mass index and obesity prevalence among public housing residents? *American Journal of Health Promotion.* 22:187–194.
69. Joshu, C.E., Boehmer, T.K., Brownson, R.C., Ewing, R. (2008) Personal, neighbourhood and urban factors associated with obesity in the United States. *Journal of Epidemiology and Community Health.* 62:202–208.
70. Lopez, R. (2004) Urban sprawl and risk for being overweight or obese. *American Journal of Public Health.* 94:1574–1579.
71. Poortinga, W. (2006) Perceptions of the environment, physical activity and obesity. *Social Science and Medicine.* 63:2835–2846.
72. Li, M., Dibley, M.J., Sibbritt, D., Yan, H. (2008) Factors associated with adolescent's overweight and obesity at community, school and household levels in Xi'an City, China: results of hierarchical analysis. *European Journal of Clinical Nutrition.* 62:635–643.
73. Giles-Corti, B., Macintyre, S., Clarkson, J.P., Pikora, T., Donovan, R.J. (2003) Environmental and lifestyle factors associated with overweight and obesity in Perth, Australia. *American Journal of Health Promotion.* 18:93–102.
74. Boehmer, T.K., Hoehner, C.M., Deshpande, A.D., Ramirex, L.K.B., Brownson, R.C. (2007) Perceived and observed neighbourhood indicators of obesity among urban adults. *International Journal of Obesity.* 31:968–977.
75. Catlin, T.K., Simoes, E.J., Brownson, R.C. (2003) Environmental and policy factors associated with overweight among adults in Missouri. *American Journal of Health Promotion.* 17:249–258.
76. Evenson, K.R., Scott, M.M., Cohen, D.A., Voorhees, C.C. (2007) Girl's perceptions of neighbourhood factors on physical activity, sedentary behaviour, and BMI. *Obesity.* 15:430–445.
77. Boehmer, T.K., Lovegreen, S.L., Haire-Joshu, D., Brownson, R.C. (2006) What constitutes an obesogenic environment in rural communities. *American Journal of Health Promotion.* 20:411–421.
78. Wilson, D.K., Ainsworth, B.E., Bowles, H. (2007) Body mass index and environmental supports for physical activity among active and inactive residents of a U.S. Southeastern County. *Health Psychology.* 26:710–717.
79. Liu, G.C., Wilson, J.S., Qi, R., Ying, J. (2007) Green neighbourhoods, food retail and childhood overweight: differences by population density. *American Journal of Health Promotion.* 21(Suppl. 4):S317–S325.
80. Petticrew, M. Cummins, S., Ferrell, C., Finday, A., Higgins, C., Hoy, C., Kearns, A., Sparks, L. (2005) Natural experiments: an underused tool for public health? *Public Health.* 119:751–757.
81. Ramanathan, S., Allison, K.R., Faulkner, G., Dwyer, J.J.M. (2008) Challenges in assessing the implementation and effectiveness of physical activity and nutrition policy interventions as natural experiments. *Health Promotion International.* 23:290–297.
82. Handy, S.L., Cao, X., Mokhtarian, P.L. (2006) Self-selection in the relationship between the built environment and walking. *Journal of the American Planning Association.* 72:55–74.
83. Giles-Corti, B., Knuiman, M., Timperio, A., Van Nielc, K., Pikora, T.J., Bull, F.C.L., Shilton, T., Bulsara, M. (2008) Evaluation of the implementation of a state government community design policy aimed at increasing local walking: design issues and baseline results from RESIDE, Perth Western Australia. *Preventive Medicine.* 46:46–54.
84. Brownson, R.C., Kelly, C.M., Eyler, A.A., Carnoske, C., Grost, L., Handy, S., Maddock, J., Pluto, D., Ritacco, B., Sallis, J., Schmid, T. (2008) Environmental and policy approaches for promoting physical activity in the United States: a research agenda. *Journal of Physical Activity and Health.* 5:488–503.
85. Active Living Research and Healthy Eating Research. (2008) Building Evidence to Prevent Childhood Obesity. 2008 Call for Proposals – Rapid-Response Grants. Retrieved November 13, 2008 from: http://www.activelivingresearch.org/files/ALR-HER_RapidResponse_FINAL.pdf.

86. Canadian Institute of Health Research. (2007–2008) Operating Grant: Intervention Research. ARCHIVED. Retrieved December 17, 2008 from http://www.researchnet-recherchenet.ca/rnr16/viewOpportunityDetails.do?prog=399&&view=currentOpps&org=CIHR&type=AND&resultCount=25&sort=program&all=1&masterList=true.

87. Gauvin, L., Robitaille, E., Riva, M., McLaren, L., Dassa, C., Potvin, L. (2007) Conceptualizing and operationalizing neighbourhoods. *Canadian Journal of Public Health*. 98(Suppl. 1):S18–S26.

88. Boström, G., Diderichsen, F. (1997) Socioeconomic differentials in misclassification of height, weight, and body mass index based on questionnaire data. *International Journal of Epidemiology*. 26:860–866.

89. John, U., Hanke, M., Grothues, J., Thyrian, J.R. (2006) Validity of overweight and obesity in a nation based on self-report versus measured device data. *European Journal of Clinical Nutrition*. 60:372–377.

90. Nyholm, M., Gullberg, B., Merlo, J., Lundquist-Persson, C., Rastam, L., Lindblad, U. (2007) The validity of obesity based on self-reported weight and height: implications for population studies. *Obesity*. 15:197–208.

91. Spencer, E.A., Appleby, P.N., Davey, G.K., Key, T.J. (2002) Validity of self-reported height and weight in 4804 EPIC-Oxford participants. *Public Health and Nutrition*. 5:561–565.

92. Troped, P.J., Cromley, E.K., Fragala, M.S., Melly, S.J., Hasbrouck, H.H., Gortmaker, S.L., Brownson, R.C. (2006) Development and reliability and validity testing of an audit tool for trail/path characteristics: the Path Environment Audit Tool (PEAT). *Journal of Physical Activity and Health*. 3(Suppl. 1):S158–S175.

93. Bedimo-Rung, A.L., Gustat, J., Tompkins, B.J., Rice, J., Thomson, J. (2006) Development of a direct observation instrument to measure environmental characteristics of parks for physical activity. *Journal of Physical Activity and Health*. 3(Suppl. 1):S176–S189.

94. Saelens, B.E., Frank, L.D., Auffrey, C., Whitaker, R.C., Burdette, H.L., Colabianchi, N. (2006) Measuring physical environments of parks and playgounds: EAPRS instrument development and inter-rater reliability. *Journal of Physical Activity and Health*. 3(Suppl. 1):S190–S207.

4 Availability and Accessibility in Physical Activity Environments

Andy Jones and Jenna Panter

4.1 Introduction

This chapter considers the manner in which the availability and accessibility of resources may be associated with physical activity levels in the population. We begin by considering the theoretical underpinnings of work that has examined the relationship between the provision of resources and their utilisation, before moving on to discuss the importance of both perceived and objectively measured indicators of accessibility and how they can tell us rather different things about underlying causal processes. We then examine how disparities in the provision, and consequent accessibility, of facilities may be patterned by socio-economic concerns before looking at how this may translate into disparities in use. The chapter concludes by highlighting the importance of utilising the research evidence base for the design of interventions and the development of planning regulations.

4.2 The concept of availability and accessibility

The terms 'accessibility' and 'availability' are often used interchangeably; yet, whilst they are undoubtedly related, they are not the same. The availability of a resource simply describes whether or not it is *potentially* available. In other words, does it exist? Accessibility, on the other hand, is concerned with the ease by which those that wish to do so are able to make use of it, and hence it is a measure of actual availability. The concept of accessibility is perhaps grounded most strongly in the field of health service delivery planning. Here, Gutmann[1] (p. 543) defines the principle of access as 'every person who shares the same type and degree of health need must be given an equally effective chance of receiving appropriate treatment of equal quality so that treatment is available to anyone'. This definition encompasses two subtle yet distinct components. Firstly, it highlights the desirability of matching accessibility with need; a resource which has good accessibility does not necessarily need to be equally accessible to all, but instead accessibility should equate to demand. When considering the links between levels of physical activity and the characteristics of the environment, a far from exhaustive list of relevant resources includes parks and greenspaces, bicycle trails and walking paths. A second key component of this definition is the use of the term 'quality', which emphasises that accessibility is more than just the ease at which the resource can be obtained, but also that the concept of value is important. Hence, both ease and satisfaction are important components of how accessible something is.

In a perfect society, we might envisage that all citizens would have excellent access to the services that they require. Of course, no such utopian vision actually exists. Therefore, we are left to try and identify and ameliorate what are known as barriers of access, or factors that lead to certain population groups finding it difficult to access the services they need. These barriers are invariably linked with issues of resource allocation, priority setting or 'rationing'.[2] We might all like to have a well-staffed sports complex available in our neighbourhood, complete with long opening hours and free entry or low entry fees, but a combination of the profit motives of capitalism and the limited finances available to state providers, often rules this out. Nevertheless, whilst barriers of access are usually complex and multifaceted, they can be usefully simplified into three broad socio-economic, geographical and organisational components. The hierarchy of these components is depicted in Figure 4.1.

Socio-economic barriers revolve around the premise that richer, more influential members of society will have easier access to the goods and services they require, with restricted access for the poor. Issues of culture, ability to pay and competence in effectively utilising resources are pivotal here. Over two decades ago, Joseph and Phillips[3] argued that the most pervasive influence on utilisation behaviours for health facilities was not necessarily need, but rather the socio-economic

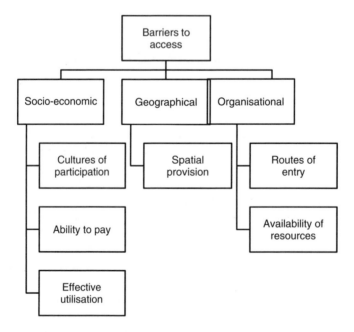

Figure 4.1 The varied nature of barriers of access.

status of the consumer. The general pattern of evidence suggests that the more socio-economically disadvantaged members of all societies exhibit lower than expected utilisation of potentially health enhancing resources, including those that can be used by individuals to be physically active, despite the fact that their need is arguably the greatest.[4] The causal pathways that underlie these observations are undoubtedly complex, yet revolve around a number of key components. One concerns cultures of participation, or rather non-participation, where certain groups may feel that facilities in their neighbourhood have not been provided for them.[5] Ability to pay is also an important determinant of resource utilisation, particularly where the management of facilities is driven by profit motives. Panter et al.[6], for example, have recently shown how the provision of private gym facilities may be best in inner-city areas where they are most available for those working in central business district employment locations. Yet, the permanent residents of these areas are often least able to afford gym entry or membership fees. There is also evidence, particularly from the field of health services research, that even if members of more socio-economically deprived populations do initiate use of a resource, their interactions may be less effective and the benefits obtained fewer.[7]

Although much of the published research investigating issues of service utilisation has been focused on individual determinants, almost three decades ago Wennberg and Gittlesohn[8] suggested that the utilisation of a service may also be more determined by organisational concerns. Brown and Barnett[9] have since proposed that delivery organisations can influence availability and accessibility through the supply of resources that are made available, the organisational structures that are put in place and the beliefs and attitudes that underpin them. In essence, variations in supply will lead to variations in the availability of resources and these in turn will influence accessibility. For example, policy-driven variations in the provision of facilities for cyclists have long been used to explain international disparities in the prevalence of cycling, with countries such as the Netherlands often being cited as examples of places where good provision of accessible and convenient facilities acts to stimulate demand.[10] Of course, the appropriate direction of causality is difficult to determine and it could be argued that good provision of facilities, in many cases, is simply meeting prior demand that is itself driven by historical cultures of participation, rather than by individuals being encouraged to actually take-up cycling by high prior levels of facility provision. Yet, Giles-Corti et al.[11] have, amongst others, strongly argued how any initiatives to increase the prevalence of physical activity in the population should be accompanied by the provision of a supportive environment, and it is difficult to see how the many observed associations between such supportiveness and physical activity reported in this chapter can be purely the result of reverse causality.

The third, and perhaps the best-researched component, is geographical, and hence concerns distance and the associated time and monetary costs of travel. Shannon and Denver[12] noted that interest in the concept of distance as a barrier to seeking healthcare has been documented as far back as the mid-19th century in the literature, although until the mid-1960s, a period known as the 'quantitative revolution' in geography when computers were beginning to be used in geographical studies, the importance of spatial patterns of service provision was largely ignored. Now there is substantial evidence that the use of many services and facilities is strongly influenced by locational factors.[13] Here, issues of rurality can come to the fore, and in the mid-1970s the term *centrism* was coined to describe the tendency of facilities to be concentrated in larger urban centres.[14]

The causal process by which distance may affect utilisation of a resource is multifaceted. Firstly, it could be that the physical problems of reaching something amongst those living further away are of a sufficient magnitude to discourage use. Relevant considerations here include the costs and availability of transportation, or the time required for the journey relative to the perceived availability of time. Alternatively, it could be that proximity acts to generate new demand amongst local populations. Those living close to an urban park, for example, may see it on a daily basis and this familiarity may generate a demand for recreational use of the park. This demand may not be observed in those living more distant as their lack of familiarity with the resource means that their desire to use it has never been stimulated. Either way, the numerous studies that have examined the effects of distance since the late 1960s have highlighted the phenomenon of 'distance decay' where use of a resource declines with distance in an often highly predictable manner.[15] Figure 4.2 provides a graphical representation of this distance decay effect.

Interpreting the significance of distance decay is not without problems. A simple view would be that its presence signifies some form of inequity, whereby those living furthest away are being denied use. Yet, given the wide variety of contexts in which physical activity may be undertaken, distance decay in the use of a particular resource may not signify unmet need but rather the fact that the less proximal are making use of alternative locations or types of resource instead. For example, rural residents typically live further from formal parks or greenspaces, yet poorer access

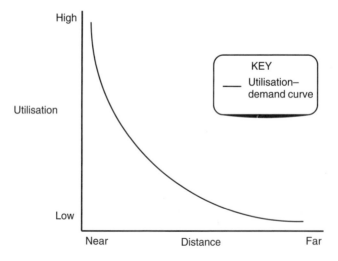

Figure 4.2 Utilisation behaviours are typically subject to distance decay where levels of use decline with increasing distance.

to these facilities may be more than adequately compensated for by the informal opportunities to be active provided by the rural environment.

All the above considerations mean that the relationships between need, utilisation, availability and access are complex. Nevertheless, considerations surrounding accessibility are an important component of the environmental influences on physical activity and, given the focus on the physical environment here, it is this spatial component that warrants particular attention and hence forms the bulk of the evidence reviewed in this chapter. Spatial considerations have certainly driven much of the recent literature, and the recent heightened interest in the spatial determinants of physical activity has, at least in part, been driven by the continued development and widespread adoption of Geographical Information Systems (GISs) and their associated databases. A good definition of GIS is that of Dueker and Kjerne (p. 8)[16] who define it as 'a system of hardware, software, data, people, organisations, and institutional arrangements for collecting, storing, analysing, and disseminating information about areas of the earth'. The high uptake of GIS in academia over the last decade has allowed researchers to undertake the often complex data manipulations and calculations required for the determination of spatial accessibility with relative ease and this, coupled with an increasing interest in the environmental determinants of physical activity, has acted to stimulate a wide range of new research programmes and initiatives. We now move on to consider the research evidence that they have generated.

4.3 Perceived and objective measures of the physical activity environment

Within the field of physical activity research there are two superficially similar, but in fact very different, means of assessing the environment; the use of either perceived or objective measurements. The first captures self-reported perceptions provided by study subjects, and is hence subjective in nature. Studies utilising perception-based measures commonly employ survey instruments that elicit information regarding the respondent's perceived proximity to amenities such as shops, parks, sports facilities or places of employment[17] or the presence of facilities such as those to assist with walking and cycling.[18] In contrast, objective assessments seek to quantify the measured characteristics of the environment. These typically use on-the-ground street audits or employ spatial referenced geographical data stored and analysed in a GIS. Accessibility may be captured in terms of the distance between destinations, either using straight-line or road distances[19] or the connectivity of the street network in an area.[20] We move on to discuss and compare the research evidence from studies that have examined perceived and observed measures, respectively, as determinants of physical activity.

4.3.1 Perceived measures of the environment

In general, the earliest works that examined the influence of the environment on physical activity levels focused on perceptions of access,[21] sometimes alone and sometimes in combination with other measures of the environment.[17] This early focus is largely a result of the only relatively recent mainstream availability of GIS. In reality, the association between perceived and objectively measured components of accessibility may not be strong. This is because, as much as anything, perceptions are largely a function of awareness of the presence of facilities, and it may only be if people perceive that facilities are available or accessible that they will actually use them. As a result, some authors have stressed the particular importance of perceptions,[22] an issue we shall return to.

Results from a recent meta-analysis indicated that environmental perceptions have a modest but significant influence on overall physical activity. The investigators found that proximity to facilities for physical activity, sidewalks and shops and services were both consistently and positively associated with physical activity.[23] In particular, perceived access to destinations appeared especially important. This appears to be the case for destinations at which physical activity can be undertaken, such as parks or sports facilities, and also for places such as shops, libraries and other community resources. For example, in a sample of women in the United States, King et al.[24] reported that shorter perceived distances to a range of non-physical activity related destinations, such as convenience stores, were associated with higher overall levels of activity. In their meta-analysis, Duncan et al.[23] also noted that access to shops and services actually explained a higher proportion of reported variances in physical activity than did access to physical activity facilities themselves. This may reflect the fact that individuals who perceive such destinations to be more accessible will be more likely to walk or cycle to reach them and will hence be more active. Alternatively, individuals who are more active may simply form a different view of what is accessible, and hence their threshold for classifying distances as more or less accessible may vary.

The potential causal mechanisms underlying the repeated observation that perceptions of better access to facilities in which to undertake physical activity are associated with higher levels of actual activity are rather more readily apparent. Studies that have reported a positive association with physical activity have been based on a variety of measures, including access to places for informal physical activity such as parks[25] as well as indoor and outdoor sports facilities.[26–28] In common with the broader literature on the environmental determinants of physical activity, most of these studies have been conducted in the United States or Australia. This limits their wider applicability as the nature of urban areas in those countries is somewhat distinctive, both in terms of street patterns and the physical location of facilities, and of the particularly high levels of reliance on motorised transportation. Nevertheless, similar findings have been reported in one large-scale analysis using a sample of participants from European member states.[29] Participants in that study who reported higher levels of physical activity were more likely to agree with the statement that the area they lived in offered many opportunities to be physically active.

Some research has specifically investigated associations with perceived access to facilities and physical activity levels in children. In their review article, Davison and Lawson[30] illustrate how inconsistent associations are mostly seen between levels of physical activity in children and perceived good access to playgrounds, although the perceived availability of recreational facilities, measured according to the self-reports of both parents and children, shows consistent positive associations with children's total physical activity.

Given that walking is the only form of moderate intensity physical activity that most able-bodied individuals regularly engage in, it is unsurprising that there has been a particular focus on the activity. The accessible nature of walking promotes social equity and it generates social interaction within communities.[31] In addition, it is relatively easy to build into daily routines for transportation purposes and is hence a significant potential contributor to overall physical activity levels.[32] Studies have considered the influence of perceived accessibility on walking for different purposes including for recreation,[19] for transport,[33] walking undertaken solely within the neighbourhood[34] and total walking.[35] Findings suggest that the importance of access to facilities varies according to purpose. In general, better perceived accessibility of destinations has been positively associated with walking for transport in American cohorts[32,36] and in men.[36] For example, when regular walking was considered in a sample of British participants by Foster et al.,[35] men who reported having a park within walking distance were also more likely to report walking for at least two and a half hours per week. Likewise, work on an Australian cohort by Giles-Corti and Donovan[37] showed an association with perceived access to a public open space, with those who reported having good access being almost 50% more likely to walk at recommended levels compared to those with the poorest access. Humpel et al.[34] also found that women who lived in a coastal location were more likely to report walking in their neighbourhood than their counterparts living further from the coast.

4.3.2   Objective measures of the environment

From the available research evidence, objectively generated measures of access to facilities have shown rather less consistent associations with physical activity than those based on perceptions. This is perhaps surprising if objective measures are taken to represent environmental 'realities', and we discuss the possible reasons for this observation later in the chapter. Nevertheless, better objectively measured access to facilities has been associated with a higher likelihood of meeting overall recommended physical activity levels[38] and greater levels of transport-related physical activity.[39,40] Two studies have examined the relationship between access to the coast or a beach and physical activity.[19,41] Both reported a positive association whereby those with better access were more physically active, although in one, the measure of accessibility used was a proxy based on postal codes,[41] whilst Giles-Corti and Donovan[19] computed actual distances. Furthermore, two studies have demonstrated the positive associations between physical activity levels and the presence of parks and recreation areas.[42,43] Although rather less work has been undertaken in children compared to adults, positive associations have been reported between children's physical activity and objectively measured access to parks and playgrounds[44] and recreational facilities.[45,46]

In contrast to the above studies, other researchers have found no associations with objectively measured access to facilities. Both Hillsdon et al.[47] and Giles-Corti et al.[48] failed to find any associations between access to public parks and greenspaces and physical activity, for example. The presence of inconsistent findings may result at least in part from the way that objective measures of access have been defined and how the prevalence of physical activity has been computed. For example, the use of dichotomous measures of access (e.g. accessible or not) versus continuous measures of distance (e.g. kilometres to the nearest facility) or the application of different thresholds for the identification of individuals as being active (e.g. five sessions a week vs. meeting health recommendations by minutes of participation) may provide divergent results. A further issue concerns the degree of specificity by which outcome measures are matched with resources to which accessibility is being calculated. For example, in their recent Australian study, McCormack et al.[49] found no association between access to vigorous physical activity levels and destinations to visit such as news agents, shops and post offices. Yet, this is perhaps unsurprising given that a higher prevalence of walking or cycling to visit these facilities would only contribute to levels of moderate activity.

Given the importance of walking, we again consider the outcome separately here. Giles-Corti and Donovan[37] have reported that better accessibility to greenspaces and to beaches are associated with higher levels of walking. In addition, good access to the non-residential destinations such as shops and public transport and other facilities has been associated with more walking for transport.[49,50] Two studies have found evidence of a dose–response relationship, whereby the number of destinations in a neighbourhood has been proportionally associated with levels of walking for transport[49] and walking and cycling for transport.[50] McCormack et al.[49] concluded, for example, that the availability of each additional destination within 400 m of a home resulted in an additional 12 minutes spent walking each fortnight.

The majority of the studies discussed above have used GIS to characterise accessibility and availability. However, there is a range of audit tools that can be used by auditors working in a neighbourhood to characterise the local environment. As reviewed by Moudon and Lee,[51] some of these tools include measures of access or availability. Yet, in many of the published works that have made use of such audits, the specific components of the environment have not been reported separately. As a consequence, the association between physical activity behaviour and accessibility or availability as identified through audits has not been extensively tested. For example, Craig et al.[52] did not report associations with individual components of their audit, although they did find that the overall walkability score that the tool produced, which included a measure of accessibility, was positively associated with levels of walking to work in their sample of Canadian residents. The study by Pikora et al.[53] is one of the few studies to separately report specific associations with accessibility and levels of walking. In their work using the SPACES audit tool amongst a sample of adults in Perth, Australia, they found that the accessibility of destinations such as shops and transit stops were significantly correlated with walking for transport, but not recreation, suggesting that the relationship may be causal and highlighting the importance of maintaining specificity in the measures used.

4.4 Comparing perceived and objective measures

If perceptions of accessibility simply act as a true surrogate for objective measures, then a moderate to strong association between both sets of indicators might be expected. Authors such as Owen *et al.*[54] thus argue that key elements of the future research agenda should include improving the reliability and validity of environmental indicators and developing better conceptual models to link them to physical activity outcomes. The use of standardised, reliable self-report measures in multiple studies would help this research field to advance more rapidly, facilitating comparisons of environmental influences across a variety of locations and populations. If possible, both rated and self-reported environmental attributes should be objectively verifiable, either by independent observation or by objective indices derived from GIS databases. If strong patterns of concordance emerged between perceived and objective measures of the accessibility of the same environmental attributes, this would provide support for the validity of the self-reported measures of perceived environment. However, the research evidence available to date suggests that high levels of accordance may not be easily achievable and indeed may not be desirable.

Research studies that have compared perceived and objective estimates of distance to destinations report correlations between the two sets of measures that range between $r = 0.3$[55] and $r = 0.46$.[39] Similarly, low agreements have been found by other authors,[38,56–59] although in their study of 1540 women residing in Melbourne Australia, Ball *et al.*[57] noted that the agreement for a measure of access to the coast was generally higher than for other types of destinations (kappa statistic 0.66). This is likely due to the relative ease with which the location of such a significant feature may be identified.

Interpreting the reason for the generally poor degree of association between perceived and objective measures of accessibility is problematic due to the paucity of gold standards against which comparisons can be made. Objective measures, whilst providing a seemingly definitive set of indicators, can be fraught with error. Chin *et al.*[60] have recently shown, for example, that failure to consider off-road pedestrian cut throughs, a type of feature that rarely appears on maps, can significantly underestimate the ease with which individuals are able to move through a locality. On the other hand, it is entirely plausible that perceptions will be influenced as much by the awareness of an individual as by the actual characteristics of the environment in which they operate. Indeed, Kirtland *et al.*[56] noted that in their study, the agreement between objective and perceived distances were higher for those participants who were more active, suggesting that this group made greater use of their local environment and in doing so gained a greater awareness of its characteristics. This may explain why studies that have examined associations between perceived accessibility and utilisation have generally found stronger associations than those using objective measures.

4.5 Relationships with utilisation

An important research question revolves around the degree to which the accessibility of resources is associated with their use. Indeed, cross-sectional associations detected between physical activity behaviours and the accessibility or availability of facilities may be misleading if they are not accompanied by evidence that those populations with better provision actually make more use of them. However, rather few studies have explored how facility accessibility relates to use. Of those, only one study found no evidence of an association; in their study of 3,000 Canadian residents, Riva et al.[61] reported that the number of physical activity facilities in an area was not associated with the likelihood of participants reporting local facility use. Most of the remaining studies have found positive associations of varying strength and significance, with attributes varying according to facility type. Using both objective and self-reported measures, Troped et al.[39] found that those who lived further from a cycle path were less likely to report path use. Similarly, those reporting the best perceived access to recreational facilities[62] and to parks and trails combined[40] have also been found to exhibit a higher prevalence of facility use as well as being more active.

Observations that better accessibility is associated with higher levels of recreational facility use have also been made by Addy et al.[63] in a US population and by Giles-Corti et al.[48] in a sample of Perth residents. Interestingly, Giles-Corti et al.[48] failed to find any association between simple measures of facility proximity and overall levels of physical activity in their study of access to urban greenspaces. However, when they computed accessibility measures that were weighted according to greenspace size and quality, they found that study participants who had very good access to large, attractive open spaces were 50% more likely to meet walking volume recommendations compared to those with poorer accessibility. The finding highlights the importance of considering the attributes of destinations in addition to how accessible they may be, something which is intuitively sensible given that destination choice will often be governed by quality considerations. This may be especially so in more mobile populations where travel effort is not a major limitation. Indeed, evidence of the importance of such additional considerations also comes from the work of McCormack et al.[49] who examined correlates of distance travelled against the use of a range of different types of facilities. They found that those who participated in vigorous physical activity generally travelled further than non-vigorous exercisers to use the same type of facility (i.e. to use parks, beaches and rivers). This observation suggests that the definition of a common set of thresholds against which 'good' and 'poor' accessibility and availability can be measured may not be sensible, particularly for those activities for which travel may be particularly behaviourally specific.

So far, we have examined the evidence supporting associations between perceived and objectively measured access to facilities and levels of physical activity in populations. We now move on to consider the manner by which the patterning of facility availability and accessibility may differ according to population characteristics, and how this may influence socio-demographic disparities.

4.6   Equity of access and facility provision

An understanding of the social distribution or patterning of environmental amenities is an important component of research into the environmental determinants of physical activity. Given the known disparities in morbidity and mortality from diseases associated with physical inactivity, coupled with consistent research evidence that poorer populations and those containing a high number of minority groups exhibit a higher prevalence of inactivity,[64] the need to better understand how these health-related disparities may be driven by disparities in the provision and accessibility of resources for physical activity is clear. This is particularly so given the emerging research evidence[49] that access to facilities shows a distance-related dose–response relationship with the form of physical activity that has the highest levels of participation – walking for transport. Indeed, recent decades have seen increased recognition that biases within environmental policy-making and regulatory processes, combined with discriminatory market forces, may lead to disproportionate exposures to environmental disamenities, or disparities in access to environmental amenities, amongst certain population groups. In the context of examining such discrepancies, the terms environmental equity and environmental justice are sometimes used synonymously,[65] although distinctions can be made.

Extended discussion of the general concept of equity is given by Harding and Holdren.[65] Lavelle[66] suggests that environmental equity implies an equal sharing of risk burdens, such as exposure to air pollution, or access to environmental 'goods' such as public parks or recreational facilities. Cutter,[67] however, argues that environmental justice implies much more, including remedial action to correct an injustice imposed upon a specific subgroup of society. Perlin et al.[68] further advocate that environmental justice should achieve adequate protection from harmful environments, or adequate access to healthy ones for everyone, regardless of ethnicity, age or socio-economic status. In reality, the exact definition of 'equity' is often context specific. Crompton and Wicks,[69] Marsh and Schilling[70] and Wicks and Backman[71] discuss different approaches to defining or ensuring equity in a planning context, and Crompton and Lue[72] and Nicholls[73] use the case study of urban park usage to consider how equity may be defined, and which definitions are likely to be practicable and preferred by the public. For the purpose of this chapter, equity is defined simply as the equality of access between social groups. In the research literature, these groups are commonly delineated according to socio-economic status, ethnicity or a mixture of the two.

Research regarding equity of access and provision of facilities for physical activity has particularly focused on parks and greenspaces. Perhaps this is unsurprising given that the establishment of the urban public park movement over a century ago had its origins in the social ideal of providing pleasant open spaces that were free at the point of access, and as such these places have always been intended to be equally available for different social groups. Hence urban public parks, a venue for urban residents to undertake physical activity[47] were originally developed, at least in part, to provide a place where rich and poor could meet on an equal footing.[74]

It is noteworthy that almost all the research evidence concerning equity with regard to public parks comes from the United States. Many of the early findings suggested that more disadvantaged populations had poorer access to parks and greenspaces. Talen[75] considered ethnic differences in the provision of public parks in two towns. They noted the total park acreage within set distances (one or two miles along the road network) of distinct populations (located by Census tract centre points). Inequities were considered in relation to race, age, overcrowded housing, single-adult households, median house value and vacant or owner-occupied housing. In Macon, Georgia, Talen[75] found that high access corresponded with white, high-income suburban locations, although in the other town (Pueblo, Colorado) there was little evidence of relationships. In a small US city, Estabrooks et al.[76] identified the location of a diverse range of physical activity resources, including 112 public parks, leisure centres, walking trails and other facilities. They concluded that communities with lower socio-economic status had inferior provision of such resources, and that this was likely to have detrimental effects on their physical health.

A number of recent studies have examined equity in accessing pay-to-use facilities such as sports centres and gymnasiums. Given that these are generally provided with profit motives in mind, it is perhaps unsurprising that they are likely to be located in areas that provide the most convenient access for clients with an ability to pay. These might be close to places of employment or in more affluent neighbourhoods (Figure 4.3). In their study of the relationship between the provision of indoor

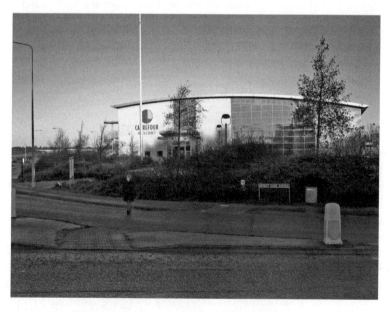

Figure 4.3 Pay-to-use facilities such as commercial gymnasiums are commonly located close to major employment centres rather than in residential neighbourhoods.

physical activity facilities and area deprivation across England, Hillsdon et al.[77] found that facility availability showed a negative association with area deprivation. In our own research examining associations between household income, access to sports facilities and gyms and physical activity amongst a sample of residents in the city of Norwich, England,[6] we found that for all facility types except gyms, the mean income was lowest amongst study participants living furthest away. Compared to those with the lowest incomes, the most affluent participants lived on average just over 0.5 km closer to a facility of any type, 1 km closer to a sports facility but 900 m further from a gym (all $p < 0.001$). In general, those living further from facilities reported that they were less active although they did not tend to report a desire to exercise more.

Findings such as those detailed above led Macintyre et al.[78] to coin the term deprivation amplification, a process by which disadvantages arising from poorer quality environments (for example, poor access to facilities) amplify individual disadvantages (often associated with poverty) in ways which are detrimental to health. Nevertheless, more recent work, particularly that concerning access and provision of free-to-use facilities such as public parks, suggests that such amplification may not be as strong as previously thought, and indeed the direction of disparities has sometimes been found to be the reverse of that hypothesised. For example, Macintyre[79] reviews how recent studies suggest outdoor play facilities for children were more likely to be provided in poorer areas in Amsterdam, Edmonton and Boston.[80-82] Furthermore Giles-Corti and Donovan[83] found that poorer members of their study population in Perth, Western Australia, have better objectively measured access to facilities for physical activity.

In addition to spatial considerations, the argument that quality should be more frequently captured in research studies is persuasive. For example, Ellaway et al.[84] reported that the provision of children's playgrounds was better in more deprived areas of the city of Glasgow, but they also reported anecdotal evidence that those in more affluent areas were of a higher quality. Similarly, Smoyer-Tomic et al.[81] found that playgrounds in deprived areas of Edmonton, Canada, were rated as poorer quality than those in more affluent neighborhoods. Hence, whilst the existence of evidence that better provision of free-to-use facilities might be compensating for poorer provision of market-based resources in some settings is reassuring, whether such compensatory measures are still apparent after quality has been accounted for is not well understood. Certainly, increasing pressures on land for development in the United Kingdom mean that newly created parks and greenspaces are generally less well resourced, smaller, and more poorly maintained than those provided in the heyday of urban parks at the end of the 19th and beginning of the 20th centuries. A comparison of Figures 4.4 and 4.5 illustrates how the quality of provision may be declining with increasing land prices and decreasing availability.

Despite the equivocal nature of some more recent findings, the research evidence available to date suggests that the accessibility, provision and quality of facilities in which physical activity can be undertaken is generally poorest amongst the most socio-economically disadvantaged groups in society. This is of particular concern given that it is these groups that show the lowest levels of physical activity, and the highest prevalence of diseases associated with inactivity. Nevertheless, criticisms

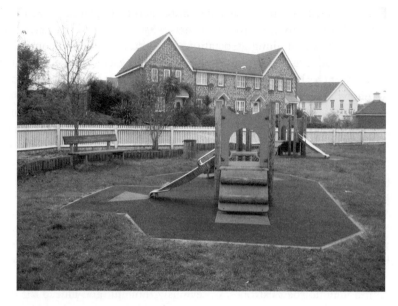

Figure 4.4   Areas of greenspace provided in modern housing developments are often small and may not be designed for a wide variety of uses.

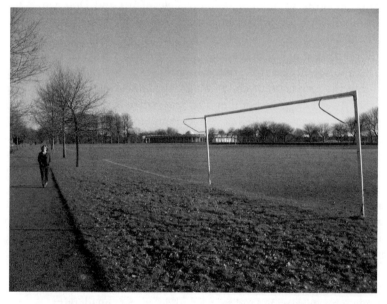

Figure 4.5   Eaton Park in Norwich, UK, is typical of the large multi-use greenspaces constructed for the residents of towns and cities in the late 19th and early 20th centuries.

have been levelled at studies that have claimed the presence of inequities is a particular cause for concern. Pearce[85], for example, contended that environmental equity studies are often flawed, because they ignore a fundamental aspect of capitalism that the rich have the ability to pay for a nicer place to live. He took an economic perspective, arguing that equity could only be properly assessed with respect to how much each community paid for a benefit (or to avoid a disamenity), and whether their benefits or costs were commensurate with those payments. Pearce's arguments are supported by many North American studies,[86,87] which suggest that many inequities arise as a result of the in-migration of poorer people to areas with a poorer environment but which benefit from lower house prices, rather than pre-existing socio-demographic disparities in facility planning and construction.

Despite the limitations of the literature, the argument that adequate accesses to facilities in which physical activity can be undertaken form a basic right, and is one that should be enjoyed by all irrespective of the ability to pay, is compelling. Further work is needed though to better determine how the extent of observed social gradients in physical activity may be associated with inequities in access to resources, as well as the degree by which the accessibility of one type of facility may be compensated for by the provision of others.

4.7 Conclusions

In this chapter, we have reviewed the current evidence around physical activity and accessibility and provision in a variety of population settings. However, in common with the wider research based on obesogenic environments from which the literature is drawn, the quality of evidence is compromised by a number of common study limitations. Perhaps the greatest is the lack of standardised research designs, leading to different methods being used to measure physical activity and varied definitions of accessibility and availability being adopted. This may be responsible for the equivocal nature of some of the research findings. It is certainly the case that accessibility is a conceptually important influence on walking or cycling behaviour if local journeys to accessible facilities are made on foot or by bicycle, but it is less clear how access might be associated with walking for recreation or physical activity in general, unless the facilities being studied are actually those at which the activity might take place. Hence, from a planning point of view, it is perhaps useful to separately consider access to general destinations, such as shops and services, which may be a component of the walkability of a neighbourhood, and access to those facilities at which activity may occur, as they may be outside of the neighbourhood and visited via private transport as opposed to an active form of travel.

A further limitation with the evidence is that the majority of published studies are cross-sectional and, therefore, causality cannot be assumed. It is, therefore, not clear if higher levels of utilisation and associated physical activity amongst residents of areas with better access or provision of facilities is a result of the opportunities that the facilities provide, or rather that these individuals have chosen to locate in areas which match their preferences for activity. To confirm the roles of access and availability as influences on physical activity, there is a need for more studies that explore in detail the interactions between people and places besides more clearly defining the hypothesised relationships between access to facilities, facility use and levels of physical activity. The potential to evaluate natural experiments, where changes in physical activity may be either an intended or unintended consequence of changes made to the environment, holds particular promise. This is especially so in cases where those modifications are expected to lead to alterations in the accessibility of resources for which a hypothesised relationship with physical activity has already been defined.

Despite the above caveats, it is clear from this review that both objective and perceived measures of access and provision are generally associated with higher levels of facility use and also show associations between both walking behaviours and overall physical activity, even though these associations are not consistent. It is reassuring that walking generally shows a stronger association than that observed for overall activity, as it is that behaviour that theoretical models suggest should be most strongly influenced by access. Yet, there is also some evidence that the accessibility and provision of facilities in which physical activity can be undertaken is socially patterned with generally better provision amongst socio-economically disadvantages populations. Worryingly, there is also evidence that suggests those populations who are poorly served also exhibit lower levels of physical activity.

Even where profit motives are not involved, human environments cannot be designed to provide completely equitable levels of access and availability as any service which has a spatial component to its provision cannot serve all members of a population equally. Indeed, it is inevitable that, where facilities are provided for profit motives, they will tend to be located so that they are most accessible to those populations which are best able to afford them. Nevertheless, if suitable land is available, these market driven inequities may be at least partly compensated for by the provision of fee-free resources such as public parks or community gymnasiums in places where affordable commercial facility provision is poor. Of course, such resources come at a cost that is associated with their construction and maintenance, and it is important that any facilities are fit for their purpose and are of an acceptable quality; otherwise, they may not be well used. However, where legislation allows, planning permissions for construction of commercial facilities may be issued in such a way that some of the costs are borne by private developers. Given the research evidence of inequities in access to places for physical activity, such interventions into free markets may be worthwhile if they go some way to reducing the burden of health inequalities associated with diseases related to physical inactivity.

References

1. Gutmann, A. (1981) For and against equal access to health care. *Health and Society.* 59(4):542–560.
2. Gatrell, A.C. *Geographies of Health.* Oxford, Blackwell Publishers, 2002.

3. Joseph, A.E., Phillips, D.R. *Geographical Perspectives on Health Care Delivery*. London, Harper and Row, 1984.
4. Cerin, E., Leslie, E. (2008) How socio-economic status contributes to participation in leisure-time physical activity. *Social Science & Medicine*. 66(12):2596–2609.
5. Cummins, S., Findlay, A., Petticrew, M., Sparks, L. (2005) Healthy cities: the impact of food retail-led regeneration on food access, choice and retail structure. *Built Environment*. 31(4):288–301.
6. Panter, J., Jones, A.P., Hillsdon, M. (2008) Equity of access to physical activity facilities in an English city. *Preventive Medicine*. 46(4):303–307.
7. Stirling, A.M., Wilson, P., McConnachie, A. (2001) Deprivation, psychological distress, and consultation length in general practice. *British Journal of General Practice*. 51(467): 456–460.
8. Wennberg, J., Gittlesohn, A. (1982) Variations in medical care among small areas. *Scientific American*. 246:100–111.
9. Brown, L.J., Barnett, J.R. (1992) The influence of bed supply and health care organisation on regional and local patterns of diabetes related hospitalisation.
10. Ministerie van Verkeer en Waterstaat. *Cycling in the Netherlands*. Den Haag, Ministerie van Verkeer en Waterstaat, 2007.
11. Giles-Corti, B. (2006) People or places: what should be the target? *Journal of Science and Medicine in Sport*. 9(5):357–366.
12. Shannon, G.W., Denver, G.E. *Health Care Delivery: Spatial Perspectives*. New York, NY, McGraw Hill, 1974.
13. Higgs, G. (2004) A literature review of the use of GIS-based measures of access to health care services. *Health Services and Outcomes Research Methodology*. 5(2):119–139.
14. Low, N. (1975) Centrism and the provision of services in residential areas. *Urban Studies*. 12:177–191.
15. Krizek, K.J., El-Geneidt, A., Thompson, K. (2007) A detailed analysis of how an urban trail system affects cyclists' travel. *Transportation*. 34(5):611–624.
16. Dueker, K.J., Kjerne, D. *Multipurpose Cadastre Terms and Definitions*. Bethesda, MD, American Society of Photogrammetry and Remote Sensing and American Congress on Surveying and Mapping, 1989.
17. Saelens, B., Sallis, J.F., Black, J., Chen, D. (2003) Neighbourhood based differences in physical activity: an environment scale evaluation. *American Journal of Public Health*. 93(9):1552–1558.
18. Leslie, E., Saelens, B., Frank, L., Owen, N., Bauman, A., Coffee, N., *et al.* (2005) Residents' perceptions of walkability attributes in objectively different neighbourhoods: a pilot study. *Health & Place*. 11:227–236.
19. Giles-Corti, B., Donovan, R.J. (2002) The relative influence of individual, social and physical environment determinants of physical activity. *Social Science & Medicine*. 54(12): 1793–1812.
20. Frank, L., Schmid, T.L., Sallis, J.F., Chapman, J.E., Saelens, B.E. (2005) Linking objectively measured physical activity with objectively measured urban form findings from SMARTRAQ. *American Journal of Preventive Medicine*. 28(2S):117–125.
21. Sallis, J.F., Hovell, M.F., Hofstetter, R.C., Faucher, P., Elder, J.P., Blanchard, J., *et al.* (1989) A multivariate study of determinants of vigorous exercise in a community sample. *Preventive Medicine*. 18(1):20–34.
22. Abbott, R., Jenkins, D., Haswell-Elkins, M., Fell, K., MacDonald, D., Cerin, E. (2008) Physical activity of young people in the Torres Strait and Northern Peninsula Region: an exploratory study. *Australian Journal of Rural Health*. 16(5):278–282.
23. Duncan, M.J., Spence, J., Mummery, K. (2005) Perceived environment and physical activity: a meta-analysis of selected environmental characteristics. *International Journal of Behavioral Nutrition and Physical Activity*. 2(11). doi:10.1186/1479-5868.
24. King, W.C., Brach, J.S., Belle, S., Killingsworth, R., Fenton, M., Kriska, A.M. (2003) The relationship between convenience of destinations and walking levels in older women. *American Journal of Health Promotion*. 18:74–82.

25. Booth, M.L., Owen, N., Bauman, A., Clavisi, O., Leslie, E. (2000) Social–cognitive and perceived environment influences associated with physical activity in older Australians. *Preventive Medicine*. 31(1):15–22.
26. Brownson, R.C., Baker, E.A., Houseman, R.A., Brennan, L.K., Bacak, S.J. (2002) Environmental and policy determinants of physical activity in the United States. *American Journal of Public Health*. 91(12):1995–2002.
27. Huston, S.L., Evenson, K.R., Bors, P., Gizlice, Z. (2003) Neighborhood environment, access to places for activity, and leisure-time physical activity in a diverse North Carolina population. *American Journal of Health Promotion*. 18(1):58–69.
28. Parks, S., Housemann, R., Brownson, R. (2003) Differential correlates of physical activity in urban and rural adults of various socioeconomic backgrounds in the United States. *Journal of Epidemiology and Community Health* 57(1):29–35.
29. Rutten, A., Abel, T., Kannas, L., von Lengerke, T., Luschen, G., Diaz, J.A.R., *et al.* (2001) Self reported physical activity, public health, and perceived environment: results from a comparative European study. *Journal of Epidemiology and Community Health*. 55(2):139–146.
30. Davison, K., Lawson, C. (2006) Do attributes in the physical environment influence children's physical activity? A review of the literature. *International Journal of Behavioral Nutrition and Physical Activity*. 3(19). doi:10.1186/1479-5868.
31. Appleyard, D. *Livable Streets*. Berkeley, CA, University of California Press, 1982.
32. Cole, R., Leslie, E., Bauman, A., Donald, M., Owen, N. (2006) Socio-demographic variations in walking for transport and for recreation or exercise among Australian adults. *Journal of Physical Activity and Health*. 3:164–178.
33. Handy, S., Clifton, K. (2001) Local shopping as a strategy for reducing automobile travel. *Transportation*. 28:317–346.
34. Humpel, N., Owen, N., Iverson, D., Leslie, E., Bauman, A. (2004) Perceived environment attributes, residential location and walking for particular purposes. *American Journal of Preventive Medicine*. 26(2):119–124.
35. Foster, C., Hillsdon, M., Thorogood, M. (2004) Environmental perceptions and walking in English adults. *Journal of Epidemiology and Community Health*. 58(1):924–928.
36. Suminski, R., Poston, W., Petosa, R., Stevens, E. (2005) Features of the neighborhood environment and walking by U.S. adults. *American Journal of Preventive Medicine*. 28(2): 149–155.
37. Giles-Corti, B., Donovan, R.J. (2003) Relative influences of individual social environmental and physical environmental correlates of walking. *American Journal of Public Health*. 93(9):1583–1589.
38. Sallis, J.F., Hovell, M.F., Hofstetter, R.C., Elder, J., Hackley, M., Casperson, C., Powell, K. (1990) Distance between homes and exercise facilities related to frequency of exercise among San Diego residents. *Public Health Reports*. 105(2):179–185.
39. Troped, P., Saunders, R.P., Pate, R., Reininger, B., Ureda, J., Thompson, S. (2001) Associations between self-reported and objective physical environment factors and use of a community rail trail. *Preventive Medicine*. 32:191–200.
40. Hoehner, C., Brennan Ramirez, L., Elliott, M., Handy, S., Brownson, R. (2005) Perceived and objective environmental measures and physical activity among urban adults. *American Journal of Preventive Medicine*. 28:105–116.
41. Bauman, A., Smith, B., Stoker, L., Bellew, B., Booth, M. (1999) Geographical influences upon physical activity participation: evidence of a 'coastal effect'. *Australian and New Zealand Journal of Public Health*. 23(3):322–324.
42. Wendel-Vos, W.G.C., Schuit, A.J., de Niet, R., Bossuizen, H.C. (2004) Factors of the physical environment associated with walking and bicycling. *Medicine and Science in Sports and Exercise*. 36(4):725–730.
43. Duncan, M., Mummery, K. (2005) Psychosocial and environmental factors associated with physical activity among city dwellers in regional Queensland. *Preventive Medicine*. 40(1):363–372.

44. Gomez, J.E., Johnson, B.A., Selva, M., Sallis, J.F. (2004) Violent crime and outdoor physical activity among inner-city youth. *Preventive Medicine.* 39(5):876–881.
45. Brodersen, N.H., Steptoe, A., Williamson, S., Wardle, J. (2005) Sociodemographic, developmental, environmental, and psychological correlates of physical activity and sedentary behavior at age 11 to 12. *Annals of Behavioral Medicine.* 29(1):2–11.
46. Norman, G., Nutter, S.K., Ryan, S., Sallis, J.F., Calfas, K.J., Patrick, K. (2006) Community design and access to recreational facilities as correlates of adolescent physical activity and body mass index. *Journal of Physical Activity and Health.* 3(1):118–128.
47. Hillsdon, M., Panter, J.R., Jones, A.P., Foster, C. (2006) The relationship between access and quality of urban green space with population physical activity. *Public Health.* 120(12):1127–1132.
48. Giles-Corti, B., Broomhall, M.H., Knuiman, M., Collins, C., Douglas, K., Lange, A., Donovan, R.J. (2005) Increasing walking: how important is distance to, attractiveness, and size of public open space? *American Journal of Preventive Medicine.* 28:169–176.
49. McCormack, G.R., Giles-Corti, B., Bulsara, M. (2008) The relationship between destination proximity, destination mix and physical activity behaviors. *Preventive Medicine.* 46: 33–40.
50. Cerin, E., Leslie, E., Toit, L.D., Owen, N., Frank, L.D. (2007) Destinations that matter: associations with walking for transport. *Health & Place.* 13(3):713–724.
51. Moudon, A., Lee, C. (2003) Walking and bicycling: an evaluation of environmental audit instruments. *American Journal of Health Promotion.* 18(1):21–37.
52. Craig, C., Brownson, R., Cragg, S., Dunn, A. (2002) Exploring the effect of the environment on physical activity: a study examining walking to work. *American Journal of Preventive Medicine.* 23(2):36–43.
53. Pikora, T., Giles-Corti, B., Knuiman, M., Bull, F., Jamrozik, K., Donovan, R.J. (2006) Neighborhood environmental factors correlated with walking near home: using SPACES. *Medicine and Science in Sports and Exercise.* 38(4):708–714.
54. Owen, N., Humpel, N., Leslie, E., Bauman, A., Sallis, J.F. (2004) Understanding environmental influences on walking; review and research agenda. *American Journal of Preventive Medicine.* 27:67–76.
55. Tilt, J., Unfried, T., Roca, B. (2007) Using objective and subjective measures of neighbourhood greeness and accessible destinations for understanding walking trips and BMI in Seattle, Washington. *American Journal of Health Promotion.* 21(4):371–379.
56. Kirtland, K.A., Porter, D.E., Addy, C.L., Neet, M.J., Williams, J.E., Sharpe, P.A., *et al.* (2003) Environmental measures of physical activity supports perception versus reality. *American Journal of Preventive Medicine.* 24:323–331.
57. Ball, K., Jeffery, R.W., Crawford, D.A., Roberts, R.J., Salmon, J., Timperio, A.F. (2008) Mismatch between perceived and objective measures of physical activity environments. *Preventive Medicine.* 47(3):294–298.
58. Macintyre, S., Macdonald, L., Ellaway, A. (2008) Lack of agreement between measured and self-reported distance from public green parks in Glasgow, Scotland. *International Journal of Behavioral Nutrition and Physical Activity.* 5(1):26.
59. McCormack, G., Cerin, E., Leslie, E., Du Toit, L., Owen, N. (2008) Objective versus perceived walking distances to destinations: correspondence and predictive validity. *Environment and Behavior.* 40(3):401–425.
60. Chin, G.K.W., van Niel, K., Giles-Corti, B., Knuiman, M. (2008) Accessibility and connectivity in physical activity studies: the impact of missing pedestrian data. *Preventive Medicine.* 46(1):41–45.
61. Riva, M., Gauvin, L., Richard, L. (2007) Use of local area facilities for involvement in physical activity in Canada: insights for developing environmental and policy interventions. *Health Promotion International.* 22:227–235.
62. Kruger, J., Carlson, S.A., Kohl, H.W. III. (2007) Fitness facilities for adults: differences in perceived access and usage. *American Journal of Preventive Medicine.* 32(6):500–505.

63. Addy, C., Wilson, D.K., Kirtland, K.A., Ainsworth, B.E., Sharpe, P. (2004) Associations of perceived social and physical environmental supports with physical activity and walking behaviour. *American Journal of Public Health*. 94(3):440–443

64. Marshall, S.J., Jones, D.A., Ainsworth, B.E., Reis, J.P., Levy, S.S., Macera, C.A. (2007) Race/ethnicity, social class, and leisure-time physical inactivity. *Medicine and Science in Sports and Exercise*. 39:44–51.

65. Harding, A.K., Holdren, G.R. (1993) Environmental equity and the environmental professional. *Environmental Science and Technology*. 27:1990–1993.

66. Lavelle, M. *The 1994 'Information Please' Environmental Almanac*. (Ed. World Resources Institute) Boston, MA, Houghton-Mifflin, 1994.

67. Cutter, S. (1995) Race, class and environmental justice. *Progress in Human Geography*. 19:111–122.

68. Perlin, S., Setzer, R., Creason, J, Sexton, K. (1995) Distribution of industrial air emissions by income and race in the United States: an approach using the toxic release inventory. *Environmental Science & Technology*. 29:69–80.

69. Crompton, J.L., Wicks, B.E. (1988) Implementing a preferred equity model for the delivery of leisure services in the US context. *Leisure Studies*. 7(3):287–304.

70. Marsh, M.T., Schilling, D.A. (1994) Equity measurement and facility location analysis: A review and framework. *European Journal of Operational Research*. 74(1):1–17.

71. Wicks, B.E., Backman, K.F. (1994) Measuring equity preferences: a longitudinal analysis. *Journal of Leisure Research*. 26(4):386–401.

72. Crompton, J.L., Lue, C.C. (1992) Patterns of equity preferences among Californians for allocating park and recreation resources. *Leisure Studies*. 14:227–246.

73. Nicholls, S. (2001) Measuring the accessibility and equity of public parks: a case study using GIS. *Managing Leisure*. 6:201–219.

74. Young, T. (1996) Social reform through parks: the American Civic Association's program for a better America. *Journal of Historical Geography*. 22(4):460–472.

75. Talen, E. (1997) The social equity of urban service distribution: an exploration of park access in Pueblo, Colorado and Macon, Georgia. *Urban Geography*. 18(6):521–541.

76. Estabrooks, P.A., Lee, R.E., Gyurcsik, N.C. (2003) Resources for physical activity participation: does availability and accessibility differ by neighbourhood socioeconomic status? *Annals of Behavioural Medicine*. 25(2):100–104.

77. Hillsdon, M., Panter, J., Foster, C., Jones, A.P. (2007) Equitable access to exercise facilities. *American Journal of Preventive Medicine*. 32(6):506–508.

78. Macintyre, S., Maciver, S., Sooman, A. (1993) Area, class and health; should we be focusing on places or people? *Journal of Social Policy*. 22:213–234.

79. Macintyre, S. (2007) Deprivation amplification revisited; or, is it always true that poorer places have poorer access to resources for healthy diets and physical activity? *International Journal of Behavioral Nutrition and Physical Activity*. 7(4):32.

80. Karsten, L. (2002) Mapping childhood in Amsterdam: the spatial and social construction of children's domains in the city. *Tijdschrift voor Economische en Sociale Geografie*. 93(3):231–241.

81. Smoyer-Tomic, K.E., Hewco, J.N., Hodgson, M.J. (2004) Spatial accessibility and equity of playgrounds in Edmonton, Canada. *Canadian Geographer* 48(3):287–302.

82. Cradock, A.L., Kawachi, I., Colditz, G.A., Hannon, C., Melly, S.J., Wiecha, J.L., *et al.* (2005) Playground safety and access in Boston neighbourhoods. *American Journal of Preventive Medicine*. 28(4):357–363.

83. Giles-Corti, B., Donovan, R.J. (2002) Socioeconomic status differences in recreational physical activity levels and real and perceived access to a supportive physical environment. *Preventive Medicine*. 35(6):601–611.

84. Ellaway, A., Kirk, A., Macintyre, S., Mutrie, N. (2007) Nowhere to play? The relationship between the location of outdoor play areas and deprivation in Glasgow. *Health & Place*. 13(2):557–561.

85. Pearce, D. (2003) The distribution of benefits and costs of environmental policies: conceptual framework and literature survey. Paper given at OECD *Environment Directorate Workshop on the distribution of benefits and costs of environmental policies*, Paris, France, March 2003.
86. Mitchell, J., Thomas, D.S.K., Cutter, S.L. (1999) Dumping in Dixie revisited: the evolution of environmental injustices in South Carolina. *Social Science Quarterly.* 80(2): 229–243.
87. Szasz, A., Meuser, M. (2000) Unintended, inexorable: the production of environmental inequalities in Santa Clara County, California. *American Behavioral Scientist.* 43(4): 602–632.

5 Defining and Mapping Obesogenic Environments for Children

Kimberley L. Edwards

5.1 Children's obesogenic environments

Increasing interest in the role of the 'obesogenic environment' is necessitating inter-disciplinary approaches to our research, as argued in Chapter 2 by Townshend *et al*. Geographers address the obesogenic environment supposition from the perspective of space and place, quintessentially questioning whether the effect is compositional, contextual or a combination of the two. This leads to many different aspects of the environment that may affect childhood obesity, from physical attributes to social factors, and individual characteristics. This chapter summarises the advantages of using mapping techniques to objectively analyse obesogenic environments, before covering the key issues with data representation and the special problems with spatial data. Progressive techniques in classifying obesogenic environments and considering the relationship with obesity are encapsulated, ahead of highlighting the key spatial analysis techniques for examining relationships in georeferenced data.

The escalation in obesity prevalence in recent decades has fuelled the environmental, rather than genetic, causation argument. This line of reasoning has led to increasing interest in the role of the 'obesogenic environment' on obesity; the classic definition being 'the sum of influences that the surroundings, opportunities or conditions of life have on promoting obesity in individuals or populations' (p. 564).[1] This is an expansive definition as it encompasses all of the different factors that may influence health behaviour to make obesity more likely to occur. In such an environment, obesity occurs in some (and worryingly, an increasing proportion of) individuals, because although our bodies are able to efficiently safeguard against excessive exhaustion of energy reserves, our physiological make-up is not so proficient at inhibiting the build up of a superfluity of energy reserves.[2]

Geographers address the obesogenic environment supposition from the perspective of space and place. Is the effect compositional, whereby particular locations attract obese people to come together? Or is the effect contextual, whereby residents of a place become obese due to its particular characteristics? Answers to these fundamental questions would help to solve the puzzle of why some people are more obese than others. Whilst evidence for both compositional and contextual effects of the environment on obesity prevalence exists, it is likely that the answer is a complex combination of both theories, as reviewed in Chapter 12 by Pearce and Day. Environmental stimuli on obesity prevalence must be impacted to some degree by individuals' (diet and activity) behaviours, as ultimately these are what lead to chronic positive energy imbalance and thus to obesity.

The obesogenic environment for children will have subtle differences as compared to that for adults. Children have much less control over their environments (increasing control as they age) than adults. What they eat and do will be strongly influenced by their home and school environments; for example, if their parents are vegetarians, they are likely to be vegetarians too. Similarly, if their parents never exercise, the children are less likely to be physically active.[3] The timeline is also much reduced in children; adults may take decades to become obese, although obese children are likely to become obese young adults.[4] The consideration of the impact of the environment on obesity is facilitated in children as generally they have migrated less than the average adult (simply due to a much shorter time in which to move around), thus their immediate location is likely to have been important in whether they developed obesity or not.

It has been shown that neighbourhood characteristics, such as deprivation, impact behaviours that affect health.[5] Deprivation is commonly associated with obesity, although the relationship is not straightforward, depending on the timing of the outcome measure of obesity (i.e. whether it is in childhood or adulthood).[6–9] Overcrowding, poverty, migration, pollution, housing and employment can all create environmental changes that may initiate the breakdown of community factors that adversely impact health. This is encapsulated in the term *urbanisation*, which relates to the concentration of populations into towns/cities and the corresponding changes associated with this – migration, transformation of the economic and physical organisation of the city, changes in behaviour of populations due to 'urban-living'.[10] It is likely that these behavioural changes affect health behaviours and so the probability of developing a disease. This potential role of urbanisation in the aetiology of obesity also needs to be considered in light of urban regeneration and whether this supposedly positive urban change impacts on health.[11] In this vein, levels of urban sprawl (i.e. the amount of developed land for a given constant population), which is a relatively recent phenomena and reduce accessibility of work, school and social activities by foot, have been shown to be positively associated with obesity in the USA[12] where walkability is more of a concern than in the United Kingdom (see also Chapter 3 by Robertson-Wilson and Giles-Corti). Poor access to affordable, healthy food is considered to be a contributory factor to poor diet, poor health and obesity. Some studies have argued that these 'food deserts' exist (e.g. Refs 13–15), although the evidence is inconclusive. Likewise, the relationship between greenspace and obesity/health[16,17] as well as the impact of road safety issues[18] has been considered in previous studies.

The choice of what variables to include within the definition of 'obesogenic environment' is both key and wide-reaching. Examining the interdisciplinary features of a place, such as culture, politics, sociology and economics, facilitates understanding it. In the context of the environment, this includes the physical attributes, such as is there a high 'walkability' factor; does urbanisation increase likelihood of obesity; are facilities (such as supermarkets, leisure facilities, greenspaces, fast food outlets located conveniently (in terms of proximity, distance, time or density); ease of availability of car parking versus public transportation links and frequency; are schools located close to community centres thereby encouraging walking/biking to school; low crime rates; low traffic flows/pedestrian safety; area level deprivation. However, social factors are very important and also affect individual behaviours, for instance, do residents perceive the neighbourhood is safe and/or that facilities are easy to access; what impact does social capital have; are there school or community level pressures to lead healthy or unhealthy lifestyles? Further, individual attributes such as access to own car and household income level may also affect whether the area is obesogenic for an individual. For example, whether the nearest shop selling affordable healthy food is 1 mile or 20 miles away will have more impact on families without a car than those with one. However, when developing a model of obesogenic environments inevitably, it will be necessary to discard some apparently extraneous detail in the process of generalisation. Accordingly, it is necessary to carefully consider what variables are, and are not, included in the model and to use the most appropriate spatial scale for the research question. In addition, multivariate analyses will be more realistic than univariate analyses, as environmental factors do not operate to shape our health behaviours in isolation.

5.2   Advantages of mapping obesogenic environments in children

Geographic information systems (GISs) and spatial analysis techniques can be used to model the obesogenic environment. This is particularly useful as obesity is such a complex interaction between biophysical, social, environmental and psychological factors.[19] Understanding spatial patterns of obesogenic environments allows socio-economic, demographic, environmental and health behaviours, at specific times and locations, to be identified. This enables us to predict the impact (or otherwise) on the population's obesity following changes in these constructs.

Coarsely aggregated, imprecise models are too far removed from the actuality of real life and do not aid the cause in the same way as a detailed small area level model. Analysing data at coarse geographic levels unrealistically assumes that populations are homogeneous within these long boundaries, which leads to inhibition of within-area variations. Trends and patterns within these areas are concealed from view and thus ignored. The coarser the geographic scale of analysis the greater the likelihood that material detail has been generalised over and lost. Equally, it is possible to be excessively engrossed with highly detailed qualitative data on individuals, which does not serve to evidence the whole picture, nor to provide a system-wide understanding of the environment and its potential relationship with obesity. Small area level models offer the best compromise between these two methodologies allowing compact problem areas of high risk to be identified and analysed whilst taking into account local features of importance.

The use of GIS and mapping facilitates both insightful and reasoned analyses of data, enabling critical analyses and problem solving. It allows numerous data points to be considered simultaneously and also with awareness of adjacency of relationships, which is not apparent in a table of data. Further, multiple layers of data (i.e. different types of obesogenic variables) can be considered concurrently. Together, this enables complex relationships over space to be visualised. The complete picture can be inferred and relationships between the data can be appreciated. In addition, the use of GIS permits rapid and easy interrogation of the data. Large data sets can quickly be summarised by any one variable of interest, either by geographic unit (such as obesity prevalence per area) or by obesogenic variable (such as obesity prevalence per food outlet density categorisation or by mean deprivation per obesity categorisation). Disparate data sets can be joined by a common field, such as the area name, maximising the number of attributes available for analyses. It is not being suggested that small area GIS analyses are the panacea for obesity research, rather that it is a highly useful and important tool whose use should be maximised.

5.3 How to map obesogenic environments – data representation

The most commonly used method for visualising areal-based data, and thus of mapping obesity, is a choropleth map. In this type of map each area is shaded with a different colour to represent a different category of the value of a particular attribute under investigation, for example, darker shading may indicate a higher prevalence of obesity (see Figure 5.1a). Alternative map representations include using a graduated symbol methodology, where the relative size of the symbol on the map indicates the attribute under investigation, for example, larger bar or circle indicates higher obesity prevalence (Figure 5.1b and c), or a dot density representation could be used, where each dot represents the number of people with the disease per given number of population (Figure 5.1d). The example maps discussed here were put together using hypothetical data for the city of Leeds, UK. Actual data were not used due to ethical considerations of mapping sensitive information at detailed scales; care should always be taken regarding the potential identification of individuals. The choropleth system is preferable are point data is also going to be overlaid on top, such as the location of supermarkets, leisure facilities and parks. Further, the underlying shading need not be disease related, but could be potential causation factors such as degree of walkability for the area.

When creating a map, disease data should not be displayed as absolute numbers. This is because the underlying base population can vary from area to area; using absolute numbers could be misleading. We would expect to have more people with a particular disease in a more populated area than in a sparsely populated area: urbanisation needs to be controlled for. That is, areas with the highest number of people with disease are not necessarily the areas with the highest number of disease per 100,000 population. Accordingly, it is normally more meaningful to display the information as a rate (rather than simply count data), although other formats can also be useful, such as z-scores (e.g. when considering childhood obesity using a body mass index standard deviation score). As an example, consider a hypothetical region with four small areas. Table 5.1 summarises the attributes of these areas.

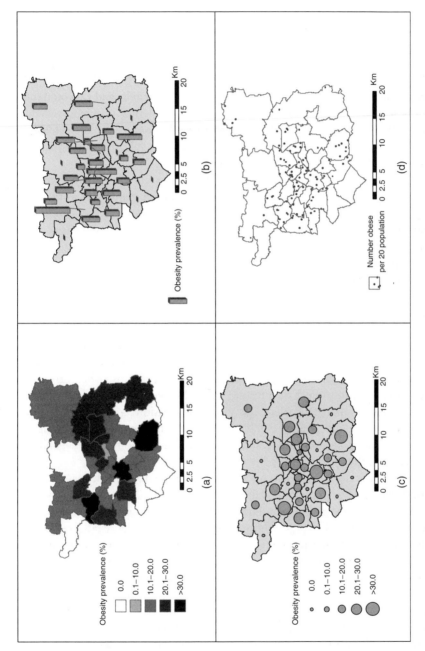

Figure 5.1 Examples of different types of maps (using hypothetical data for the city of Leeds, UK). (a) Choropleth map: darker shading indicates a higher prevalence of obesity. (b) Bar chart map: a larger bar indicates higher obesity prevalence. (c) Graduated symbol map: a larger circle indicates higher obesity prevalence. (d) Dot density map: each dot represents 1 obese person per 20 population.

Table 5.1 Summary of attributes of four hypothetical census areas.

Ward	Population	Obese	% Obese
A	100	25	25%
B	50	15	30%
C	25	10	40%
D	200	20	10%

If we were to map the absolute number of obese people, areas A and D would have the most obese people. However, this would mask the actual problem, which is that nearly half of the population in area C are obese. If we calculate the rate of the population that are obese and map this instead, it will be clear that the prevalence of obesity is lower in area D than all other areas.

When considering data displayed in a map, it is important that the mapmaker's perspective when they prepared the map is questioned, in the same way as critically appraising a journal article, not inexorably taking the authors' conclusions at face value. The techniques employed to integrate data and depict the results are crucial as they can influence the interpretations. Caution is required when making different data sets compatible with each other (data integration) as if done badly, it can make any analyses void. This predicament is due to several factors, for instance, locational errors or differences in temporal coverage or spatial referencing systems,[20] while maps may also mislead people into wrong conclusions.[21] A classic example is that geographical boundaries on a choropleth map are not necessarily representative of the underlying population; so a large sparsely populated rural area can look more prominent and more important than a smaller but highly populated urban area. There are ways around this problem, such as using cartograms, where areas are resized according to the subject of interest,[22] but this technique is not commonly used. Another factor that can affect the visual impression is how the data are categorised and how many categories have been used. Changes to these dimensions may alter the 'pattern' in the data,[23] but careful consideration of the legend can help to understand the impact of this.

The choice of spatial scale is also an important factor to consider, as different patterns of disease and/or associations in disease may be evident at different spatial scales.[24] The area used could be at a large scale, like counties, or a much smaller scale, like postcode areas. The larger the area that the data are aggregated to, the less specific the results are to that population (a lack of external accuracy), but equally there are then less problems with small number bias and imprecision, improved due to a reduction in sampling error.[25] Inevitably, a compromise is required that best suits the needs of the research questions being investigated. For the purpose of examining childhood obesogenic environments, balance is required between going into precise detail about an individual's residential/school environment and retaining sufficiently large numbers of measured and obese children in the study area to produce statistically meaningful results.

As the spatial scale of the data reduces, by using a finer geography for analysis, researchers using health data can run into confidentiality problems. It is essential to ensure that data are anonymised and extreme sensitivity is required over maps published to ensure that children cannot be identified. If individual-level health data are available, acceptable levels of confidentiality may be retained if the centroid of each child's full postcode is used as an approximation of location, albeit introducing an element of measurement error. The difference for small areas (e.g. urban postcodes) is likely to be minimal (e.g. the middle of a street rather than the right end of the street), but could be significant where the underlying area is larger (e.g. rural postcode areas, wards, etc.). However, concern over subject confidentiality means that data tend to be aggregated to areal units instead of using individual point data, which leads to corresponding data aggregation problems, the principal ones being the modifiable areal unit problem (MAUP) and ecological fallacy.

5.4   Problems with spatial data

Analysing data spatially is not without its problems, but is a negotiable minefield. Some of the specific problems relate to the inherent lack of independence in spatial data, some simply to epidemiological data, and some to the scale of analysis or use of aggregated rather than individual data. The key problems to watch out for are discussed below.

A map of disease prevalence or incidence (the former being more useful for slow developing, chronic conditions like obesity) may demonstrate geographic patterns or clusters, which can provide evidence about the aetiology of the disease or its relationship with covariates. This patterning is spatial autocorrelation – it is present when the locality of a disease case is dependent on the locality of other disease cases. For example, assuming obesity was due to a deficit of walkability in an area, then all inhabitants of districts with low walkability can be expected to be similarly impacted. Spatial autocorrelation does not exist where the composition of values is entirely random. Where comparable values populate bordering positions, we observe positive spatial autocorrelation; likewise, where divergent values inhabit neighbouring locations we observe negative spatial autocorrelation. It is clear that the finer the spatial resolution (the smaller the geographic units) the more chance that nearby geographic units are dependent. Since many statistical techniques assume data are independent, this inherent dependence in spatial data affects the choice of statistical techniques available to examine relationships in the data. Ignoring the existence of spatial autocorrelation would lead to an overestimate in the confidence in the risk relationships, producing inaccurate (too small) p-values, thus demonstrating 'statistically significant' results invalidly (i.e. when none are present).[26]

Additionally, it may be that any apparent pattern in a map, and any association between the variables, is due to chance. An example of this confounding could be that a map may suggest a relationship between obesity and say greenspace, but both of these may be associated with another variable, such as ice cream consumption (see Figure 5.2). Confounding is a concept that is central to both epidemiology and spatial epidemiology, representing 'one of the most fundamental impediments to

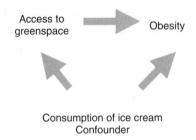

Figure 5.2   Coincidental visual correlations in maps may be due to confounding.

the elucidation of causal inferences from empirical data' (p. 173).[27] It is a mixing of effects between exposure and a second 'auxiliary' variable.

Over and above the standard sources of bias that impact individual-level data (e.g. selection bias, observation bias, interviewer bias, recall bias), aggregated areal data also suffer with the problem of 'ecological fallacy'. This is where heterogeneity within the areal units leads to the population/community level (ecological) estimates not being a true reflection of the individual-level (biological) data.[28] Thus, results from areal data can lead to incorrect conclusions about individual/household level relationships.[29] The MAUP can cause further trouble when mapping disease data. This occurs when the relative location of cases of a disease can be changed depending on the configuration of the areal units. In other words, the MAUP occurs when analysing point data aggregated to areal units and different results are achieved depending on how the areal units are constructed; namely, where the boundaries are drawn, which is a relatively arbitrary choice, that is, areal units are 'modifiable'.[30]

The size of areal units is important: smaller areas are more homogenous and allow for more detailed, localised analyses, but can have small numbers of data that can cause problems. Where there is a small number of the population at risk, then risk estimates can be misclassified – leading to excessive risk estimates for areas with small numbers of cases or small populations[24] and large standard errors. With small area level investigations, where there are a limited number of cases per area, then disease risk estimates become unstable, because the elimination or supplement of even one case can seriously impact the estimate. For example, in Table 5.1 the population of ward D is 8 times higher than ward C. When an area has a very low population, a very small change in the absolute number of illness can have a much bigger impact on the rate. Also, where data numbers are small the impact on mean data can be greater. For example, if income and tenure were being considered in a predominantly homeowner area, a few wealthy people renting homes would have a greater impact on mean rental-household income than a few wealthy homeowners would have on mean homeowner-household income in the same area.[21] Accordingly, the small number problem is essentially a problem of scale, because as the size of the areal units increases, so does the number of cases/population within the unit. Thus micro-level analyses, by definition, are prone to small number problems: a small area with a small population is more likely to have a small number of events (e.g. cases of obesity).

Gatrell[24] suggests a number of solutions to minimise the effect of this small number problem and to increase precision. The first option is to aggregate data where feasible, either by working at a coarser spatial scale (albeit not helpful if the investigation is deliberately at the small area level) or by lengthening data collection over many years. Another option is to draw on statistical shrinkage techniques that contract unstable disease estimates in the direction of the population mean rate, for example, by using Empirical Bayes estimators. Empirical Bayes estimation is a 'smoothing' technique that produces risk estimates derived from the variation in the data itself, producing a mean risk value pooled from the areal unit and that of nearby areas,[31] thereby averting unwarranted attention being directed to areas with small numbers. The technique takes effect by 'borrowing strength' from areas with substantial numbers measured in order to impart more stable estimates in areas with few numbers measured. There are four Empirical Bayes smoothing algorithms: a global method that smoothes rates based on all zones (i.e. using the mean for the whole study area) and the three local smoothing methods that limit zones included in the smoothing algorithm to a subset of the study area's zones based on a different criterion, founded on population limits, distance or a specific field in the data set. The characteristics of the data and the requirements of the investigation influence the choice of the appropriate algorithm.

Migration can also be a potential problem when dealing with patterns of, particularly chronic, disease, such as obesity. The latency period of diseases, between pathogen exposure and emergence of symptoms, can be decades. As such, present health status may be due to where the individual previously resided, perhaps a long time ago, rather than their present abode. Given that people in lower socio-economic groups tend to move home over only small distances,[32,33] this problem is more significant when examining small area data, particularly in areas with low homeowner occupancy. Accurate personal histories would be required to attaining dependable results, but this is not feasible in epidemiological research, being too expensive, protracted and impractical. Fortunately, in the case of children, their intrinsic young age means migration is less likely to be an issue.

In conclusion, there are multiple potential difficulties with analysing data spatially. However, with a considered selection of statistical techniques and reasonably homogenous areal units to investigate, mapping and spatially analysing health data can add important information about the location of hot spots of high prevalence of disease and about disease causation and relationships with covariates. Spatial analysis can also help to inform policy and to target resources to the high-risk populations.

5.5 Spatial analysis techniques

As part of the process of defining obesogenic environments for children, it is necessary to interrogate the data in order to understand the relationship between environmental factors and obesity. For example, the research question may want to consider how many children live or go to school within 300 m of a fast food outlet; which children live within 10 minutes of a park or play area; whether areas with more parks have fewer obese children; whether an area has better walkability after allowing for a preference for some walkways over others; to consider the relation between childhood obesity and the provision of services; where it would be best to place a new skate park in order to improve access for high-risk children or for those with limited access to park space facilities. Four important techniques to undertake this analysis are use of buffers, density measures, spatial interaction models and location–allocation modelling. Each technique is addressed in turn below. We then move on to address spatial statistical techniques to identify hot spots of high prevalence of obesity and regression analysis for spatial data.

In a GIS, it is possible to add a buffer zone of any size (whether in distance or time) to a point feature, such as a food outlet or gym. Then, assuming data are available, it is possible to calculate which children live in this buffer zone and how many of them are obese or otherwise. This technique can be used to address many different research questions relevant to the analysis of obesogenic environments, such as the relationship between food outlet proximity and income,[34] or other socio-economic markers[35]; or to examine the buffer zones around schools for particular attributes such as type of food advertising and outlets.[36] Similarly, the relationship between environmental variables and childhood overweight and obesity (or diet and physical activity behaviours) can be considered, including obesogenic variables such as distance or travel time from children's home to the nearest fast food outlet or public playground, and crime rates in the residential neighbourhood.[37–40] Little work has been undertaken linking distance/time to obesogenic/leptogenic variables, such as fast food outlets or gyms and individual diet and physical activity behaviours, although recent work in New Zealand showed no association between aspects of diet, such as fruit and vegetable intake, and proximity to food outlets,[41] which is also discussed in Chapter 12 by Pearce and Day.

If only the child data are available at an aggregated level, rather than individual point data, it would only be possible to estimate the population living in the buffer zone based on the population of each areal unit within the buffer. This also means that if any part of the areal unit falls within the buffer zone, the entire population in that unit will be counted, although it is possible that children living at the far edge of a large unit that just touches the buffer boundary have farther than the buffer limit to get to that outlet. In this case, the smaller the areal units used the better, so the buffers would provide more meaningful estimates. Alternatively, it is possible to calculate the likely population within the buffer by calculating the percentage area under the buffer in each areal unit, and calculating the corresponding percentage of the unit's population to get an estimate of the percentage population in each unit within the buffer. However, this assumes that the population is evenly distributed throughout the unit. Sometimes, boundary data come with population weighted centroids, which indicate where the population centre of each polygon lies. This can be used to estimate the population distribution and again calculate the percentage of the area that falls within the buffer.

Density analysis is generally a matter of calculating the number of point locations (e.g. food outlets) in a given area, either as an absolute number, per square kilometre, or more usually per capita, depending on the research question. In relation to obesogenic environments, this technique has principally been used to consider the relation between fast food outlet density and different markers of socio-economic status, although it can obviously apply to other potentially obesogenic/leptogenic data, such as gym facilities, road traffic, crime rates, parks and greenspace.

Studies have predominantly used an ecological design using residential (or school) areas as neighbourhoods. Those that limited their analyses to franchise fast food outlet density have shown a relationship between density and area measures of socio-economic status, such as ethnicity,[42] income[34,43] or more broadly using a combination of socio-economic measures,[44–46] although when a more expansive 'all out-of-home fast food outlet' definition is used, no such association was found.[47] Similarly, no association was found between obesity and shop density.[48] Few studies have used a geocoding design to capture individual data (rather than summary area measures) or considered the relationship between outlet density and actual obesity data. One longitudinal study has done so using home and school neighbourhood locations, but no association with food outlet density was found.[49] Recent work in Australia has shown a positive relationship between fast food outlet density/proximity and actual consumption of fast food[50] but more work is required in this area.

Buffer and density calculations permit basic analyses on simple proximity (calculating nearest outlet) or relative availability (number of outlets) to be considered but do not allow for any weighting of comparative appeal or preference for specific outlets (which may be constrained by size, brand, car availability, etc.). Spatial interaction models permit this extra dimension to be added.[13,51] They can be used to address questions about access to outlets or services more comprehensively and realistically than the simple accessibility measurements. For example, these models have been used to calculate access to GP services in relation to health care analyses,[52] and could be used to address similar style questions pertinent to the obesogenic environment.

Similarly, location–allocation models can be used to calculate the optimal location for the provision of particular services given the locality of demand, which may be the residential or school location of obese children. Optimisation works by minimising travel distance or time for all persons with 'demand' (e.g. those who are obese), allowing for reduced uptake of services with increased distance (whether straight-line or road network distances) or time to travel, as well as to vary preferences with socio-economic factors (such as car availability and income levels) as these factors may influence take-up of services. A good example of their use is in the determination of where to allocate smoking cessation clinics for most effective provision of services for people who wish to stop smoking,[53] and this clearly has applications for obesogenic environment investigations. A number of different algorithms can be used depending on the problem to be described. The 'p-median model' (originally described by Hakimi[54]) is most often used and allocates each obese person (demand site) to just one facility (say a park or food outlet). A 'location set covering problem' algorithm is more appropriate if the analysis requires the supply outlets (e.g. park facilities) to be located within a specified distance or travel time of a set number of obese people (demand sites).[55] A 'maximal covering problem' algorithm is a combination of the previous two algorithms and is useful where the demand sites are allocated to a set of supply sites, for instance, with provision of care from the emergency services.[56]

Given the inherent lack of independence of spatial data, basic assumptions underlying 'normal' regression analyses methods often fail. Additionally, aggregation of spatial data to coarser, global scales can lead to incorrect conclusions about the underlying relationships. Accordingly, it is important to ensure that appropriate spatial analyses techniques are utilised, otherwise results will be unreliable and may be inaccurate. Identifying hot spots of high prevalence of disease by investigating geographic clusters of data (rather than simply clusters of data) are actually searching for local spatial autocorrelation in the data.[57] These spatial clusters of high disease prevalence can be identified by using spatial scan statistic techniques, such as spatial scan statistic (SaTScan),[58] FleXScan[59] or WinBUGs[60] (the software for each is freely available from the Internet, see refs. 61–63, respectively). These spatial scan statistics detect and evaluate clusters by applying a continually moving circular window (SaTScan, WinBUGS), or flexible cluster shape (e.g. disease following the course of a river) (FleXScan), across time and/or space and comparing the quantity of observed and expected observations in the windows at each location, whilst adjusting for the underlying population distribution (as clustering is obviously going to occur in highly populated areas).[26] The cluster(s), least likely to be due to chance, are identified and p-values assigned. It is possible to run different types of probability model in order to best suit the data under examination. For example, a Bernoulli model can be used when the data consist of individuals with or without the disease in question (i.e. obesity or obesity and overweight – and normal weight individuals would be the controls); a normal model is suitable for continuous data that can be of positive or negative values (i.e. mean body mass index standard deviation score).

Geographically weighted regression (GWR) is another useful spatial regression technique that permits parameter estimates to vary across space (i.e. location dependent results), whereas 'normal' non-geographic regression models assume that processes are stationary and thus that parameter estimates are constant over space (i.e. location independent results). That is, this model assumes the relationships being modelled are the same across the entire study area. Conversely, a local model is a spatial disaggregation of a global model, and the results are, accordingly, location specific; a local model allows the processes under investigation to vary spatially. Spatial non-stationary exists when the same stimulus provokes a different response in different parts of the study region. Accordingly, use of GWR techniques can highlight potentially important local variations in relationships that would not otherwise be as easily apparent, but possible to calculate by mapping the residuals from a global model or calculating the autocorrelation statistics of the residuals.[64] The main output from GWR is a set of local parameter estimates for each relationship, which can be mapped to provide information on non-stationarity in the relationships being examined. The extent of the spatial variability of any relationship can be ascertained by comparing the range of the local parameter estimates with a confidence interval around the global estimate of the equivalent parameter.[65] Accordingly, GWR analyses will permit spatial variations in relationships in the data to be investigated, for example, considering whether any non-stationary relationships between obesity and obesogenic predictor variables exist.[66] GWR analysis also allows the spatial autocorrelation that is inherent in the data to be accounted for.

5.6 Conclusion

Tackling the obesity epidemic, particularly in children, remains high up the (UK) government's agenda. The United Kingdom has seen a shift in government health policy away from considering isolated disease groupings towards a population approach that considers the determinants of health. Furthermore, whilst it may be possible to identify individual-level determinants of health, very often it is not possible to modify these factors or behaviours. Accordingly, interventions need to occur at a higher level (the 'upstream' factors), changing the cultural, social and physical factors that also affect health, thereby considering the determinants of health at the population level rather than individual-level.

It can be reasoned that the health (or ill-health) of an area is composed of a combination of the health profiles and health behaviours of the residents together with environmental factors of the locality, such as access to greenspace, number of primary health care facilities, pollution levels, etc. This issue of compositional or contextual effects of the environment on a population's health can be elucidated by establishing the extent of spatial variation of obesity in an area. Individual-level variation in disease is less likely to be explained by contextual effects where there is minimal spatial variation, but if there is significant spatial variation then it is possible to consider the contextual effects and, whether or how such variation is explained by place.[67] Accordingly, it is preferable that analyses would contain data on both community and individual attributes, modelling the two simultaneously in order to glean the most information about health determinants. It is necessary to appreciate how both populations and individuals relate to their environments in terms of obesogenic behaviours.[68] In addition, importantly, it is at the contextual level where public health measures can be most effectively introduced, rather than trying to change the behaviour of individuals directly.

There is a strong case for relationships existing between different aspects of the environment and obesity. Obesity studies employing spatial analysis methods do not necessarily indicate causality; nevertheless they do provide more detail about correlations between environmental factors and obesity and also suggest that overcoming social and economic challenges would facilitate the reduction of health inequalities. Furthermore, the consideration of environmental patterns, rather than single socio-economic variables, more closely simulates the real world and real environments in which people live and work. Environmental factors cannot, and do not, operate in isolation. As such, a combined effect needs to be considered. A nutritional analogy is looking at dietary patterns (such as a Mediterranean diet, traditional British diet, etc.) rather than individual nutrients. Rather than focusing on the 'downstream' outcomes of individual behaviours or lifestyles, better understanding of the 'upstream' factors that tip environments into obesogenic environments is required, and whether any trigger points or thresholds exist.

Illuminating how people react and interact with the environment to the benefit or detriment of their health may not provide a complete solution to understanding the obesity problem, but it does provide an enhanced platform for analysis, evaluation and decision making in health planning. Furthermore, as public health embraces the micro-level spatial analysis concept and moves to a more local approach, this will facilitate more focused and detailed health planning. It enables governments and health professionals to respond to local differences in health behaviours, and to develop and implement more targeted interventions and health policies for prevention. This is a time when many different literatures are coming together, and through this combination of expertise the field of obesity prevention has much to gain with some innovative thinking and challenging of traditional analysis. Looking forward, mapping and spatially analysing obesity and obesogenic environment data should have a role in improving our knowledge about the aetiology of obesity (i.e. 'spatial epidemiology' works alongside, not instead of, traditional epidemiology). These are additional erudite ways of conceptualising and devising population-level and place-level interventions and health policies to help prevent obesity, which may assist in transforming the propensity of interventions that focus too much on individual-level activities.

5.7 Acknowledgements

The boundary data used in this chapter are Crown copyright produced by the Office for National Statistics (ONS). Licensed for academic use by the Economic and Social Research Council (ESRC) with the support of the Joint Information Systems Committee (JISC), which funded free access to the data for researchers in the United Kingdom. The data service providers are the Census Geography Data Unit (UK Boundary Outline and Reference Database for Education and Research Study: UKBORDERS) via Edinburgh University Data Library (EDINA). The 2001 Census Ward Boundaries are Crown copyright 2003 where Crown copyright material is reproduced with the permission of the Controller of HMS. http://edina.ac.uk/ukborders

References

1. Swinburn, B., Egger, G., Raza, F. (1999) Dissecting obesogenic environments: the development and application of a framework for identifying and prioritizing environmental interventions for obesity. *Preventive Medicine.* 29:563–570.
2. Yeung, J., Hills, A.P. Introduction. In: *Children, Obesity and Exercise: Prevention, Treatment and Management of Childhood and Adolescent Obesity.* (Eds. Hills, A.P., King, N.A., Byrne, N.M.) Chapter 1. Routledge, Abingdon, 2007 pp. 1–10.
3. Steinbeck, K.S. (2001) The importance of physical activity in the prevention of overweight and obesity in childhood: a review and an opinion. *Obesity Reviews.* 2:117–130.
4. Guo, S.S., Roche, A.F., Chumlea, W.C., Gardner, J.D., Siervogel, R.M. (1994) The predictive value of childhood body mass index values for overweight at age 35 years. *American Journal of Clinical Nutrition.* 59(4):810–819.
5. Ross, C.E. (2000) Walking, exercising, and smoking: does neighbourhood matter? *Social Science & Medicine.* 51:265–274.

6. Parsons, T.J., Power, C., Logan, S., Summerbell, C.D. (1999) Childhood predictors of adult obesity: a systematic review. *International Journal of Obesity*. 23 (Suppl. 8):S1–107.

7. Hardy, R., Wadsworth, M., Kuh, D. (2000) The influence of childhood weight and socio-economic status on change in adult body mass index in a British national birth cohort. *International Journal of Obesity*. 24(6):725–734.

8. Okasha, M., McCarron, P., McEwen, J., Durnin, J., Davey Smith, G. (2003) Childhood social class and adulthood obesity: findings from the Glasgow Alumni Cohort. *Journal of Epidemiology and Community Health*. 57:508–509.

9. Monden, C.W.S., van Lenthe, F.J., Mackenbach, J.P. (2006) A simultaneous analysis of neighbourhood and childhood socio-economic environment with self-assessed health and health-related behaviours. *Health & Place*. 12(4):394–403.

10. Asthana, S., Curtis, S., Duncan, C., Gould, M. (2002) Themes in British health geography at the end of the century: a review of published research 1998–2000. *Social Science & Medicine*. 55:167–173.

11. Curtis, S., Cave, B., Coutts, A. (2002) Is urban regeneration good for health? Perceptions and theories of the health impacts of urban change. *Environment and Planning C-Government and Policy*. 20(4):517–534.

12. Vandegrift, D., Yoked, T. (2004) Obesity rates, income, and suburban sprawl: an analysis of US states. *Health & Place*. 10:221–229.

13. Clarke, G.P., Eyre, H., Guy, C. (2002) Deriving indicators of access to food retail provision in British cities: studies of Cardiff, Leeds and Bradford. *Urban Studies*. 39(11):2041–2060.

14. Whelan, A., Wrigley, N., Warm, D., Cannings, E. (2002) Life in a 'food desert'. *Urban Studies*. 39(11):2083–2100.

15. Wrigley, N. (2002) 'Food deserts' in British cities: policy context and research priorities. *Urban Studies*. 39(11):2029–2040.

16. Liu, G.C., Cunningham, C., Downs, S.M., Marrero, D.G., Fineberg, N. (2002) A spatial analysis of obesogenic environments for children. *Proceedings of the AMIA Annual Symposium*:459–463.

17. Coen, S.E., Ross, N.A. (2006) Exploring the material basis for health: characteristics of parks in Montreal neighbourhoods with contrasting health outcomes. *Health & Place*. 12:361–371.

18. Timperio, A., Salmon, J., Telford, A., Crawford, D. (2005) Perceptions of local neighbourhood environments and their relationship to childhood overweight and obesity. *International Journal of Obesity*. 29:170–175.

19. Foresight Report. (2007) Tackling obesities: future choices, http://www.foresight.gov.uk/OurWork/ActiveProjects/Obesity/Obesity.asp, accessed September 09.

20. Fischer, M., Scholten, H.J., Unwin, D., eds. *Spatial Analytical Perspectives of GIS*. London, Taylor & Francis, 1996.

21. Sinton, D.S., Lund, J.J. *Understanding Place: GIS and Mapping Across the Curriculum*. Redlands, CA, ESRI, 2007.

22. Dorling, D. (1995) The visualization of local urban change across Britain. *Environment and Planning B: Planning & Design*. 22(3):269–290.

23. Monmonier, M. *How to Lie with Maps*. 2nd Edition, Chicago, University of Chicago Press, 1996.

24. Gatrell, A.C. *Geographies of Health: An Introduction*. Oxford, Blackwell publishers, 2002.

25. Wilkinson, P., Grundy, C., Landon, M., Stevenson, S. In: *GIS and Health*. (Eds. Gatrell, A., Löytönen, M.) Chapter 11. Taylor & Francis, London, 1998.

26. Kulldorff, M. (2006) *SaTScan User Guide for version 7.0*. Available at: http://www.satscan.org/.

27. Pearl, J. *Causality: Models, Reasoning and Inference*. Cambridge, Cambridge University Press, 2000.

28. Rothman, K.J., Greenland, S. *Modern Epidemiology*. 2nd Edition, Philadelphia, PA, Lippincott-Raven publishers, 1998.

29. Wrigley, N., Holt, T., Steel, D., Tranmer, M. Analysing, modelling, and resolving the ecology fallacy. In: *Spatial Analysis: Modelling in a GIS Environment*. (Eds. Longley, P., Batty, M.) Chapter 2. Geoinformation International, Cambridge, 1996 pp. 25–31.

30. Openshaw, S. The modifiable areal unit problem. *Concepts and Techniques in Modern Geography*. Volume 38. Environmental publications, Norwich, 1983, http://qmrg.org.uk/files/2008/11/38-maup-openshaw.pdf.
31. Leyland, A.H., Davies, C.A. (2005) Empirical Bayes methods for disease mapping. *Statistical Methods in Medical Research*. 14(1):17–34.
32. Halfacree, K.H., Flowerdew, R., Johnson, J.H. (1992) The characteristics of British migrants in the 1990s: evidence from a new survey. *Geographic Journal*. 158(2):157–169.
33. Vandersmissen, M.H., Séguin, A.M., Thériault, M., Claramunt, C. (2009) Modelling propensity to move after job change using event history analysis and temporal GIS. *Journal of Geographic Systems*. 11(1):37–65.
34. Block, J.P., Scribner, R.A., DeSalvo, K.B. (2004) Fast food, race/ethnicity, and income: a geographical analysis. *American Journal of Preventive Medicine*. 27(3):211–217.
35. Smoyer-Tomic, K.E., Spence, J., Raine, K.D., Amrhein, C., Yasenovsky, V., Cutumisu, N., Hemphill, E., Healy, J. (2008) The association between neighbourhood socioeconomic status and exposure to supermarkets and fast food outlets. *Health & Place*. 14:740–754.
36. Maher, A., Wilson, N., Signal, L. (2005) Advertising and availability of 'obesogenic' foods around New Zealand secondary schools: a pilot study. *New Zealand Medical Journal*. 118(1218), http://www.nzma.org.nz/journal/118-1218/1556/.
37. Burdette, H.L., Whitaker, R.C. (2004) Neighbourhood playgrounds, fast food restaurants and crime: relationships to overweight in low income preschool children. *Preventive Medicine*. 38:57–63.
38. Jeffery, R.W., Baxter, J., McGuire, M., Lende, J. (2006) Are fast food restaurants an environmental risk factor for obesity? *International Journal of Behavioural Nutrition and Physical Activity*. 3:2–8.
39. Pearce, J., Blakely, T., Witten, K., Bautre, P. (2007) Neighbourhood deprivation and access to fast food retailing. *American Journal of Preventive Medicine*. 32(5):375–382.
40. Tucker, P., Irwin, J.D., Gilliland, J., He, M., Larsen, K., Hess, P. (2008) Environmental influences on physical activity levels in youth. *Health & Place*. 15:357–363.
41. Pearce, J., Hiscock, R., Blakely, T., Witten, K. (2008) A national study of the association between neighbourhood access to fast-food outlets and the diet and weight of local residents. *Health & Place*. 15:193–197.
42. Kwate, N.O.A., Yau, C.-Y., Loh, J.-M., Williams, D. (2008) Inequality in obesogenic environments: fast food density in New York City. *Health & Place*. 15:364–373.
43. Reidpath, D.D., Burns, C., Garrard, M., Mahoney, M., Townsend, M. (2002) An ecological study of the relationships between social and environmental determinants of obesity. *Health & Place*. 8:141–145.
44. Cummins, S.C.J., McKay, L., MacIntyre, S. (2005) McDonald's restaurants and neighbourhood deprivation in Scotland and England. *American Journal of Preventive Medicine*. 29(4):308–310.
45. MacDonald, L., Cummins, S., MacIntyre, S. (2007) Neighbourhood fast food environment and area deprivation – substitution or concentration? *Appetite*. 49:251–254.
46. Hemphill, E., Raine, K., Spence, J.C., Smoyer-Tomic, K.E. (2008) Exploring obesogenic food environments in Edmonton, Canada: the association between socioeconomic factors and fast-food outlet access. *American Journal of Health Promotion*. 22(6):426–432.
47. MacIntyre, S., McKay, L., Cummins, S., Burns, C. (2005) Out-of-home food outlets and area deprivation: case study in Glasgow, UK. *International Journal of Behavioral Nutrition and Physical Activity*. 2:16.
48. Winkler, E., Turrell, G., Patterson, C. (2006) Does living in a disadvantaged area mean fewer opportunities to purchase fresh fruit and vegetables in the area? Findings from the Brisbane food study. *Health & Place*. 12:306–319.
49. Sturm, R., Datar, A. (2005) Body mass index in elementary school children, metropolitan food prices and food outlet density. *Public Health*. 119:1059–1068.
50. Thornton, L., University of Melbourne, personal communication (September, 2008).
51. Fotheringham, A.S., Nakaya, T., Yano, K., Openshaw, S., Ishikawa, Y. (2001) Hierarchical destination choice and spatial interaction modelling: a simulation experiment. *Environment and Planning A*. 33:901–920.

52. Morrissey, K., Clarke, G., Ballas, D., Hynes, S., O'Donoghue, C. (2008) Examining access to GP services in rural Ireland using microsimulation analysis. *Area*. 40(3):354–364.
53. Tomintz, M.N., Clarke, G.P., Rigby, J.E. (2008) The geography of smoking in Leeds: estimating individual smoking rates and the implications for the location of stop-smoking services. *Area*. 40(3):341–353.
54. Hakimi, S.L. (1964) Optimum locations of switching centres and the absolute centres and medians of a graph. *Operations Research*. 12(3):450–459.
55. Toregas, C., Swain, R., ReVelle, C., Bergman, L. (1971) The location of emergency service facilities. *Operations Research*. 19(6):1363–1373.
56. Church, R.L., ReVelle, C.S. (1974) The maximal covering location problem. *Papers of the Regional Science Association*. 32:101–118.
57. Rigby, J.E., Gatrell, A.C. (2000) Spatial patterns in breast cancer incidence in NW Lancashire. *Area*. 32:71–78.
58. Kulldorff, M. (1997) A spatial scan statistic. *Communications in Statistics: Theory and Methods*. 26:1481–1496.
59. Tango, T., Takahashi, K. (2005) A flexibly shaped spatial scan statistic for detecting clusters. *International Journal of Health Geographics*. 4:11.
60. Cowles, M.K. (2004) Review of WinBUGS 1.4. *American Statistician*. 58(4):330–336.
61. Kulldorff, M., Information Management Services Inc. (2005) SaTScanTM v6.0: Software for the spatial and space-time scan statistics, http://www.satscan.org/.
62. Takahashi, K., Yokoyama, T., Tango, T. *FleXScan v1.1: Software for the Flexible Scan Statistic*. Japan, National Institute of Public Health, 2005, http://www.niph.go.jp/soshiki/gijutsu/index_e.html.
63. Spiegelhalter, D.J., Thomas, A., Best, N.G., Lunn, D. *WinBUGS Version 1.4 User Manual*. Cambridge, MRC Biostatistics Unit, 2002, http://www.mrc-bsu.cam.ac.uk/bugs Software available from http://www.mrc-bsu.cam.ac.uk/bugs/winbugs/contents.shtml.
64. Brunsdon, C.A., Fotheringham, A.S., Charlton, M.E. (1998) Geographically weighted regression - modelling spatial nonstationary. *Statistician*. 47:431–443.
65. Fotheringham, A.S., Brunsdon, C., Charlton, M. *Geographically Weighted Regression: The Analysis of Spatially Varying Relationships*. Chichester, John Wiley & Sons, Ltd, 2002.
66. Procter, K.L., Clarke, G.P., Ransley, J.K., Cade, J. (2008) Micro-level analysis of childhood obesity, diet, physical activity, residential socio-economic and social capital variables: where are the obesogenic environments in Leeds? *Area*. 40(3):323–340.
67. Yiannakoulias, N., Rowe, B.H., Svenson, L.W., Schopflocher, D.P., Kelly, K., Voaklander, D.C. (2003) Zones of prevention: the geography of fall injuries in the elderly. *Social Science & Medicine*. 57:2065–2073.
68. Lake, A., Townsend, T. (2006) Obesogenic environments: exploring the built and food environments. *Journal of the Royal Society of Health*. 126(6):262–267.

6 Objective Measurement of Children's Physical Activity in the Environment: UK Perspective

Ashley Cooper and Angie Page

6.1 UK policy and research context

There has been a significant shift in UK public health policy to recognise that changes in the environment and individual approaches are required to increase population-level physical activity and attempt to halt the rapid increase in obesity. The influential Foresight Report concluded that 'the obesity epidemic cannot be prevented by individual action alone and demands a societal approach' (p. 3)[1] and that the consequences on society would be grave if we did not tackle the obesogenic environment (p. 3).[2] More recently, 7 of the 15 recommendations included in the UK National Institute for Clinical Excellence (NICE) guidelines for promoting physical activity, active play and sport for young people[3] relate to how various sectors can shape the environment to increase physical activity. This complements earlier NICE guidelines on physical activity and the environment[4] which were the first national, evidence-based recommendations on how to improve the physical environment to encourage physical activity. One of the recommendations was that planning processes for new developments should prioritise the need for routine physical activity along with the needs of cyclists and pedestrians when developing or maintaining roads. The wide-ranging Children's Plan[5] by the UK Department for Children, Schools and Families includes significant commitment to improve the outdoor physical activity environment to provide enhanced opportunities for play. Specifically, it pledges to offer funding that would allow up to 3500 playgrounds to be rebuilt or renewed and to create 30 new supervised adventure playgrounds for 8- to 13-year-olds in disadvantaged areas in England. The publication of the Children's Plan prompted the recent Play Strategy[6] which includes Governmental aims that 'local neighbourhoods are, and feel like, safe, interesting places to play, routes to children's play space are safe and accessible for all children and young people and that parks and open spaces are attractive and welcoming to children and young people' (p. 1). Collectively, these recent documents signal a shift in UK policy that recognises the importance of improvements in the physical environment to encourage physical activity and the need to evaluate how they impact on the public's health. However, there is limited specific UK empirical evidence on which this policy is based.

Contemporary literature on young people's physical activity and the physical environment is dominated by evidence from North America and Australia.[7] It is unclear to what extent these findings are generalisable to countries such as the United Kingdom where urban structure is very different to that found in studies based, for example, in the United States.[7,8] There are strong contributions to the obesogenic environment literature from the United Kingdom, but these have tended to focus more on neighbourhood deprivation[9] and the food environment.[10,11] More recent studies have investigated the availability of indoor and park facilities in relation to physical activity but included only adult samples.[12–15] Relevant literature does exist in young people but it is largely restricted to small school-based UK intervention examples[16,17] and some recent promising qualitative work.[18] As Jones *et al.*[8] point out, research in this area is in its infancy but they further comment that in the United Kingdom, a number of new studies are underway. The three examples they cite are summarised below. It is acknowledged that these are not the only contemporary studies in this area but they are included here as they have used objective measures of the physical environment in relation to objective measures of physical activity in young people. They are used as a platform to discuss how objective measures can help overcome some of the significant methodological limitations inherent in much of the physical activity literature in this area.

6.2   A brief review of current studies in the United Kingdom

6.2.1   CAPABLE: Children's Activities, Perceptions and Behaviour in the Local Environment

The aim of CAPABLE was to understand the nature and structure of routes, spaces and networks as used and perceived by children, the extent to which the local environment met the needs of children and their activities and to develop a better understanding of the impact of the local environment on children's behaviour and spatial understanding, particularly in terms of independent travel.[19] It built upon an earlier project in which the impact of car use upon children was investigated, and combined accelerometer, Global Positioning System (GPS) and diary data to explore children's travel patterns.[20] In one part of CAPABLE 330 primary school children (8- to 11-year olds) were recruited from two schools in Hertfordshire, England, and asked to complete a questionnaire about their use of the environment. Data were collected in winter 2005–2006 for a subgroup of 162 children. These children wore GPS receivers, accelerometers and kept travel diaries for 4 days to investigate how they interacted with the environment, including the effects of being allowed out independently.[21]

6.2.2   SPEEDY: Sport, Physical activity and Eating behaviour: Environmental Determinants in Young people

The SPEEDY study was established by a multidisciplinary collaborative group at the Medical Research Council Epidemiology Unit in Cambridge and the University of East Anglia in Norwich. Its aim was to examine physical activity levels and dietary behaviour in a large population-based sample of British 9- to 10-year old children, and to investigate the individual and collective factors associated with these behaviours. Schools in the county of Norfolk, East England, were sampled purposively to achieve heterogeneity in location; 92 schools agreed to participate and were visited for a measurement session during the 12-week summer term of 2007. All year 5 children (aged 9–10 years) at these schools were invited to participate ($N = 3619$). Only children with a fully completed consent form (signed by both a parent/guardian and the child) on the day of measurement were included in the study. A total of 2064 children participated (57.0% response rate). Teams of two or more research assistants visited the schools for the measurement sessions. Data collected include physical activity over 7 days measured by ActiGraph accelerometer and self-reported physical activity, anthropometry (height, weight, waist circumference and body fat percentage), food choice and a food diary, and child and parent self-reported questionnaires on potential behavioural determinants. Head teachers also completed a questionnaire about potential school-level determinants and a school audit was administered to objectively assess the school grounds. Using the exact location of participants' homes and schools, a range of GIS-based measures of the objective physical characteristics of the residential environment was computed for each participant from residential density, proximity of greenspace and food outlets through to crime and transport infrastructure. All children were invited 1 year later for follow-up measurements of physical activity (using ActiGraph accelerometers) and potential determinants in which 999 children participated (48.4% response rate).[22] In an additional small pilot study during the summer holiday of 2007 designed to help gain greater insight into the levels and patterns of activity in different locations, a sample of 100 SPEEDY children wore a GPS receiver at the same time as accelerometers on four consecutive days including the weekend, and also completed an activity diary recording times and reasons when they needed to remove the monitors.

6.2.3 PEACH: Personal and Environmental Associations with Children's Health

The PEACH project is a longitudinal study, based at the University of Bristol, which is designed to investigate the environmental and personal determinants of physical activity, diet and obesity in young people across the transition between primary and secondary school. This transition is known to coincide with the start of a progressive decline in children's physical activity. A sample of 23 state primary schools in Bristol were recruited, selected on the basis of transition rates above 40% to one of eight urban state funded secondary schools. The secondary schools were selected by geographic location and index of multiple deprivation (IMD) to be representative of the city. All children in their final year of school (year 6; aged 10–11 years) were invited to participate ($N = 1899$), and 1340 provided written parental consent (70.5%). Of these, 1307 children were present in school on measurement days. Almost 1000 of these children were followed up 1 year later in their first year of secondary school. Data were collected between September 2006 and July 2009 and measurements took place throughout the school year to allow for seasonality. At baseline and follow-up simple anthropometric measures were taken, physical activity was measured for 7 days with an ActiGraph accelerometer and children also wore a GPS receiver and completed an activity diary for 4 days. A computerised questionnaire was used to investigate the correlates of physical activity and eating behaviours and data were also collected from parents via a self-report questionnaire.

These three studies were each designed to address limitations in the understanding of environmental influences on children's physical activity. Although differing in design and the range of questionnaire measures used, these studies have in common the use of objective measures of physical activity (accelerometry) and location (GPS).

6.3 Objective measurement in physical activity research

Understanding which characteristics of the physical environment may encourage or inhibit young people's physical activity is central to identifying targets for change[23] but little is known about where children or adolescents spend time outside their homes and school. The limited understanding of activity taking place in the built environment is partly due to methodological difficulties in identifying physical activity within different contexts and locations. This issue was identified by Jones et al. in their review[8] who noted that the majority of studies relied upon self-reported physical activity and thus have the possibility of inaccuracy and bias. They also identified, in common with other reviews of the environmental correlates of physical activity in children,[24,25] a need for more studies using objective measurements based on the use of accelerometers and GPS in order to better understand children's physical activity in the physical environment. This would allow more accurate assessment of what behaviour is occurring, how much movement it produces and the location of that behaviour. Methods are now becoming available which will allow us to address these issues. Accelerometry, the measurement of vertical accelerations of the body, has become a standard method for the measurement of physical activity in children.[26,27] In contrast, the use of GPS to investigate children's mobility in the built environment is a novel but rapidly emerging methodology. There is substantial potential for these techniques, both separately and in combination, to improve our understanding of how the environment may influence children's physical activity, and these methods are reviewed below.

6.3.1 Motion sensors

Physical activity, defined as any bodily movement requiring energy expenditure, is a complex behaviour, subject to frequent changes in intensity and mode (e.g. sitting, standing, walking), that takes place in a range of contexts and locations. There are also many different types of everyday physical activity – activity at work (occupational), exercise, sport/recreation, travel and 'other' (non-sport, non-occupational). It is thus not surprising that measurement of physical activity by self-report methods is generally imprecise, since individuals have difficulty in recalling their past activity behaviour and tend to remember structured, higher intensity activities more accurately than those of low intensity or that are more sporadic in nature (recall bias). These limitations are particularly marked in children where the majority of their physical activity is sporadic and unstructured[28]; it is, therefore, not surprising that associations between self-report and criterion methods are particularly weak in children.[29] The various methods used to measure physical activity and the limitations of these methods have been extensively reviewed.[30,31] Many of the limitations of self-report methods have been overcome by the use of motion sensors to measure physical activity, and in recent years use of these instruments has moved from the domain of a few investigators to a method that is now widely used even in population surveys.[32]

Motion sensors fall into two main types: pedometers and accelerometers. Pedometers are simple devices that usually consist of a horizontal spring-suspended lever arm that moves with the vertical acceleration of the body and provides a simple measure of the number of steps taken. These instruments can provide a measure of total ambulation with great accuracy, although the accuracy of different models varies substantially. Pedometers are generally cheaper than accelerometers and thus more widely used, but most models only store the total number of steps taken, not the time over which these were accumulated. Consequently, it is difficult to provide time-resolved data from pedometers, and thus any measure of activity intensity, even though new models allow recording to be segmented over at least 7 days. However, as walking is the major physical activity that most individuals take, pedometers can provide a good estimate or overall physical activity, and they have been used successfully in a number of population studies in youth.[33]

Accelerometers are substantially more sophisticated instruments which sample accelerations of the body with high frequency (30 times per second for the commonly used ActiGraph GT1M). The majority of accelerometers in current use are uniaxial, and are usually worn on a belt around the waist where they measure vertical accelerations of the trunk. A number of accelerometers (e.g. the RT3 used in CAPABLE) also measure accelerations in other axes, and although theoretically this should improve the precision of activity estimates, particularly in children due to the sporadic and varied nature of their activities, to date this has not been demonstrated. The acceleration data are digitally filtered to a band-limited frequency range of 0.25–2.5 Hz. This frequency range detects normal human movement but excludes motion from other sources, such as vehicles. The output signal from the digital filter responds linearly to changing accelerations and is thus proportional to movement speed so that, for example, an individual's walking speed will be linearly related to the accelerometer output. The frequent sampling of accelerations means that physical activity can be described not only in terms of overall amount (similar to a pedometer) but also as intensity (light, moderate or vigorous) and pattern of activity, and these data can be recorded over a period of up to 2 weeks.

Accelerometer data are usually expressed as 'counts', an arbitrary value that is often not comparable between monitor brands. To aid interpretation, the counts recorded every 0.03 seconds are summed over a user-defined period commonly called an 'epoch'. A 1-minute epoch is most often used, though with the higher memory capacity of recent accelerometers this is increasingly being reduced to 10–15 seconds or less, in order to try and capture the short, intense nature of children's movements. Counts per epoch are then summarised to describe physical activity volume in terms of accelerometer counts per unit of time (usually minute or hour) for the period of interest (e.g. day/week). To give a broader meaning to accelerometer output, data are often expressed in terms of activity intensity, that is, amount of time spent in light, moderate or vigorous activity. Most commonly, practitioners are interested in the amount of moderate-to-vigorous physical activity (MVPA) accumulated to allow comparison with public health guidelines (30 minutes for adults or 60 minutes for children daily of MVPA).[34] However, the interpretation of accelerometer output as a measure of activity intensity is a topic of substantial debate.[26,27] A number of studies have reported accelerometer values (counts per minute) that differentiate light, moderate and vigorous activity (known as 'cut points'), but these estimates vary substantially, particularly in children, and to date there is no consensus regarding the appropriate cut points for either adults or children. Use of different cut points has a substantial impact on the proportion of individuals meeting guidelines – in one study of children from an inner city British school, the proportion meeting guidelines was between 7.2% and 100% depending on the cut point chosen.[35]

In addition to the issues around the validity of cut points, accelerometers have a number of other limitations. When worn around the waist, they do not record upper movements of the body, but they poorly record activity during cycling (since the participant is seated and movements of the hips are small), and they are usually removed for water-based activity or in vigorous contact sports. In addition, although accelerometers can provide a good estimate of energy expenditure in steady walking, they are limited in their ability to provide a reliable estimate of energy expenditure in free-living individuals due to the diversity of activities carried out. Nonetheless, despite these limitations accelerometers have provided a major step forward in the measurement of physical activity in free-living individuals, and have proved to be an important tool in improving our understanding of the association between physical activity and health. Such instruments are now being used in many major studies and have started to be introduced into population surveys.

Although the accelerometers used in most studies provide highly time-resolved data, few investigators have looked at temporal patterns of activity. However, such data can provide important information on when differences in physical activity between active or less active groups occur, for example, between obese and non-obese children[36] or between active and passive travellers.[37] In the latter example, accelerometers used in conjunction with activity diaries identified substantially higher levels of physical activity for several hours after school in children walking to school, and this was reflected in more time spent in self-reported outdoor play.[38] These findings suggest that children's use of the outdoor physical environment may be facilitated by active travel to school. Researchers are also starting to use accelerometry in combination with measures of neighbourhood environmental variables to investigate whether features such as access/proximity to parks or leisure centres are associated with objectively measured physical activity. Neighbourhoods with a greater proportion of park area, higher housing density or more pleasant sidewalk characteristics (e.g. presence of trees, lighting) have been positively associated with higher physical activity in some, but not all, studies.[39–41] These studies have been based in the United States and Australia, and to our knowledge, no UK data have been published at the time of writing. Further investigation of these associations and the potential role of active travel in facilitating outdoor physical activity requires measurement methods that are able to identify both the location and level of physical activity during defined periods of the day; a potential solution that is gaining interest is the use of the GPS.

6.3.2 Use of GPS to investigate children's spatial mobility

GPS technology measures location, distance travelled and speed based upon the signal received from a network of satellites. GPS technology has been used within the transport field to augment survey data by allowing the recording of trip origins and destinations, and also routes travelled. Health researchers have begun to realise the potential of GPS to describe individual behaviour and the way in which individuals may interact with the physical environment. In the last few years, personal wearable GPS receivers have become readily available that allow position to be recorded to within 15–20 m and are thus sufficiently precise to track participants' movements.[42] At present, very few studies have used this technology in free-living children. The journey to school has been investigated in 11-year old children, where the distance between home and school was found to be comparable when measured directly by GPS receivers worn during the journey and when computed using GIS shortest route analysis.[43] However, the travel routes described by the two methods were substantially different, with the GIS computed routes crossing significantly more busy streets than the actual routes taken, indicating that children seek out routes that avoid busy streets, where possible.

GPS-enabled mobile phones have been used in two recent studies. In the United States, 15 adolescent women were asked to carry phones for a week, with location data automatically recorded at 5-minute intervals using the cell phone network and subsequently enhanced using satellite communication.[44] Researchers were able to reliably track participant locations, finding that most participants had variable paths, often extending beyond their immediate neighbourhoods. In addition, the phones used were able to record diary information, allowing the possibility that this technology might not only be able to provide in-depth information about location but also to provide context-specific data on other behaviours. More recently, Mikkelsen and Christensen[45] used GPS combined with mobile phone tracking to investigate independent mobility in children. Higher levels of independent mobility have been related to higher levels of both self-reported[46] and objectively measured[47] physical activity in children. Mikkelsen and Christensen[45] piloted a portable GPS unit with 32 Danish children who were 10–13 years old along with a mobile phone survey sent 5 times a day to document where children were, who they were with, how they got there, etc. These data were used to determine children's use of their neighbourhood, whether they spent most of their time inside or outside, who they were with and the means they used to get from place to place. GPS data were interpreted via GIS to produce two types of maps, the 'itinerary map' and the 'sojourn map'. The itinerary map was based on the track-logs of the GPS to represent the mobility pattern of every respondent. The sojourn map, based on the time interval between the single GPS points, was used to evaluate the time spent in each 100 m^2 grid cell. The locations in which the children spent their time were categorised into three different scales: the local area around the home and the school, the municipality and nationwide, and both individual and collective maps were generated. The latter were structured according to gender and showed that girls' outdoor play took place predominantly in the garden or in the vicinity of the home, whereas boys played near the home and also took more trips, often with friends, into the wider neighbourhood.

GPS has potential for investigating more complex patterns of physical activity in relation to the physical environment where traditional techniques, even in-depth diaries, have struggled to accurately represent the diverse range of children's behavioural choices. One important time to focus on is the period after school. This period has been identified in a number of studies as important for children to be physically active[48,49] and is a time where differences in objectively measured physical activity between groups of children have been reported.[36,37] However, interpreting data from this period is complex since children leave school at variable times depending on participation in after-school activities, and have a wide range of possible activity patterns which may be influenced by a range of physical and social factors. Providing objective data on where children are during key periods of the day will help identify why some youth are more active than others and where strategies might be most effectively implemented to increase physical activity in less active youth.

Using GPS to record children's journeys produces a dataset that is highly detailed but also highly complex to interpret when there are more than a few participants, and most studies have been limited to a small number of individuals. A potential use of GPS, that does not require tracking of participants within a GIS, is to provide an objective measurement of time outside, regardless of specific location. Time spent outside is a consistent correlate of children's physical activity[50] and is associated with objectively measured physical activity in 10- to 12-year-old children in cross-sectional and longitudinal analyses.[51] However, the magnitude of the association between time outside and accelerometer-measured physical activity is relatively small, which may be due to the limitations of the parental proxy method often used to assess time outside. Since GPS receivers do not record a signal indoors, GPS may provide a feasible objective method of assessing time outside that could be used in a large sample of children to investigate how the amount of time young people spend outdoors relates to overall physical activity and other health parameters. This approach has been taken in preliminary analyses of PEACH data which show that the more active children record higher amounts of GPS data (presumed to be time outdoors) and that the amount of GPS data was a significant independent predictor of children's physical activity, after adjustment for other potential explanatory factors in regression analyses. Although preliminary, these data support the idea that GPS wear time may be a useful objective measure of time spent outside that is associated with physical activity levels in children.

6.3.3 Combining GPS and accelerometry

As described above, GPS is now being used to provide information on where young people live, travel and interact. In addition, accelerometry has become an accepted method of physical activity measurement in youth. Combining these methods to provide a simultaneous assessment of free-living physical activity and location will allow us to learn more about the environmental context of objectively measured physical activity and to quantify physical activity duration and intensity during different travel trips. An example is shown in Figure 6.1, where the combined accelerometer and GPS data for a single child are visualised using GIS. The data

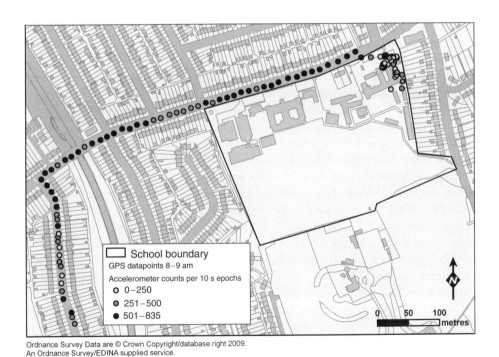

Ordnance Survey Data are © Crown Copyright/database right 2009.
An Ordnance Survey/EDINA supplied service.

Figure 6.1 An example of integrated GPS and accelerometry track showing the intensity and duration (in 10-second epochs) of the journey to school for one child.

are sampled at 10-second intervals and show the route taken to school and time spent in the school playground at the end of the journey. The accelerometer data allow the activity level associated with each GPS reading to be visualised in counts per 10-second-epoch, in this case illustrating that the physical activity during the journey (above 250 counts per 10 seconds) is higher than that within the playground (generally below 250 counts per 10 seconds).

This is a research area which is still in its infancy, and to date, very few studies have been published. In a pilot study in adults, combined accelerometer and GPS data showed that participants who obtained most of their MVPA in their neighbourhoods lived in areas of high population density, housing density and street connectivity and with more public parks.[42] Taking another approach in adults, GPS data have been used in combination with accelerometry to try and discriminate between different types of physical activities.[52] As described above, a limitation of accelerometers is that they do not record activity mode and a supporting diary/log is required to capture what a participant is doing, limiting the identification of activity mode in free-living conditions. Researchers are beginning to develop complex statistical methods for use with accelerometer data that are able to discriminate between different activity modes with a degree of success.[53] Combined data may be a useful alternative/additional method to discriminate between sedentary and active modes of travel (e.g. travelling by car and bicycle) where speeds can be similar but physical activity differs, or between activities where accelerometer values may be similar but speed differs (e.g. walking and in line skating). Being able to discriminate between different activities will help to more accurately understand the nature of activities that take place in different environments, for example, on a cycle path.

At the time of writing, very little has been published describing the use of combined accelerometer and GPS data in children. In the CAPABLE study, combined data have been used to investigate children's independent movement, suggesting that children's walking behaviour (speed and directness) is influenced by whether they are accompanied by an adult.[21] In SPEEDY, matched accelerometer and GPS data were overlaid with a detailed land cover dataset developed in a GIS to identify the types of environment supporting bouts of MVPA. The results showed that urban children tended to be active close to their home and that gardens and streets were the most commonly used environments for MVPA.[54] In PEACH, combined accelerometer and GPS data have been used to investigate physical activity taking place around the journey to school with location of outdoor activity identified in GIS.[55] In this study, the time before school was categorised as 'unmatched' (accelerometer but no GPS data), 'journey' (combined accelerometer and GPS data; outside the school playground) and 'playground' (combined data within the playground). Activity during the journey was 2.5 times higher than in unmatched data, with activity levels in the playground being half those of the journey. These data are consistent with a picture of light intensity domestic activity taking place in the home before school, a purposeful walk to school of moderate or greater intensity and a short time spent in the playground during which activity levels are in general light/moderate before classes start. They demonstrate that combined accelerometer and GPS data can describe the location and level of children's outdoor physical activity, and support suggestions that the journey to school can potentially be a significant contributor to children's daily activity.

Although GPS shows great promise for understanding how individuals interact with the environment, there are a number of technical and practical limitations to be overcome. GPS signals may be blocked by tree cover or buildings, causing loss of data or may be reflected from buildings (multipath error) causing inaccurately located data points. Similarly, the time taken for the receiver to connect to the satellite network on leaving a building may result in loss of data. Practical concerns include the relatively limited battery life of current personal GPS receivers (approximately 16 hours) requiring frequent recharging and the participant to turn the instrument off when not in use (e.g. indoors) in contrast to accelerometers which have a continuous on-time of 2 weeks or more. These limitations result in increased participant burden in studies, introduce the possibility of participant error in using the instruments and potentially lower compliance. Combining GPS and accelerometer data may be used to improve estimates of journey time by accounting for short periods of GPS drop-out. When considering multiple journeys, a method is required to discriminate drop-out which occurs during a journey (and should thus be considered as part of the journey) and that which represents the end of one journey and the start of another. Methods for imputing location data across short gaps in GPS recordings are now being described, but combining GPS with accelerometer data, with the accelerometer as a reference time stamp, may allow the accelerometer data to be used to impute activity for these missing periods. Further investigation is required of the maximum duration over which it is valid to impute missing data and the impact of different sampling frequencies to data integrity. A number of practical limitations of using GPS will doubtlessly be resolved by advances in battery and receiver technology, and it is likely that instruments with combined accelerometer and GPS will shortly be available.

6.4 Conclusion

The role that the environment may play in contributing to the obesity epidemic has recently been recognised by the UK government, and has led to a shift in emphasis in public health policy. One key area in which environmental factors may negatively influence energy balance and potentially impact development of obesity is in restricting or reducing levels of physical activity. This may occur through a number of mechanisms, but a physical infrastructure that does not encourage or actively inhibits children's walking, cycling or outdoor play is likely to be a key driver. Reviews of the evidence base for the way in which the environment may impact children's physical activity have identified very few examples from the United Kingdom, with most data originating from the United States or Australia, although a number of major UK studies, reviewed in this chapter, are underway to address this issue.

In order to accurately quantify the relationship between the physical environment and physical activity, levels and patterns of activity and how children interact with the outdoor environment need to be measured as accurately as possible. This has led to a call in most reviews for greater use of objective methods of measurement. Within physical activity research, there has been a substantial shift over the last decade towards using instruments (pedometers and accelerometers) that greatly improve precision of measurement over self-report methods, and which have led to a better understanding of the association between physical activity and health outcomes. In contrast, measures of the environment generally have a substantial subjective component. However, the rapid advance of GPS technology, with widespread public familiarity through vehicle satellite navigation systems, has led to the availability and acceptability of small personal GPS receivers. These instruments may be used in a number of ways to investigate individual mobility and time spent in the outdoor environment, and offer great opportunities for understanding the location and levels of children's physical activity and how physical environments may encourage or inhibit physical activity. Advances in technology, the development of instruments combining an accelerometer with a GPS receiver, development of methods to analyse and interpret the data and greater use of these methods among the research community will doubtlessly lead to a rapid growth of understanding in this field. These data will enable the development of interventions to modify aspects of the environment in order to attempt to increase the physical activity of young people, and could also be used to monitor and evaluate the impact of these interventions. The results of such interventions are likely to significantly inform and impact public health policy and in the long term may lead to infrastructural change to encourage greater physical activity in the population.

This chapter has provided examples demonstrating how GPS and accelerometry, alongside other objective measures, can be used to help us understand how children actually use their local and wider environment; this information is for the first time being consistently related to health behaviours, including physical activity. This should help improve a currently weak evidence base to inform policy in relation to how the environment can be manipulated to increase children's physical activity levels.

References

1. Government Office for Science. *Foresight. Tackling Obesities: Future Choices – Summary of Key Messages.* London, HMSO, 2007.
2. Government Office for Science *Foresight. Tackling Obesities: Future Choices – Project Report.* London, HMSO, 2007.
3. National Institute for Clinical Excellence. *Public Health Guidance 17: Promoting Physical Activity, Active Play and Sport for Pre-school and School-age Children and Young People in Family, Pre-school, School and Community Settings.* London, National Institute for Health and Clinical Excellence, 2009. http://www.nice.org.uk/nicemedia/pdf/PH017Guidance.pdf.
4. National Institute for Clinical Excellence. *Public Health Guidance 8: Promoting and Creating Built or Natural Environments that Encourage and Support Physical Activity.* London, National Institute for Health and Clinical Excellence, 2008. http://www.nice.org.uk/nicemedia/pdf/PH008Guidance.pdf.
5. Department for Children, Schools and Families. *The Children's Plan: Building Brighter Futures.* London, HMSO, 2007. http://www.dcsf.gov.uk/childrensplan.

6. Department for Children, Schools and Families & Culture, Media and Sport. *Fair Play – A Consultation on the Play Strategy: A Commitment from the Children's Plan*. London, HMSO, 2008.

7. Ogilvie, D., Mitchell, R., Mutrie, N., Petticrew, M., Platt, S. (2008) Personal and environmental correlates of active travel and physical activity in a deprived urban population. *International Journal of Behavioral Nutrition and Physical Activity*. 5(43). doi:10.1186/1479-5868-5-43.

8. Jones, A., Panter, J., Hillsdon., M. *Obesogenic Environments: Evidence Review. Foresight. Tackling Obesities: Future Choices – Project Report*. London, HMSO, 2007.

9. Macintyre, S. (2007) Deprivation amplification revisited; or, is it always true that poorer places have poorer access to resources for healthy diets and physical activity? *International Journal of Behavioral Nutrition and Physical Activity*. 4(32). doi:10.1186/1479-5868-4-32.

10. Cummins, S.C., McKay, L., MacIntyre, S. (2005) McDonald's restaurants and neighborhood deprivation in Scotland and England. *American Journal of Preventive Medicine*. 29(4):308–310.

11. Hackett, A., Boddy, L., Boothby, J., Dummer, T.J., Johnson, B., Stratton, G. (2008) Mapping dietary habits may provide clues about the factors that determine food choice. *Journal of Human Nutrition and Dietetics*. 21(5):428–437.

12. Hillsdon, M., Panter, J., Foster, C., Jones, A. (2006) The relationship between access and quality of urban green space with population physical activity. *Public Health*. 120(12):1127–1132.

13. Dawson, J., Hillsdon, M., Boller, I., Foster, C. (2007). Perceived barriers to walking in the neighborhood environment: a survey of middle-aged and older adults. *Journal of Ageing and Physical Activity*. 15(3):318–335.

14. Stafford, M., Cummins, S., Ellaway, A., Sacker, A., Wiggins, R.D., Macintyre, S. (2007) Pathways to obesity: identifying local, modifiable determinants of physical activity and diet. *Social Science and Medicine*. 65(9):1882–1897.

15. Panter, J.R., Jones, A.P. (2008). Associations between physical activity, perceptions of the neighbourhood environment and access to facilities in an English city. *Social Science and Medicine*. 67(11):3.

16. Stratton, G., Mullan, E. (2005) The effect of multicolor playground markings on children's physical activity level during recess. *Preventive Medicine*. 41(5-6):828–833.

17. Ridgers, N.D., Stratton, G., Fairclough, S.J., Twisk, J.W. (2007) Children's physical activity levels during school recess: a quasi-experimental intervention study. *International Journal of Behavioral Nutrition and Physical Activity*. 4(19). doi:10.1186/1479-5868-4-19.

18. Pearce, A., Kirk, C., Cummins, S., Collins, M., Elliman, D., Connolly, A.M., Law, C. (2009) Gaining children's perspectives: a multiple method approach to explore environmental influences on healthy eating and physical activity. *Health and Place*. 15(2):614–621.

19. University College London (2008) About CAPABLE. Available at http://www.casa.ucl.ac.uk/capableproject.

20. Mackett, R.L., Gong, Y., Kitazawa, K., Paskins, J. (2007) Children's local travel behaviour – how the environment influences, controls and facilitates it [online]. Available at www.casa.ucl.ac.uk/capableproject/download/WCTR06Mackett.pdf

21. Mackett, R., Brown, B., Gong, Y., Kitazawa, K., Paskins, J. (2007) Children's independent movement in the local environment. *Built Environment*. 33(4):454–468.

22. van Sluijs, E.M., Skidmore, P.M., Mwanza, K., Jones, A.P., Callaghan, A.M., Ekelund, U., Harrison, F., Harvey, I., Panter, J., Wareham, N.J., Cassidy, A., Griffin, S.J. (2008) Physical activity and dietary behaviour in a population-based sample of British 10-year old children: the SPEEDY study (Sport, Physical activity and Eating behaviour: environmental Determinants in Young people). *BMC Public Health*. 8:388.

23. Giles-Corti, B., Timperio, A., Bull, F., Pikora, T. (2005) Understanding physical activity environmental correlates: increased specificity for ecological models. *Exercise and Sports Sciences Review*. 33(4):175–181.

24. Davison, K.K., Lawson, C.T. (2006) Do attributes in the physical environment influence children's physical activity? A review of the literature. *International Journal of Behavioral Nutrition and Physical Activity*. 19(3):3. doi:10.1186/1479-5868-3-19.

25. Ferreira, I., van der Horst, K., Wendel-Vos, W., Kremers, S., van Lenthe, F.J., Brug, J. (2007) Environmental correlates of physical activity in youth – a review and update. *Obesity Reviews*. 8:129–154.

26. Corder, K., Brage, S., Ekelund, U. (2007) Accelerometers and pedometers: methodology and clinical application. *Current Opinion in Clinical Nutrition and Metabolic Care*. 10:597–603.

27. Reilly, J.J., Penpraze, V., Hislop, J., Davies, G., Grant, S., Paton, J.Y. (2008) Objective measurement of sedentary behaviour: review with new data. *Archives of Disease in Childhood*. 93:614–619.

28. Bailey, R.C., Olson, J., Pepper, S.L., Porszasz, J., Barstow, T.J., Cooper, D.M. (1995) The level and tempo of children's physical activities: an observational study. *Medicine and Science in Sports and Exercise*. 27(7):1033–1041.

29. Corder, K., van Sluijs, E.M., Wright, A., Whincup, P., Wareham, N.J., Ekelund, U. (2009) Is it possible to assess free-living physical activity and energy expenditure in young people by self-report? *American Journal of Clinical Nutrition*. 89(3):736–737.

30. Welk, G.J., Corbin, C.B., Dale, D. (2000) Measurement issues in the assessment of physical activity in children. *Research Quarterly for Exercise and Sport*. 71(2 Suppl):S59–S73.

31. Ekelund, U., Yngve, A., Sjöström, M. (1999) Total daily energy expenditure and patterns of physical activity in adolescents assessed by two different methods. *Scandinavian Journal of Medicine and Science in Sports*. 9(5):257–264.

32. Troiano, R.P. (2009) Can there be a single best measure of reported physical activity? *American Journal of Clinical Nutrition*. 89(3):736–737.

33. Duncan, E., Scott, D.J., Schofield, G. (2008) Pedometer-determined physical activity and active transport in girls. *International Journal of Behavioral Nutrition and Physical Activity*. 5(2). doi:10.1186/1479-5868-5-2.

34. Department of Health. *At Least Five a Week. Evidence on the Impact of Physical Activity and its Relationship to Health. A Report from the Chief Medical Officer.* London, Department of Health, 2004.

35. Trayers, T., Cooper, A.R., Riddoch, C.J., Ness, A.R., Fox, K.R., Deem, R., Lawlor, D.A. (2006) Do children from an inner city British school meet the recommended levels of physical activity? Results from a cross sectional survey using objective measurements of physical activity. *Archives of Disease in Childhood*. 91:175–176.

36. Page, A., Cooper, A.R., Stamatakis, E., Foster, L.J., Crowne, E.C., Sabin, M., Shield, J.P.H. (2005) Physical activity patterns in non obese and obese children assessed using minute-by-minute accelerometry. *International Journal of Obesity and Related Metabolic Disorders*. 29:1070–1076.

37. Cooper, A.R., Page, A.S., Foster, L.J., Qahwaji, D. (2003) Commuting to school: are children who walk more physically active? *American Journal of Preventive Medicine*. 25(4):273–276.

38. Cooper, A.R., Page, A.S. Childhood obesity, physical activity and the environment. In: *Childhood Obesity: Contemporary Issues*. Symposia of the Society for the Study of Human Biology no. 45. (Eds. Cameron, N., Norgan, N.G., Ellison, T.H.), Taylor & Francis Group, Boca Raton, FL, 2006 pp. 119–134.

39. Jago, R., Baranowski, T., Zakeri, I., Harris, M. (2005) Observed environmental features and the physical activity of adolescent males. *American Journal of Preventive Medicine*. 29(2):98–104.

40. Roemmich, J.N., Epstein, L.H., Raja, S., Yin, L., Robinson, J., Winiewicz, D. (2006) Association of access to parks and recreational facilities with the physical activity of young children. *Preventive Medicine*. 43:437–441.

41. Timperio, A., Giles-Corti, B., Crawford, D., Andrianopoulos, N., Ball, K. (2008) Features of public open spaces and physical activity among children: Findings from the CLAN study. *Preventive Medicine*. 47:514–518.

42. Rodriguez, D.A., Brown, A.L., Troped, P.J. (2005) Portable global positioning units to complement accelerometry-based physical activity monitors. *Medicine and Science in Sports and Exercise*. 37(11):S572–S581.

43. Duncan, M.J., Mummery, W.K. (2007) GIS or GPS? A comparison of two methods for assessing route taken during active transport. *American Journal of Preventive Medicine*. 33(1):51–53.

44. Wiehe, S.E., Carroll, A.E., Liu, G.C., Haberkorn, K.L., Hoch, S.C., Wilson, J.S., Fortenberry, J.D. (2008) Using GPS-enabled cell phones to track the travel patterns of adolescents. *International Journal of Health Geographics*. 7:22.
45. Mikkelsen, M.R., Christensen, P. (2009) Is children's independent mobility really independent? A study of children's mobility combining ethnography and GPS/mobile phone technologies. *Mobilities*. 4(1):37–58.
46. Prezza, M., Pilloni, S., Marabito, C., Sersante, C., Alparone, F.R., Giuliani, M.V. (2001) The influence of psychosocial and environment factors on children's independent mobility and relationship to peer frequentation. *Journal of Community and Applied Social Psychology*. 11:435–450.
47. Page, A.S., Cooper, A.R., Griew, P., Davis, L., Hillsdon, M. (2009) Independent mobility in relation to weekday and weekend physical activity in children aged 10–11 years: the PEACH Project. *International Journal of Behavioral Nutrition and Physical Activity*. 6(2). doi:10.1186/1479-5868-6-2.
48. Tudor-Locke, C., Lee, S.M., Morgan, C.F., Beighle, A., Pangrazi, R. (2006) Children's pedometer-determined physical activity during the segmented school day. *Medicine and Science in Sports and Exercise*. 38(10):1732–1738.
49. Trost, S.G., Rosenkranz, R.R., Dzewaltowski, D. (2008) Physical activity levels among children attending after-school programs. *Medicine and Science in Sports and Exercise*. 40(4):622–629.
50. Sallis, J.F., Prochaska, J.J., Taylor, W.C. (2000) A review of correlates of physical activity of children and adolescents. *Medicine and Science in Sports and Exercise*. 32(5):963–975.
51. Cleland V., Crawford, D., Baur, L.A., Hume, C., Timperio, A., Salmon, J. (2008) A prospective examination of children's time spent outdoors, objectively measured physical activity and overweight. *International Journal of Obesity and Related Metabolic Disorders*. 32(11):1685–1693.
52. Troped, P.J., Oliveira, M.S., Matthews, C.E., Cromley, E.K., Melly, S.J., Craig, B.A. (2008) Prediction of activity mode with global positioning system and accelerometer data. *Medicine and Science in Sports and Exercise*. 40(5):972–978.
53. Pober, D.M., Staudenmayer, J., Raphael, C., Freedson, P.S. (2006) Development of novel techniques to classify physical activity mode using accelerometers. *Medicine and Science in Sport and Exercise*. 38(9):1626–1634.
54. Jones, A., Coombes, E., Griffin, S., van Sluijs, E. (2009) Environmental supportiveness for physical activity in English schoolchildren: a study using Global Positioning Systems. *International Journal of Behavioral Nutrition and Physical Activity*. 6(42). doi:10.1186/1479-5868-6-42.
55. Cooper, A.R., Page, A.S., Wheeler, B.W., Griew, P., Davis, L., Hillsdon, M.H., Jago, R. (2010) Mapping the walk to school using accelerometry combined with Global Positioning System. *American Journal of Preventive Medicine*. 38(2):178–183.

7 Physical Activity and Environments Which Promote Active Living in Youth (US)

*H. Mollie Greves Grow
and Brian E. Saelens*

7.1 Introduction

Changes in built environments have interacted with changes in social environments to affect the availability and quality of settings for youth physical activity in the United States. Research to date has explored associations between different settings (e.g. neighbourhood, schools) and environmental characteristics (e.g. presence of amenities) that facilitate or hinder youth physical activity. More recently, ecological studies explored changes in youth physical activity after environment changes were made. This chapter reviews research on environments which promote or hinder physical activity in youth with a focus on research conducted in the United States and discusses research and community action needed to improve environments for youth physical activity.

7.1.1 Background

Physical and social environment changes in the United States over the past 50 years have rapidly altered the landscape for youth physical activity. Frumkin *et al.*[1] note that a shift away from agricultural occupations and the development of land around cities (suburbs) have transformed the environments of many youth, impacting on opportunities and space for physical activity. Perhaps the most dramatic impact has been more cars on the road, the need to move cars faster and more efficiently, and multi-lane streets with higher traffic speeds and large intersections, making it difficult for children to safely walk or bicycle.[1]

Physical environment changes have interacted with and impacted social changes.[2] Parents report increased fear about the safety of their neighbourhoods, in part due to higher traffic and fewer children playing outside and also due to 24-hour widespread news coverage of child abductions, despite their relative rarity. A dramatic rise in sedentary activities that are attractive to children, less parental role modelling for physical activity, and policies to cut back physical education (PE) and recess in schools have occurred.[3,4] Finally, structured activities for youth after school have changed, with team sports often highly competitive and limited among youth of lower socio-economic status (SES).[5]

7.2 Case examples

The following case examples illustrate some of the background context described above and are drawn from a qualitative study recently conducted in a mid-sized Midwestern US city. For this study, youth and parents were interviewed about physical activity spaces in their neighbourhood.[6]

> *David is 11 years old, has school PE once per week, and does not play any organised sports. He walks about ¼ mile to the school bus stop. Away from school, David plays with peers his age in his neighbourhood. His parents allow this because they consider the neighbourhood safe. However, parental rules restrict his crossing busy arterial streets within ¾ mile of home. He mostly plays in the street, including football and tag, and in his friends' driveways and yards. Some private property he and his friends avoid, based on owners' requests, but he otherwise feels the neighbourhood is 'open' for active play. He loves this sense of independence.*

David's physical activity is associated with his neighbourhood's physical and social environment; without this particular mix of factors, he would likely not be as active, at least in the same way. David's situation illustrates the importance of (1) accessible play environments (streets, sidewalks, yards, driveways), (2) adequate safety or parent perception of safety, for children to be free to play outside and (3) similarly aged peers or siblings with whom to play. David's physical activity and related physical and social environment contrasts with Stephanie's:

> *Stephanie, who is 14 years old and lives within ½ mile of David. Unlike David's parents, Stephanie's mom is very concerned about child abductions and does not allow Stephanie to be outside alone. Her mom is concerned about her inactivity, but does not know what to do. Stephanie used to play volleyball as part of a school-based team, but quit after an injury and the team became too competitive. She has infrequent PE and is driven to school, more than 10 miles away from home. There is no community recreation centre near home and she does not use local parks because she has no friends to go with her. If her mom felt safer about the neighbourhood, Stephanie says she would enjoy being in her neighbourhood. Stephanie says being at home is "bor-ing."*

Stephanie's situation exemplifies a relatively common phenomenon of parental concern for safety in and around their neighbourhood that limits children's physical activity, especially for youth not engaged in school or recreational team sports. Despite living in the same neighbourhood, how David's and Stephanie's parents differently *perceive* the environment impacts physical activity. Other children may indeed live in unsafe neighbourhoods and their access to opportunities in that environment will also be limited; however, the parents may help overcome that in some way, depending on the parents' ability/commitment to do so. For example:

> *Jennifer is 15 years old and lives in a neighbourhood that would be considered "walkable" (e.g., many close-by shops and restaurants), but the neighbourhood is lower income and considered by Jennifer's mom to be very unsafe. Jennifer is not allowed to walk alone anywhere in her neighbourhood. Jennifer has no friends in her neighbourhood. But Jennifer still gets plenty of physical activity, because her mom (who feels guilty about Jennifer not being able to be active in the neighbourhood) spends 1–2 hours per day driving her daughter to soccer practice, games and tournaments. Jennifer is driven to a better school outside her neighbourhood, where she has PE every other day.*

Jennifer's case illustrates how youth obtain adequate physical activity not necessarily based on their neighbourhood environments, but dependent on supportive social environments where parents commit time and resources to organised sports. For youth without this social environment or interest or skills for competitive organised sports, the physical environment is likely to be much more influential on physical activity. Our conceptual model (Figure 7.1) illustrates how physical and social environment factors could operate together to allow youth to be active, or remain inactive. Outdoor-specific play/physical activity is more likely to be influenced by built environment, particularly in neighbourhoods, and is distinguished from overall physical activity, which may or may not be as influenced by built environment (dotted lines).

This chapter reviews the current research on environment and youth physical activity in and around the main settings of schools and child care, and community settings, including the home/neighbourhood. The chapter focuses primarily on the

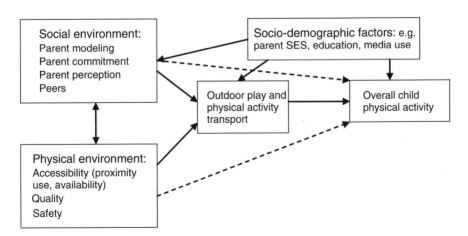

Figure 7.1   A conceptual model of how physical and social environments and socio-demographic factors interact to influence youth physical activity in outdoor settings and overall settings.

physical environment, particularly outdoor settings, where most evidence exists and highlights the important interaction between physical and social (adult and peer) contexts that determine youth physical activity.

7.3   School and child care

7.3.1   Active transport to school

Active transport to school (i.e. walking, biking or other non-motorised transport) is perhaps the best studied topic in the examination of associations between environment and youth physical activity. While the benefits of active transport for youth to obtain physical activity have been described in several studies,[7–9] active transport to school in the United States has declined in the past 30 years.[10] Saelens and Handy[11] reviewed the built environment correlates of walking for children and found that all but one study reviewed examined walking to school specifically. The predominant factors associated with more walking to school were closer proximity to school, greater population density, and good pedestrian infrastructure and traffic safety on the walk-to-school route; however, these factors were not universally found to be associated with more walking to school.[11]

Given the strong association between school proximity and walking to school, the decline in part reflects decreased school accessibility due to schools being built further apart in suburban areas where land was less expensive[1] and where districts could meet school location requirements.[12] Ham et al.[13] compared US data from the 2001 National Household Transportation Survey to the 1969 National Personal Transportation Survey and found that in 2001, fewer 5–18-year-old students lived within 1 mile of their school (19.4% vs. 34.7%) and fewer students walked or biked any distance to school (16.2% vs. 42.0%). By parent report, distance to school has been cited as the single largest barrier for children walking/biking to school in the United States.[10] By contrast, more children walk/bike to school in higher density neighbourhoods and in schools that have smaller pupil populations (presumably due to smaller size of closer neighbourhood schools).[14]

The safety of the *physical infrastructure* of the route to school, such as sidewalks and street crossings, is another factor influencing whether youth walk and bike to school. Interventions in the environment to improve the physical safety of the route to school and thereby promote active transport to school have shown some promising findings in small-scale evaluations. In California, children who used routes on which Safe Routes to School (SR2S) projects were completed were more likely to have increased walking or biking (by parent report) than were children who did not use routes impacted by such projects (15% vs. 4%).[15] Another study in Marin County, CA,[16] showed that a promotion program which included built environment changes – more sidewalks and improved intersection crossings – resulted in a 64% increase in walking to school. In Texas, an evaluation of SR2S projects funded by the state beginning in 2002 found school districts making progress in implementing SR2S infrastructure improvements; however, few programs had been fully implemented, due to funding limitations some sites still had hazardous conditions on walking routes to schools.[17] No data were available in Texas on how funding or infrastructure changes improved rates of children's walking or biking, or overall physical activity. Nationally, the Federal Highway Administration (FHWA) allocated $612 million in 2005 to establish SR2S programs for children in kindergarten to eighth grade across the United States. To date, only limited voluntary evaluation, with almost no research on health outcomes, has been conducted by the state and local communities receiving funds. Therefore, the impact of this funding to improve physical environments and increase child walking/biking to school remains largely unknown.[18]

Beyond distance to school and pedestrian infrastructure, barriers to walk-to-school programs remain in the perceived safety of the social environments. Even among students who live within 1 mile of school in the United States, less than half walk or bike on even 1 day in the week.[19] In a national survey, parents reported lack of safety from traffic (30.4%) and from crime (11.7%) as barriers for their 5- to 18-year-old children, with even higher percentages for the 5- to 11-year-old age group.[10] Immigrant families have reported similar concerns for traffic and crime safety for their children walking to school.[20] Parents' concerns about their child being abducted or physically harmed are very high[21,22] and may reduce the likelihood of providing permission for children to walk/bike to school. McMillan[23] found that the proportion of street segments with more houses containing windows that face the street was positively related to the likelihood of walking/biking to school. It is hypothesised that this is a proxy for increased 'eyes on the street', which increase parents' perceptions of safety for their children. In a study comparing walk-to-school program strategies, authors concluded that a multidisciplinary approach to influence parent support is critical to maintain walk-to-school initiatives.[24]

Preliminary evidence suggests that positive social influence by other children and parents is associated with higher rates of walking to school[25] and that parents interested in having their children being more socially interactive had children who walked/biked more to school.[23] Indeed, opportunity for sociability is considered one of the benefits of children's walking/biking.[26] Nationally, the SR2S program has a clearing house that includes promoting walking in groups with adult supervision (i.e. 'walking school buses')[27] to remove safety barriers and promote positive social influence around active transport to school. A case–control study in New Zealand in the 1990s[28] showed that being accompanied by an adult was associated with a much lower likelihood of child injury (odds ratio 0.31) during active commuting to and from school.

In addition to safe routes improvements, school-zone improvements are advocated based on safety principles, such as separating children on foot from cars.[29] These include marked drop-off and pick-up areas separate from bus areas, school-zone speed limit enforcement at 25 miles/hour and well-trained adult crossing guards.[29] While there is little experimental data to define effectiveness of these approaches to increase walking, some evidence exists in the transportation literature about the effects of such approaches on improved pedestrian safety. For example, a study has demonstrated the benefit of trained crossing guards in improving pedestrian safety behaviours, automobile speed compliance and traffic control.[30] However, some physical environment changes to improve pedestrian safety have resulted in no change or have been associated with negative impacts. In particular, the largest study examining marked crosswalks found that crosswalks without signals were associated with increased pedestrian accidents in multi-lane roads with average daily traffic greater than 12,000 vehicles, and had no benefit or detriment on two-lane roads.[31] The area type, speed limit and type of crosswalk marking pattern had no effect on the rate of pedestrian crashes.[31]

More research is needed specifically for strategies to modify both objective and perceived safety for youth on the walk to school. Parents and other caregivers currently prioritise safety to the exclusion of physical activity.[26] There have been few attempts to modify objective or perceived safety and even fewer attempts to evaluate whether interventions led to increased safety.[21] If safety is a prominent barrier to youth walking to school or to other sites in their communities, we can extrapolate that improving safety will improve frequency of walking, but more direct evidence is needed to confirm this.

7.3.2   Within-school environments

Children in the United States spend considerable time in school. There are few studies that have documented differences in physical activity based on school design. In a theory-based paper on this topic, Gorman et al.[32] argued that school design can enhance youth physical activity and offered possible school designs incorporating more space for a broader range of activities (e.g. dance, yoga, walking trails), particularly to promote physical activity for youth not participating in traditional organised sports. Another possible design approach cited[33] was the use of more activity-promoting classroom settings, such as standing desks, and even more so, encouraging 'activity-permissive environments' in which children are much freer to move about the classroom. In a laboratory setting, Lanningham-Foster et al.[33] have tested methods of increasing non-exercise activity thermogenesis (NEAT[34]) (i.e. differences which may contribute to susceptibility towards weight gain) in classroom and workplace settings and have demonstrated increases in NEAT with designs that allowed for more frequent standing and movement compared with sitting.

In elementary schools, active schoolyards have been promoted to improve the quality of physical activity environments in actual school settings. Models considered to promote physical activity include more horizontal use of space for younger children to run between areas.[35] Among middle school girls in the Trial of Adolescent Activity for Girls (TAAG) in six cities in the United States, school ground size was found to account for 4% of all light physical activity and 16% of all metabolic equivalent (MET)-weight moderate-to-vigorous physical activity (MW-MVPA) during school hours.[36] Other studies suggest the importance of availability of more amenities and facilities that support physical activity. In TAAG, availability of active outdoor amenities accounted for 29% of all MW-MVPA during school. A recent study in Norway[37] found that a higher number of outdoor facilities at school is related to more physical activity.

Several grass roots efforts in the United States, such as the Boston Schoolyard Initiative in Boston, MA, a public–private partnership since 1985, have sought to develop models of active schoolyards.[35,38] Boston's program has been associated with higher academic test scores[39]; however, no studies are available to track changes in physical activity. In Belgium and the United Kingdom, studies have shown increased physical activity on playgrounds at recess through use of coloured markings,[40] provision of game equipment[41] and improving/updating activity structures.[42] The effect size of these changes was small, for example, game equipment increased moderate activity from 38% to 50% and vigorous activity from 10% to 11%, which was significant compared to a control group that had a decline in moderate and vigorous activity during the same time period.[41] More longitudinal studies are needed to replicate and extend these findings and to learn more about how to improve physical space for youth to be active at school. Even if the effect sizes of such interventions are small, the contribution to overall physical activity at a population level could be substantial. The types of social environments to encourage children to continue to use/interact with built environments that promote physical activity (e.g. particular equipment) are unknown.

It is challenging to determine the relative importance of more physical activity resources within and adjacent to schools compared to the effects of programs established to use such resources. Most school-based interventions in the United States have sought to improve social and programmatic environments for physical activity in PE classes, including changing curricula and teacher training, as well as use of social marketing to promote physical activity; some have also included family-based intervention. A recent international review by Salmon et al.[43] through 2006 for interventions to promote physical activity in children and adolescents reports on the most well-known interventions. One of these is the Child and Adolescent Trial for Cardiovascular Health (CATCH) program, which successfully improved the activity level of PE through more movement-based PE and teacher training; however, there was no evidence to indicate whether physical activity increased overall.[44] At 3-year[45] and 5-year follow-up,[46] the overall effects on more active PE were maintained, but were attenuated. A combined school and family-based intervention group in CATCH found no difference in behaviours for children in the combined school and family-based component; however, dose–response was demonstrated for adult participation on children's improved knowledge and attitudes.[47] Training courses to implement CATCH, now called Coordinated Approach to Child Health, continue to be offered through a licensed company. Another school-based program for elementary students (Sports, Play and Active Recreation for Kids – SPARK[48]) provided training for teachers and incorporated family components as well, such as take-home curriculum materials to stimulate parent–child interaction. This program improved physical activity for boys and girls and physical fitness outcomes for girls in the PE specialist-led classes, but, like CATCH, showed no significant differences in physical activity by accelerometer outside of school.[48]

Among adolescents, two middle school-based programs have shown modest positive effects in increasing physical activity. M-SPAN was a 2-year middle school

PE intervention[49] that improved physical activity in PE classes compared to control schools. By year 2, intervention schools increased moderate-to-vigorous physical activity (MVPA) by 18%, with large effect sizes for boys and medium effect sizes for girls[49]. The Trial for Activity in Adolescent Girls (TAAG)[50] intervention sought to expand social environment support for girls' physical activity through linking schools and community agencies, PE, health education and social marketing. The results of this 2-year, multi-site intervention showed very modest effects (only 1.6 minutes of daily MVPA, or 80 kcal per week) in improving physical activity among girls in intervention middle schools.[50] The improvement was only demonstrated in schools with a physical activity 'Program Champion'-directed intervention, which occurred after a staff-directed intervention that demonstrated no effect.[50]

7.3.3   After-school programs

Few studies have examined levels of physical activity or factors influencing physical activity in after-school programs. In a study of after-school programs for 147 third to sixth grade youth (8–12 years old) in the mid-west United States, MVPA assessed by accelerometer averaged 20 minutes per day in the programs, with 80 minutes spent in sedentary to light activity.[51] MVPA varied by gender (lower in girls) and by weight status (lower in overweight youth), as in other settings. Overall, the most notable finding was that unstructured activity had higher MVPA than structured activity in this setting, attributed to instructional time and choosing activities in which youth would be removed from games if they lost (e.g. dodgeball).[51] This suggests that directors could be better trained to facilitate physical activity for youth in after-school program settings, and to choose activities better suited to girls and overweight youth, who tend to be less active. Such coach training to promote physical activity in an after-school program has been feasible, at least in one pilot study[52] to expand the in-school CATCH program (described above in school programs), to an after-school CATCH program for elementary youth. Another after-school pilot program[53] specifically to promote physical activity and prevent obesity among African-American girls demonstrated promise, but was not funded for further development.

7.3.4   Child care settings

Child care settings have been relatively infrequently studied in terms of child physical activity, although interest is growing in recognition that more caregivers are also working; currently 60% of US mothers with preschool children are employed outside the home.[54] Observed differences in objective measures of children's physical activity in child care have been attributed to policy differences at sites, with the most variance (27%) explained not by individual child characteristics but by the culture and environment around physical activity at the site of child care.[55,56] For example, in one study, child care environments that offered more frequent physical-activity-oriented field trips and college-educated teachers were associated with higher MVPA among children.[57] Children have been observed to be largely inactive in child care, with more than 80% of observed time spent inactive.[56] Interventions to prevent obesity in child care settings, including increased physical activity, are being developed in several settings, but few results are available to date. One published program[58] focused on improving child care centres' self-assessment of policies and identification of changes needed, but found no changes in the intervention group for physical activity, although changes occurred for nutrition policies.

In summary, walking/biking to school is a potentially significant source of physical activity, but distance, lack of safe pedestrian infrastructure and other social and environmental barriers may be precluding this option for many US children. There is some evidence that modifying the programming environment of PE and providing more facilities and amenities geared towards physical activity on school grounds are related to higher physical activity in children. However, given the potential population impact, there exists a need for implementation and evaluation of physical and social-environmental changes that could occur within and around schools in order to promote physical activity.

7.4 Community settings (home/neighbourhood)

7.4.1 Young children

Few studies have examined relationships between the physical environment of communities or homes and physical activity in younger children, perhaps because younger children are not old enough to decide where they go in their community. However, resources for active play in a community may encourage caregivers to bring their young children to these resources. For instance, in one study of Mexican-American and Anglo-American preschool children, parents' reports of the number of play areas within walking distance of home were positively associated with observed levels of physical activity.[59] Another study in a US city found no association between distance to the nearest neighbourhood playground and the weight status of preschool children; however, physical activity was not measured.[60] A small study of 59 children in a slightly older age group, ages 4–7 years, found that higher neighbourhood park area and density of homes were both positively associated with greater physical activity for children.[61] The environment immediately around home and within-home may also impact young children's physical activity. Spurrier et al.[62] found that having a larger backyard and more outdoor play equipment was related to greater outside physical activity by preschool-aged children.

For young children (0–5 years), physical activity may be particularly sensitive to the interaction between social environments and physical environments, as young children require supervision in their play and have less mobility in their neighbourhoods. Regarding social environments, particularly parent perception of safety of facilities/environment and young children, Beets and Foley[63] studied a nationally representative sample of kindergarten children in the United States.

They found a positive association between kindergarteners' physical activity and parents' perceptions of neighbourhood safety, with approximately 7.6% of the variance in physical activity explained by the neighbourhood. In the same study, by comparison, the family environment, which included child–father time and family time spent doing sports together (both positively related to greater child physical activity), accounted for 19.1% of the children's physical activity variance.[63] In a separate study of 3-year-old children in a US national sample, maternal perception of neighbourhood safety was unrelated to children's outdoor physical activity by parent self-report.[64] Currently, research on environments and activity for young children is limited, but a theme emerges that access to facilities and perception of safety may influence activity in this age to some extent, perhaps through enabling or preventing parents to facilitate physical activity with their young children. Inconsistency across studies may reflect differences in study methodology and lack of specificity with the types of physical activity measured.

7.4.2 School-age children and adolescents

Reviews of environment and physical activity

Many studies, mostly cross-sectional, have examined home and neighbourhood characteristics in their relation to physical activity for school-age children. Comprehensive reviews of this literature are provided by Davison and Lawson[65] and by Ferreira *et al.*[66] Davison and Lawson[65] included 33 studies examining associations between physical activity and either perceived or objectively measured physical environment. Their summary found no consistent relationship between home environment equipment and child physical activity; only two of six studies found an association with home equipment and activity, and these were based on self-report of activity. By contrast, they found a positive association for the majority of studies for self-report of physical activity and access to public recreational facilities (including schools), with three of the studies from US samples.[67–69] Some pedestrian infrastructure and other urban form characteristics were also positively associated with school-aged children's physical activity: presence of sidewalks,[15,70] controlled intersections,[15,71] better access to destinations[68,72,73] and access to public transportation.[71] The number of studies that examined these factors were limited to between one and three studies. Transport infrastructure that was negatively associated with physical activity included number of roads to cross[71] and traffic density/speed.[71,72,74]

   The review by Ferreira *et al.*[66] included studies examining environment – including social, physical and economic – and youth physical activity through December 2004. It included 68 studies in North America; of the 150 publications reviewed, 66 studies were among children 3–12 years old and 84 with adolescents aged 13–18. For children, Ferreira *et al.*[66] reported no neighbourhood physical environments that were consistently associated with youth physical activity across studies internationally. For adolescents, the only physical environment variable reported to be consistently related to physical activity was neighbourhood crime incidence, which was negatively related to physical activity in two out of three studies.[66]

Differences between the summary findings of the two review papers reflect differences in criteria for inclusion, categorisation of environmental characteristics (e.g. Ferreira *et al.*[66] included access to equipment and facilities in the same category) and examining youth by age group (Ferreira *et al.*[66] separated the results by child and adolescent), as well as by including multivariate analyses, which were less likely to show positive results (Ferreira *et al.*[66]) versus bivariate analyses (Davison & Lawson).[65]

More recent US studies on availability of recreation facilities and older youth activity

Since these reviews were published, several US studies have documented associations between availability of local recreational facilities and older youth physical activity. Using a nationally representative sample, Gordon-Larsen *et al.*[75] showed an incremental association between weekly bouts of physical activity and an objective measure of the number of physical activity facilities within an 8-km buffer from home. In this study, lower income and higher minority youth were found to live in areas with less access to physical activity facilities and to also have lower physical activity and higher rates of obesity.[75] Another nationally representative study examined number of commercial physical activity sites and self-report of physical activity and reported a small but significant positive association; higher associations were seen for 12th grade girls and boys, representing a 6% increase in vigorous physical activity from lowest (1) to highest (8) number of recreation sites.[76]

Other studies have examined associations of availability of activity resources in the environment and physical activity, specifically for girls. A study in a population of older adolescent girls in South Carolina corroborated the association between the self-report level of activity and objectively measured number of recreational facilities near home, in this case within a 0.75-mile buffer of girls' homes.[77] The TAAG study found that for each public park within 0.5 miles of a girl's home, there was an additional 17 minutes of non-school moderate/vigorous physical activity every 6 days, which accounted for about 5% of girls' non-school physical activity.[78] Furthermore, specific features in the parks were associated with higher non-school metabolic equivalent minutes per 6 days: walking paths (13 minutes), running tracks (82 minutes), playgrounds (28 minutes) and basketball courts (30 minutes). Parks with streetlights and floodlights were also associated with higher minutes of physical activity (18 and 22 minutes, respectively).[78] Data from the same study showed that weekend accessibility of schoolyards was not related to girls' weekend physical activity, but locked schoolyards were associated with greater rates of obesity, which tended to be in lower SES neighbourhoods.[79] Perception of availability of facilities was also correlated with physical activity among the girls participating in TAAG. For each additional recreational facility perceived, the girls had 3% more metabolic equivalent minutes of MVPA.[80]

Perceived safety and physical activity

Recent studies have also documented the relation between perceived safety and youth physical activity. For 5–10-year-old children, parents in at least one study have reported lower levels of physical activity in inner city environments compared to parents in suburban environments; parents' higher anxiety about neighbourhood safety in inner city neighbourhoods was negatively correlated with their child's activity.[81] Two studies on adolescents have found similar findings. Molnar *et al.*[82] found neighbourhood disorder and lack of safety reported by adolescents correlated with decreased self-report of physical activity among 1378 youth in Chicago. Gomez *et al.*[83] found that local neighbourhood statistics for violent crime were associated with decreased report of adolescent outdoor activity among a sample consisting of mostly Mexican-American youth in San Antonio. In settings where the neighbourhood is perceived to be unsafe, the availability of home exercise equipment has been shown to be associated with higher self-report of physical activity among adolescent girls in one study, which is in contrast to prior studies where home equipment was not found to be associated with the level of physical activity.[84] This is an example where differential effects of the environment may operate depending on the overall environment context.

'Walkability' features and physical activity

Beyond neighbourhood safety and accessibility to recreation sites, additional measures of neighbourhood physical environments to assess 'walkability' include land use mix, retail density, street connectivity and residential density[85] (see also Chapter 3 by Robertson-Wilson and Giles-Corti). These have been examined primarily in adults, but a few studies are now assessing those factors among youth. Kligerman *et al.*[86] examined neighbourhood walkability using an index combining multiple factors in a 0.5-mile buffer in relationship to physical activity among 96 adolescents; they found a 4% variance of minutes of MVPA in a linear regression model based on increased walkability. Frank *et al.*[87] examined walkability, specifically residential density, intersection density, land use mix, commercial and recreation space and physical activity among 3161 youth between 5 and 20 years in Atlanta, GA. They found that the highest associations between walking and walking-promoting environments for 12- to 15-year-olds; 3.7 times greater odds of walking for adolescents in highest- versus lowest-density (tertile) areas and 2.6 times greater walking for adolescents with at least one commercial and 2.5 times greater for those with at least one recreational destination within 1 km from home.[87] In this study, the variable associated with the highest walking across age groups was access to recreation or open space.[87] We found that access to recreation facilities, measured by both proximity to facilities and accessibility by walking/biking, was related to 2–10 times higher rates of using recreation facilities among adolescents.[88] In addition, features of the built environment including traffic safety, crime threat and pedestrian infrastructure were associated with youth walking/biking to more recreation sites.[88]

7.5   Conclusions and future research

Research on physical environment and related social-environmental factors and youth physical activity has increased in recent years in response to the rapid rise in obesity and concerns about inactivity in US youth. Overall, research to date supports an association between youth physical activity and some physical environmental features, particularly greater number of nearby facilities for activity, and safe environments for walking/bicycling, especially among older children and adolescents (for a UK perspective see Chapter 6 by Cooper and Page). The effect size of the associations is generally small across these studies and associations are more likely to be seen when the assessment of physical environment and the type of physical activity are more methodologically linked (e.g. assessing proximity to parks and after-school activity, specifically, or built environment and walking, as opposed to overall physical activity). Specific features of facilities are likely to promote physical activity, such as playground markings, adequate equipment and size/layout of schools and playgrounds, but more research is needed to definitively describe how these factors influence youth activity. Furthermore, most physical environments are at least somewhat dependent on social environments, such as adequate adult supervision, or adults being assured of adequate safety, for physical environments to influence youth activity. Below, we propose directions for future research and likely policy implications.

Almost all of the studies described in this chapter are cross-sectional studies, which can demonstrate association, but not necessarily causality. There is a clear need for longitudinal studies to assess how changes to environments impact youth physical activity. One of the few studies testing an environmental impact found that offering supervised access to a school playground after school and on weekends over a 2-year period resulted in 84% higher observed physical activity among youth in the neighbourhood around the school compared to a control site.[89] The intervention was conducted in a low-income community and also resulted in a decrease in child report of sedentary activity in the intervention neighbourhood compared to the control neighbourhood. The youth playing at the schoolyard were observed to be active about 66% of the time, which was noted to be higher than in school PE programs where instruction time is required. This study represents a promising lower cost ($49,000 per year in 2003–2005) environmental intervention, addressing accessibility (opening the playground) and safety (providing supervision) that should be replicated in other sites. In particular, this study may demonstrate that children at highest risk for low activity and obesity, such as those in low-income communities, may be most impacted by the environment for physical activity. For example, children living in high SES families may not be as dependent on their immediate environment, as parents may be able to provide transportation to organised sports outside the community. Unfortunately, at this time, most research suggest that children in low-income communities in the United States have overall less access to nearby recreational facilities.

Individual demographic factors including sex, race/ethnicity and household income also likely interact with environmental factors to impact children's physical activity. In order to better target interventions, more evidence is needed to elucidate these interactions. For example, higher levels of inactivity and sedentary activities are reported for immigrant children in the United States.[90] No difference in overall levels of meeting the recommended physical activity level was reported by race/ethnicity among adolescents in a nationally representative sample; however, adolescents in higher income families were more likely to meet the recommended physical activity level.[91] How physical environment characteristics, and the interaction of social and physical environments, lead to these differences by race/ethnicity or SES is not well established. It is hypothesised that cultural norms and socio-economic factors may be predominant factors in physical activity differences observed for children in different ethnic/SES groups, but access, quality and safety of physical environment features are also likely to contribute.[90]

The need for longitudinal, ecological studies to examine changes in communities and impact on physical activity is clear and research funding will hopefully support such novel research in the future.[92] Increasing physical activity among the highest risk youth, who are likely most dependent on physical environment, will require community partnerships and infrastructure development and investment to provide access to nearby quality, safe sites for physical activity. Solutions for some communities may be as simple as schools and community recreation facilities opening up sites that are open after school and on weekends,[89] but systematically improving environments for youth physical activity more broadly will likely require comprehensive investments of resources in multiple settings where youth are affected: schools, day care, after-school programs, neighbourhoods and community settings. Such efforts should be based on sound evidence where available, but should not be delayed, so that we can begin to address the low levels of physical activity among US children, particularly adolescents.

References

1. Frumkin, H., Frank, L., Jackson, R. *Urban Sprawl and Public Health: Designing, Planning, and Building for Healthy Communities*. Washington, DC, Island Press, 2004.
2. Sallis, J.F., Glanz, K. (2006) The role of built environments in physical activity, eating, and obesity in childhood. *Future Child*. 16(1):89–108.
3. Dollman, J., Norton, K., Norton, L. (2005) Evidence for secular trends in children's physical activity behaviour. *British Journal of Sports Medicine*. 39(12):892–897; discussion 897.
4. American Academy of Pediatrics Councils on Sports Medicine and Fitness and School Health. (2006) Active healthy living: prevention of childhood obesity through increased physical activity. *Pediatrics*. 117(5):1834–1842.
5. Johnston, L.D., Delva, J., O'Malley, P.M. (2007) Sports participation and physical education in American secondary schools: current levels and racial/ethnic and socioeconomic disparities. *American Journal of Preventive Medicine*. 33(4, Suppl. 1):S195–S208.
6. Kerr, J., Saelens, B., Rosenberg, D., Norman, G., Durant, N., Eggerman, J., Sallis, J. Active Where?: Multi-region formative research to understand children's physical activity environments. *Active Living Research Annual Conference*. Coronado, CA, 2006.
7. Saksvig, B.I., Catellier, D.J., Pfeiffer, K., *et al.* (2007) Travel by walking before and after school and physical activity among adolescent girls. *Archives of Pediatrics and Adolescent Medicine*. 161(2):153–158.

8. Cooper, A.R., Andersen, L.B., Wedderkopp, N., Page, A.S., Froberg, K. (2005) Physical activity levels of children who walk, cycle, or are driven to school. *American Journal of Preventive Medicine.* 29(3):179–184.

9. Sirard, J.R., Riner, W.F., Jr., McIver, K.L., Pate, R.R. (2005) Physical activity and active commuting to elementary school. *Medicine and Science in Sports and Exercise.* 37(12):2062–2069.

10. Centers for Disease Control and Prevention. (2005) Barriers to children walking to or from school – United States, 2004. *MMWR Morbidity and Mortality Weekly Report.* 54(38):949–952.

11. Saelens, B.E., Handy, S.L. (2008) Built environment correlates of walking: a review. *Medicine and Science in Sports and Exercise.* 40(Suppl. 7):S550–S566.

12. U.S. Environmental Protection Agency. (2003) *Travel and Environmental Implications of School Siting*, EPA231-R-03-004. Vol. Available at http://www.epa.gov/smartgrowth/pdf/school_travel.pdf, last accessed September 2008. Washington, DC, U.S. EPA Office of Policy, Economics, and Innovation.

13. Ham, S.A., Martin, S.L., Kohl, H.W. *Changes in the Percentage of Students Who Walk or Bike to School - United States, 1969 and 2001.* Vol 5. Human Kinetics, Champaign, IL, 2008.

14. Braza, M., Shoemaker, W., Seeley, A. (2004) Neighborhood design and rates of walking and biking to elementary school in 34 California communities. *American Journal of Health Promotion.* 19(2):128–136.

15. Boarnet, M.G., Anderson, C.L., Day, K., McMillan, T., Alfonzo, M. (2005) Evaluation of the California Safe Routes to School legislation: Urban form changes and children's active transportation to school. *American Journal of Preventive Medicine.* 28(Suppl. 2):134–140.

16. Staunton, C.E., Hubsmith, D., Kallins, W. (2003) Promoting safe walking and biking to school: the Marin County success story. *American Journal of Public Health.* 93(9):1431–1434.

17. Goodwin, G., Soria, Y. *An Analysis of the Texas 2002 Safe Routes to Schools Program in Selected Cities.* Texas Southern University, Houston Southwest Region University Transportation Center, Houston, TX, 2008.

18. GAO. *Safe Routes to School: a Report to the Ranking Member.* U.S. Senate Committee on Environment and Public Works, Vol GAO-08-789, 2008.

19. Martin, S.L., Lee, S.M., Lowry, R. (2007) National prevalence and correlates of walking and bicycling to school. *American Journal of Preventive Medicine.* 33(2):98–105.

20. Greves, H.M., Lozano, P., Liu, L., Busby, K., Cole, J., Johnston, B. (2007) Immigrant families' perceptions on walking to school and school breakfast: a focus group study. *The International Journal of Behavioral Nutrition and Physical Activity.* 4:64.

21. Rowland, D., DiGuiseppi, C., Gross, M., Afolabi, E., Roberts, I. (2003) Randomised controlled trial of site specific advice on school travel patterns. *Archives of Disease in Childhood.* 88(1):8–11.

22. Saelens, B.E., Kerr, J. Social and contextual factors in youth physical activity and sedentary behavior: the family. In: *Youth Physical Activity and Sedentary Behavior.* (Eds. Smith, A.L., Biddle, S.J.H.) Human Kinetics, Champaign, IL, 2008.

23. McMillan, T.E. (2007) The relative influence of urban form on a child's travel mode to school. *Transportation Research Part A.* 41:69–79.

24. Fesperman, C.E., Evenson, K.R., Rodriguez, D.A., Salvesen, D. *A Comparative Case Study on Active Transport to and from School.* Vol 5. Centers for Disease Control and Prevention, 2008.

25. Zhu, X., Lee, C. Correlates of walking to school and their implications for health and equity. *Data presented at Active Living Research Conference*, April 2008. Texas A & M University, 2008.

26. Lorenc, T., Brunton, G., Oliver, S., Oliver, K., Oakley, A. (2008) Attitudes to walking and cycling among children, young people and parents: a systematic review. *Journal of Epidemiology and Community Health.* 62(10):852–857.

27. National Center for Safe Routes to School Pedestrian and Bicycle Information Center. (2008) *The Walking School Bus Guide: Combining Safety, Fun and the Walk to School.* Available at http://www.saferoutesinfo.org/resources/encouragement_walking-school-bus-guide.cfm. Accessed 2008

28. Roberts, I. (1995) Adult accompaniment and the risk of pedestrian injury on the school-home journey. *Injury Prevention*. 1(4):242–244.
29. Committee on Injury, Violence, and Poison Prevention, Council on School Health. (2007) School transportation safety. *Pediatrics*. 120(1):213–220.
30. Campbell, B.J., Zegeer, C.V., Huang, H.H., Cynecki, M.J. *A Review of Pedestrian Safety Research in the United States and Abroad*. Washington, DC, Federal Highway Administration Office of Safety Research and Development, 2004. FHWA-RD-03-042. Available at http://drusilla.hsrc.unc.edu/cms/downloads/Pedestrian_Synthesis_Report2004.pdf.
31. Zegeer, C.V., Stewart, J.R., Huang, H., Lagerwey, P. (2001) Safety effects of marked versus unmarked crosswalks at uncontrolled locations - analysis of pedestrian crashes in 30 cities. *2001 Trb Distinguished Lecture, Pt 1 - Bicycle and Pedestrian Research, Pt 2*. 1773:56–68.
32. Gorman, N., Lackney, J.A., Rollings, K., Huang, T.T.K. (2007) Designer schools: the role of school space and architecture in obesity prevention. *Obesity*. 15(11):2521–2530.
33. Lanningham-Foster, L., Foster, R.C., McCrady, S.K., Manohar, C.U., Jensen, T.B., Mitre, N.G., Hill, J.O., Levine, J.A. (2008) Changing the school environment to increase physical activity in children. *Obesity*. 16(8):1849–1853.
34. Levine, J.A., Kotz, C.M. (2005) NEAT - non-exercise activity thermogenesis – egocentric & geocentric environmental factors vs. biological regulation. *Acta Physiologica Scandinavica*. 184(4):309–318.
35. Moore, R. Playgrounds: a 150-year-old model. In: *Safe and Healthy School Environments*. (Eds. Frumkin, H., Geller, R., Rubin, I.L., Nodvin, J.) New York, NY, Oxford University Press, 2006:86–103.
36. Cohen, D., Scott, M., Wang, F.Z., McKenzie, T.L., Porter, D. (2008) School design and physical activity among middle school girls. *Journal of Physical Activity and Health*. 5(5): 719–731.
37. Haug, E., Torsheim, T., Sallis, J.F., Samdal, O. (2008) The characteristics of the outdoor school environment associated with physical activity. *Health Education Reports*. Oct 20. doi: 10.1093/her/cyn050.
38. Lopez, R., Campbell, R., Jennings, J. (2008) The Boston schoolyard initiative: a public-private partnership for rebuilding urban play spaces. *Journal of Health Politics, Policy and Law*. 33(3):617–638.
39. Teicher Khadaroo, S. (2008) Boston's newest classrooms: schoolyards. *The Christian Science Monitor*. August 20.
40. Stratton, G., Mullan, E. (2005) The effect of multicolor playground markings on children's physical activity level during recess. *Preventive Medicine*. 41(5-6):828–833.
41. Verstraete, S.J.M., Cardon, G.M., De Clercq, D.L.R., De Bourdeaudhuij, I.M.M. (2006) Increasing children's physical activity levels during recess periods in elementary schools: the effects of providing game equipment. *European Journal of Public Health*. 16(4):415–419.
42. Ridgers, N.D., Stratton, G., Fairclough, S.J., Twisk, J.W. (2007) Children's physical activity levels during school recess: a quasi-experimental intervention study. *International Journal of Behavioral Nutrition and Physical Activity*. 4:19.
43. Salmon, J., Booth, M.L., Phongsavan, P., Murphy, N., Timperio, A. (2007) Promoting physical activity participation among children and adolescents. *Epidemiologic Reviews*. 29(1):144–159.
44. Luepker, R.V., Perry, C.L., McKinlay, S.M., *et al*. (1996) Outcomes of a field trial to improve children's dietary patterns and physical activity. The child and adolescent trial for cardiovascular health. CATCH collaborative group. *JAMA*. 275(10):768–776.
45. Nader, P.R., Stone, E.J., Lytle, L.A., Perry, C.L., Osganian, S.K., Kelder, S., Webber, L.S., Elder, J.P., Montgomery, D., Feldman, H.A., Wu, M., Johnson, C., Parcel, G.S., Luepker, R.V. (1999) Three-year maintenance of improved diet and physical activity: the CATCH cohort. Child and adolescent trial for cardiovascular health. *Archives of Pediatrics and Adolescent Medicine*. 153(7):695–704.
46. McKenzie, T.L., Li, D., Derby, C.A., Webber, L.S., Luepker, R.V., Cribb, P. (2003) Maintenance of effects of the CATCH physical education program: results from the CATCH-ON study. *Health Education and Behavior*. 30(4):447–462.

47. Nader, P.R., Sellers, D.E., Johnson, C.C., Perry, C.L., Stone, E.J., Cook, KC., Bebchuk, J., Luepker, R.V. (1996) The effect of adult participation in a school-based family intervention to improve children's diet and physical activity: the child and adolescent trial for cardiovascular health. *Preventive Medicine*. 25(4):455–464.
48. Sallis, J.F., McKenzie, T.L., Alcaraz, J.E., Kolody, B., Faucette, N., Hovell, M.F. (1997) The effects of a 2-year physical education program (SPARK) on physical activity and fitness in elementary school students. Sports, play and active recreation for kids. *American Journal of Public Health*. 87(8):1328–1334.
49. McKenzie, T.L., Sallis, J.F., Prochaska, J.J., Conway, T.L., Marshall, S.J., Rosengard, P. (2004) Evaluation of a two-year middle-school physical education intervention: M-SPAN. *Medicine and Science in Sports and Exercise*. 36(8):1382–1388.
50. Webber, L.S., Catellier, D.J., Lytle, L.A., *et al.* (2008) Promoting physical activity in middle school girls: trial of activity for adolescent girls. *American Journal of Preventive Medicine*. 34(3):173–184.
51. Trost, S.G., Rosenkranz, R.R., Dzewaltowski, D. (2008) Physical activity levels among children attending after-school programs. *Medicine and Science in Sports and Exercise*. 40(4):622–629.
52. Kelder, S., Hoelscher, D.M., Barroso, C.S., Walker, J.L., Cribb, P., Hu, S. (2005) The CATCH Kids Club: a pilot after-school study for improving elementary students' nutrition and physical activity. *Public Health Nutrition*. 8(2):133–140.
53. Story, M., Sherwood, N.E., Himes, J.H., Davis, M., Jacobs, D.R., Jr, Cartwright, Y., Smyth, M., Rochon, J. (2003) An after-school obesity prevention program for African-American girls: the Minnesota GEMS pilot study. *Ethnicity and Disease*. 13(1, Suppl. 1):S54–S64.
54. Story, M., Kaphingst, K.M., French, S. (2006) The role of child care settings in obesity prevention. *Future of Children*. 16(1):143–168.
55. Pate, R.R., Pfeiffer, K.A., Trost, S.G., Ziegler, P., Dowda, M. (2004) Physical activity among children attending preschools. *Pediatrics*. 114(5):1258–1263.
56. Pate, R.R., McIver, K., Dowda, M., Brown, W.H., Addy, C.L. (2008) Directly observed physical activity levels in preschool children. *Journal of School Health*. 78(8):438–444.
57. Dowda, M., Pate, R.R., Trost, S.G., Almeida, M.J., Sirard, J.R. (2004) Influences of preschool policies and practices on children's physical activity. *Journal of Community Health*. 29(3):183–196.
58. Ward, D.S., Benjamin, S.E., Ammerman, A.S., Ball, S.C., Neelon, B.H., Bangdiwala, S.I. (2008) Nutrition and physical activity in child care: results from an environmental intervention. *American Journal of Preventive Medicine*. 35(4):352–356.
59. Sallis, J.F., Nader, P.R., Broyles, S.L., Berry, C.C., Elder, J.P., McKenzie, T.L., Nelson, J.A. (1993) Correlates of physical activity at home in Mexican-American and Anglo-American preschool children. *Health Psychology*. 12(5):390–398.
60. Burdette, H.L., Whitaker, R.C. (2004) Neighborhood playgrounds, fast food restaurants, and crime: relationships to overweight in low-income preschool children. *Preventive Medicine*. 38(1):57–63.
61. Roemmich, J.N., Epstein, L.H., Raja, S., Yin, L., Robinson, J., Winiewicz, D. (2006) Association of access to parks and recreational facilities with the physical activity of young children. *Preventive Medicine*. 43(6):437–441.
62. Spurrier, N.J., Magarey, A.A., Golley, R., Curnow, F., Sawyer, M.G. (2008) Relationships between the home environment and physical activity and dietary patterns of preschool children: a cross-sectional study. *The International Journal of Behavioral Nutrition and Physical Activity*. 5:31.
63. Beets, M.W., Foley, J.T. (2008) Association of father involvement and neighborhood quality with kindergartners' physical activity: a multilevel structural equation model. *American Journal of Health Promotion*. 22(3):195–203.
64. Burdette, H.L., Whitaker, R.C. (2005) A national study of neighborhood safety, outdoor play, television viewing, and obesity in preschool children. *Pediatrics*. 116(3):657–662.
65. Davison, K.K., Lawson, C.T. (2006) Do attributes in the physical environment influence children's physical activity? A review of the literature. *The International Journal of Behavioral Nutrition and Physical Activity*. 3:19.

66. Ferreira, I., van der Horst, K., Wendel-Vos, W., Kremers, S., van Lenthe, F.J., Brug, J. (2007) Environmental correlates of physical activity in youth - a review and update. *Obesity Reviews.* 8(2):129–154.

67. Zakarian, J.M., Hovell, M.F., Hofstetter, C.R., Sallis, J.F., Keating, K.J. (1994) Correlates of vigorous exercise in a predominantly low SES and minority high school population. *Preventive Medicine.* 23(3):314–321.

68. Norman, G.J., Nutter, S.K., Ryan, S., Sallis, J.F., Calfras, K.J., Patrick, K. (2006) Community design and access to recreational facilities as correlates of adolescent physical activity and body-mass index. *Journal of Physical Activity and Health.* 3(Suppl. 1):S118–S128.

69. Brodersen, N.H., Steptoe, A., Williamson, S., Wardle, J. (2005) Sociodemographic, developmental, environmental, and psychological correlates of physical activity and sedentary behavior at age 11 to 12. *Annals of Behavioral Medicine.* 29(1):2–11.

70. Ewing, R., Schroeer, W., Green, W. (2004) School location and student travel: analysis of factors affecting mode choice. *Transportation Research Record.* 1895:55–63.

71. Timperio, A., Crawford, D., Telford, A., Salmon, J. (2004) Perceptions about the local neighborhood and walking and cycling among children. *Preventive Medicine.* 38(1):39–47.

72. Carver, A., Salmon, J., Campbell, K., Baur, L., Garnett, S., Crawford, D. (2005) How do perceptions of local neighborhood relate to adolescents' walking and cycling? *American Journal of Health Promotion.* 20(2):139–147.

73. Mota, J., Almeida, M., Santos, P., Ribeiro, J.C. (2005) Perceived neighborhood environments and physical activity in adolescents. *Preventive Medicine.* 41(5-6):834–836.

74. Timperio, A., Ball, K., Salmon, J., Robert, R., Giles-Corti, B., Simmons, D., Baur, L.A., Crawford, D. (2006) Personal, family, social, and environmental correlates of active commuting to school. *American Journal of Preventive Medicine.* 30(1):45–51.

75. Gordon-Larsen, P., Nelson, M.C., Page, P., Popkin, B.M. (2006) Inequality in the built environment underlies key health disparities in physical activity and obesity. *Pediatrics.* 117(2):417–424.

76. Powell, L.M., Chaloupka, F.J., Slater, S.J., Johnston, L.D., O'Malley, P.M. (2007) The availability of local-area commercial physical activity-related facilities and physical activity among adolescents. *American Journal of Preventive Medicine.* 33(4 Suppl):S292–S300.

77. Pate, R.R., Colabianchi, N., Porter, D., Almeida, M.J., Lobelo, F., Dowda, M. (2008) Physical activity and neighborhood resources in high school girls. *American Journal of Preventive Medicine.* 34(5):413–419.

78. Cohen, D.A., Ashwood, J.S., Scott, M.M., Overton, A., Evenson, K.R., Staten, L.K., Porter, D., McKenzie, T.L., Catellier, D. (2006) Public parks and physical activity among adolescent girls. *Pediatrics.* 118(5):e1381–1389.

79. Scott, M.M., Cohen, D.A., Evenson, K.R., Elder, J.P., Catellier, D., Ashwood, S., Overton, A. (2007) Weekend schoolyard accessibility, physical activity, and obesity: the Trial of Activity in Adolescent Girls (TAAG) study. *Preventive Medicine.* 44(5):398–403.

80. Scott, M.M., Evenson, K.R., Cohen, D.A., Cox, C.E. (2007) Comparing perceived and objectively measured access to recreational facilities as predictors of physical activity in adolescent girls. *Journal of Urban Health.* 84(3):346–359, Mar 31.

81. Weir, L.A., Etelson, D., Brand, D.A. (2006) Parents' perceptions of neighborhood safety and children's physical activity. *Preventive Medicine.* 43(3):212–217.

82. Molnar, B.E., Gortmaker, S.L., Bull, F.C., Buka, S.L. (2004) Unsafe to play? Neighborhood disorder and lack of safety predict reduced physical activity among urban children and adolescents. *American Journal of Health Promotion.* 18(5):378–386.

83. Gomez, J.E., Johnson, B.A., Selva, M., Sallis, J.F. (2004) Violent crime and outdoor physical activity among inner-city youth. *Preventive Medicine.* 39(5):876–881.

84. Kerr, J., Norman, G.J., Sallis, J.F., Patrick, K. (2008) Exercise aids, neighborhood safety, and physical activity in adolescents and parents. *Medicine and Science in Sports and Exercise.* 40(7):1244–1248.

85. Saelens, B.E., Sallis, J.F., Frank, L.D. (2003) Environmental correlates of walking and cycling: findings from the transportation, urban design, and planning literatures. *Annals of Behavioral Medicine.* 25(2):80–91.

86. Kligerman, M., Sallis, J.F., Ryan, S., Frank, L.D., Nader, P.R. (2007) Association of neighborhood design and recreation environment variables with physical activity and body mass index in adolescents. *American Journal of Health Promotion.* 21(4):274–277.

87. Frank, L., Kerr, J., Chapman, J., Sallis, J. (2007) Urban form relationships with walk trip frequency and distance among youth. *American Journal of Health Promotion.* 21(4 Suppl):305–311.

88. Grow, H.M., Saelens, B.E., Kerr, J., Durant, N.H., Norman, G.J., Sallis, J.F. (2008) Where are youth active? Roles of proximity, active transport, and built environment. *Medicine and Science in Sports and Exercise.* 40(12):2071–2079.

89. Farley, T.A., Meriwether, R.A., Baker, E.T., Watkins, L.T., Johnson, C.C., Webber, L.S. (2007) Safe play spaces to promote physical activity in inner-city children: results from a pilot study of an environmental intervention. *American Journal of Public Health.* 97(9):1625–1631.

90. Singh, G.K., Yu, S.M., Siahpush, M., Kogan, M.D. (2008) High levels of physical inactivity and sedentary behaviors among US immigrant children and adolescents. *Archives of Pediatrics and Adolescent Medicine.* 162(8):756–763.

91. Butcher, K., Sallis, J.F., Mayer, J.A., Woodruff, S. (2008) Correlates of physical activity guideline compliance for adolescents in 100 U.S. Cities. *Journal of Adolescent Health.* 42(4):360–368.

92. Sallis, J.F., Cervero, R.B., Ascher, W., Henderson, K.A., Kraft, M.K., Kerr, J. (2006) An ecological approach to creating active living communities. *Annual Review of Public Health.* 27(1):297–322.

8 Active Travel

Roger L. Mackett

8.1 The potential for active travel

'Active travel' is travel that requires physical effort in order to move across space; the commonest forms are walking and cycling, and this chapter focuses on these. Other forms of active travel include non-motorised wheelchair, roller skating and skateboarding, but these are all very small in overall travel terms. It is important to treat walking and cycling separately because the two modes are very different: almost everybody walks, it requires no special equipment, and it costs nothing. In contrast, cycling is only participated in by a minority of the population, requires special equipment, and so costs money (but not for individual trips once a bicycle and, if desired, special clothes have been purchased). In 2006, Great Britain's 69% of the population cycled less than once a year or never.[1] Despite (or, perhaps, because of) this, cycling has a powerful lobby, such as the Cyclists' Touring Club (see http://www.ctc.org.uk), and hence often included in policy formulation and implementation. In contrast, walking tends to be much less focused on in policy terms, despite the existence of organisations such as Living Streets, formerly The Pedestrians Association (see http://www.livingstreets.org.uk).

Walking and cycling were identified as suitable ways for individuals to achieve the recommended levels of physical activity required to be healthy by the UK Chief Medical Officer in his report 'At least five a week: Evidence on the impact of physical activity and its relationship to health'.[2] Walking and cycling were regarded as suitable methods to achieve the recommended levels of activities for all seven of the different age groups identified. The UK Department for Transport[3] included the promotion of health benefits as an element in one of its five goals to develop a sustainable transport system. Attitudinal research carried out for the Department for Transport has demonstrated that very high proportions of the respondents thought that people should be encouraged to walk and cycle to help their health.[4]

Walking and cycling are forms of travel and leisure activities. For example, many children cycle in open space but do not use their bicycles to make journeys. In this chapter, the emphasis is on walking and cycling as forms of travel; walking and cycling as recreation activities have not been discussed except where they are also part of journeys.

8.2   Trends in active travel

The National Travel Survey (NTS) shows trends in travel in Great Britain, including active travel.[1] It should be noted that NTS excludes walk trips of less than 50 yards (45.7 m) and trips across open countryside, so some walk trips are excluded. Because trips are classified by the mode of travel used on the longest stage, the walking element of public transport and car trips is ignored. Notwithstanding these issues, NTS provides data that facilitate the identification of temporal trends in walking and cycling trips.

Table 8.1 shows the trends in travel by various modes of transport from 1975–1976 to 2006. The total number of trips and total distance travelled have increased, with increases in car travel. The increase in the mean trip length for all trips reflects two trends: the decentralisation of urban activities and the switch from the slower modes to the car, which means that people can travel farther within a given time. This has in turn led to greater choice of, for example, shops and schools. Both the number of trips and the distance travelled by walking and cycling have decreased. The average lengths of bicycle and car trips have increased, probably because of the greater spread of urban areas, while those for walking have remained constant.

For cycling, it is possible to go back further in time. In Britain, in 1949, the total distance travelled by pedal cycle was 23.6 billion vehicle-km.[5] This was the last year that the figure for cycling exceeded than that of cars and taxis. The total distance cycled decreased to 3.7 billion vehicle-km in 1973, after which it grew slightly up in 1982 and then it declined again in the early 1990s; since then it has grown slightly. Changes in definition in 1992–1993 mean it is difficult to make direct comparisons before and after these dates, but the NTS figures suggest that the volumes of walking have been fairly constant in recent years.

The influence of the car on levels of walking is illustrated by the fact that in 2006, people living in households with a car walked an average of 288 km a year, while those living in households without a car walked an average of 469 km.[1] Of those living in households with a car, those regarded as the main driver, walked an average of only 238 km. In 2006, of the 249 trips walked on average in a year, 21 (8%) were for commuting or business, while 44 (18%) were children walking to school or adults escorting them to school.[1] Eighty-one (33%) trips were shopping

Table 8.1   Trips and distance travelled per head in Great Britain.

	Trips per year			Distance per year in km			Mean trip length in km		
	1975/76	2006	Change %	1975/76	2006	Change %	1975/76	2006	Change %
Walk	325	249	−23	408	322	−21	1.3	1.3	0
Bicycle	30	16	−46	82	61	−26	2.7	3.8	+41
Car	429	658	+53	5,118	9,109	+78	11.9	13.8	+16
All travel	935	1,037	+11	7,584	11,413	+50	8.1	11.0	+36

Source: Department for Transport.[1]

and personal business trips, while 92 (37%) were for leisure or 'other (including 'just walk')'. This implies there is plenty of scope for increasing the volume of walk on some types of trip. For example, the 21 commuting and business trips that are walked are only 11% of all the trips in this category.

There is little doubt that the volumes of walking and cycling are considerably lower than in the 1950s. However, the levels seem to have remained fairly constant in recent years, despite the continuing rise in car ownership.

8.3   Barriers to active travel

To identify the barriers to active travel, the question that needs to be addressed is: what stops an individual who does not walk or cycle from doing so? Evidence on the reasons why people use their cars for trips of less than 8 km is provided in the research carried out by the Centre for Transport Studies at University College London for the Department for Transport.[6-8] In this work, short trips were identified in diaries that the respondents kept and then they were interviewed about these trips to investigate if they could have been made in other ways.

Table 8.2 shows the reasons that people who said that they could have walked or cycled short trips gave for using the car.[8] Many of the reasons were related to family life: 20% of the trips were giving a lift to someone else, probably a child or other household member in many cases, and 17% had heavy goods to carry, probably shopping. Others gave reasons associated with the complexity of travel: 9% needed the car for a further trip and 6% needed the car at work. Others gave less specific reasons: 15% because they were short of time, 10% said it was more convenient to use the car and 7% said it was a long way. For 21% of the trips, the respondents said that no specific action would be required to make them use modes other than the car: in other words, self-motivation would be required.[7] The constraints given by those who said that they could have cycled were similar, but with greater percentages giving shortage of time, distance and bad weather as reasons, compared to the potential walkers.

The reasons cited in the table can be summarised under the following headings:

- Lack of motivation
- Lifestyle
- Difficulty in walking and cycling

Faced with the alternative of making a (short) trip either using the car which will make the journey quick, comfortable and safe from the weather or walking (or cycling) which will take longer, require effort and involve exposure to the weather, many people will choose the car. For many people, there is no obvious motivation to walk or cycle rather than using the car.

For some people, staying at home may be more attractive than going out. Home entertainment in the form of television, social computing networks, such as Facebook, computer games, home shopping and so on, means that many of the activities people used to leave home for, such as entertainment, shopping and social

Table 8.2 Main reasons for using the car for short trips given by people who said that they could have walked or cycled the trip.

Reason for using car	Percentage who could have walked	Percentage who could have cycled
I was giving a lift to a family member or friend	20	15
I had heavy goods to carry	17	15
I was short of time	15	24
It was convenient	10	5
I needed the car for a further trip	9	9
It was a long way	7	14
The weather was bad	6	12
It was dark out	6	3
I needed my car at work	6	1
I was on a social trip	2	3
I was taking an elderly or ill person	1	0
I cannot manage without my car	1	0
I felt unwell	0	0
I was taking the dog for a walk	0	0
It was an unpleasant environment to travel through	0	0
Total	100	100
Number of cases	500	114

Source: Mackett and Ahern.[8]

contact, can be achieved in an electronic form at home, reducing the motivation for some people, particularly those who are electronically literate (often the young), to go out.[9] The need to make some local trips has been eliminated by technological innovation, thus reducing the motivation to leave the house to make such trips, which would often have been walked or cycled in the past.

Modern family life has become very complex for a number of reasons, including the increase in the number of mothers who are employed, often part-time, and the perceived need to protect younger children by not letting them out without adult supervision. This desire to supervise children based upon concerns about road safety and possible abduction has led to the shift from free play to supervised structured activities for children.[10] In the past, children were allowed out to play, alone or with friends; now children tend to go to clubs, lessons and other organised activities. This means that parents have to ensure that they can reach them, which becomes more complex when there are several children in the household. Unlike play, the structured activities are organised in specific locations (often not very close to home), and they often occur at specific times of day (such as after school), so parents tend to use the car rather than walk to take their children there.[11] The more rapid pace of modern life has led to many trips being made by car when previously they would have been walked (or cycled). Many of the reasons discussed above can be summarised under the term 'lifestyle'.

Many households have adopted a car-oriented lifestyle because they can afford enough cars to meet most of their travel needs and the range and location of activities that they have chosen to participate in are reachable by car. Some may be within walking distance, such as primary schools or local shops, and they may walk (or cycle) to them, but, in general, most of their trips are made by car. Many of the equivalent trips by their parents and grandparents would have been walked or cycled, because fewer of them would have owned a car, or the only car would have been used by the adult male of the household to travel to work and not be available during the day. This gradual transition towards a car-oriented society has been part of a two-way interaction with the decentralisation process: as cars have become more widely available, suppliers, such as retailing chains, have chosen locations best served by cars, and households have felt an increasing need for a car (or two) to help them reach the opportunities offered. This process has been fuelled by decisions by public bodies to concentrate facilities, such as schools and hospitals, into larger premises to offer economies of scale and a greater range of activity within the premises. The transport implications for users are rarely considered when planning these facilities.

There are a number of difficulties in making a walking or cycling trip:

- Physical difficulties
- Fear of going out
- Local environment is unsuitable
- Desired opportunities are far away

Some people have a well-defined disability that prevents them from walking (or cycling) and physical aids such as wheelchairs can facilitate local trips. Many others, particularly the more elderly, who make-up an increasing proportion of the population, have difficulty in walking. Whilst some assistance may be given by walking sticks and similar equipment, the distance that many elderly people can walk is often rather limited.[12] Younger people can have difficulty walking, for example, when shopping or with very young children. Many people shop in large supermarkets which provide almost all types of goods, but as a result, large volumes of shopping need to be carried home; for those who own a car, this is the most efficient way to transport the goods. Very young children cannot walk very far: many parents use pushchairs, but it may often be perceived as easier to take the child on a short car ride than a longer walk, pushing a pushchair with all the paraphernalia that is needed with very young children such as nappies, spare clothes and toys.

The media report many stories about crime. Whilst there are some places in Britain where street crime levels are high, people reading such stories may perceive their local area as being much more dangerous than it really is. They may interpret signs such as groups of young people or graffiti as indications that areas are threatening, even if there is little or no crime there. Such negative perceptions may be heightened after dark, which may cause people not to walk about, or parents to forbid their children from doing so. Instead they use their cars or stay at home, which they perceive as being safer, ignoring the increased risks to their health from lack of physical activity. People need to feel safe and comfortable in their environment when they go out. Streets with poor quality pavements, dog mess, chewing gum and so on do not make pleasant areas in which to walk. There is evidence that higher levels of greenery and lower levels of graffiti and litter in residential environments are associated with being physically active and not being overweight or obese.[13] At night, streets lacking good lighting will discourage people from walking. People making a journey in daylight but returning after dark may well choose to use the car because of the return journey, even though they might have been willing to walk the outward leg of the journey.

In recent years, urban areas have spread, as discussed in Chapter 3 by Robertson-Wilson and Giles-Corti. Suburbs have been developed with dwellings usually having one or more garages. It is usually possible to walk in more mature suburbs and, often, quite pleasant to do so, because they contain trees and other greenery, have suitable pavements and low crime rates. However, the size of the plots means that densities are fairly low, and so many people tend not to live very near to the activities they need as part of their lives, such as employment, shops, schools and leisure facilities. Since those living in the suburbs tend to have cars and the roads are usually not very busy, the usual mode of travel is the car. Over the past two decades, it might be argued that many new UK suburbs have, on the whole, become much less walkable as densities have increased, the use of disconnected 'cul-de-sac' layouts has been employed and landscaping often 'squeezed' out, resulting in a monotonous sea of housing which provides little interest to the pedestrian. The situation is rather different in the United States where suburban densities tend to be lower and have remained low and car ownership higher. Conversely, in most countries in continental Europe, urban densities are higher and walking and cycling more popular than in Britain; however, the car orientated suburb has become more widespread.

There is a further dimension, which makes it particularly difficult to increase the volumes of walking and cycling. Many households have chosen to live in places where car is the only way to reach the desired range of destinations. Many families live in different types of residential environments to their parents and grandparents: lower density, suburban or rural, poorer access to public transport and further from shops, schools and leisure activities. This works well if there is a car available, but fails if there is not. More importantly, in this context, it means that few journeys can be walked or cycled. Of course, it is possible to go out for a walk or cycle ride for pleasure or exercise, but busy lifestyles often make that difficult. Many people who feel that they ought to take more exercise join a health club paying high subscriptions to use expensive equipment, often followed by socialising that involves eating and drinking. Such places are marketed by demonstrating a lifestyle that some people aspire to. Joining a health club may be more about trying to live a particular lifestyle and socialising than about exercise.

The issues discussed so far imply that it is difficult to encourage more people to walk and cycle. It is not simply a matter of reversing the pattern of switching from active modes to the car. Many people have grown up in an environment where society is largely geared up to using the car. For them, it is the easy choice, enabling fast journeys and opening up opportunities unreachable by any other means. It enables people to continue the comfortable lifestyle that they have created. It enables them to project an image of success to their friends and neighbours. There is evidence from the United States that the levels of obesity are related to nature of the neighbourhood and the time spent in cars.[14] This car-oriented lifestyle is not true of everywhere in Britain, because there are places, for example within London, where people do manage without cars, cycle to work and walk with their children to school. There are parts of London where the percentage of trips walked to work is as high as 65%.[15] Handy[16] has suggested that in the United States 'New Urbanists' may walk more than those living in suburban areas, but recognising that the neotraditional neighbourhoods may be selected by those who wish to walk and cycle. Overall, such people are probably in the minority.

It is clear that it will not be easy to increase the volumes of walking and cycling because the trends have been in the opposite direction, and the various factors that have caused the rise in car use have reinforced one another. Some ways of increasing active travel are discussed in the next section.

8.4   Overcoming the barriers to active travel

For those not currently walking, the motivation to do so will need to be based on the intrinsic benefits of walking, such as health. This requires increasing awareness of the health risks associated with lack of physical activity. Advertising campaigns may help here, but it seems unlikely that these alone will have much impact on those who have currently chosen a sedentary lifestyle. In some cases, it may be more effective to target other members of the household who can repeat messages to their more sedentary spouses, children or parents, whenever they think it is appropriate.

For those who make short trips by car it is necessary to promote walking as more attractive relative to the car, or, putting it another way, make car use less attractive. The latter is probably easier and can involve increasing the cost of car use or increasing travel time by car. Increasing the cost of using the car is, in theory, straightforward: increasing fuel tax or charging for the use of road space can both be implemented if the government has the will to do so. Fuel tax is already high in Britain compared with some other countries; the percentage of tax on a litre of petrol and diesel was higher in Britain than any other country in the EU in 2006,[5] although this has not prevented many short trips being made by car. The nature of taxation on fuel is such that if the price increases for external reasons, the tax also increases. Large increases have induced protests in the past. The government is aware that the majority of the population live in car-owning households, and that votes may be lost if motorists feel they are being treated unfairly.

Charging for road space such as the congestion charging scheme in central London can be effective at shifting some people out of their cars. In the Western

Extension to the charging zone there is evidence of a small transfer to walking and cycling.[17] On the other hand, the reduction in congestion may have improved bus speeds to the extent that some people are attracted to switch from walking to the bus. Another way of making car use less attractive is to increase the cost of vehicle ownership by increasing vehicle excise duty. As of 2009, this is being done for environmental reasons, increasing tax for cars that use large amounts of fossil fuels and decreasing it for cars that are seen as 'green'. This may be politically acceptable, on the grounds that the public is aware of the fact that fossil fuels are finite. However, large increases in vehicle excise duty to reduce car ownership levels in order to improve physical activity levels seem unlikely to be accepted by the public.

Many of the motivations for using the car arise from meeting the requirements of children. These partly arise because of parental concern about the risks to children by allowing them to walk or cycle without an adult. Hence, one need is to increase parental confidence in letting children out without an adult; this may involve making the streets safer and convincing parents that this is the case.

Methods of overcoming the barriers associated with the difficulties of walking and cycling are relatively easy to identify. Improving the walking environment by investing in better and wider pavements, installing better quality street lighting, putting in more benches and paying staff to clear up litter and dog mess are straightforward. Similar improvements can be made for cycling. Whether they actually encourage more people to walk or cycle is another matter, which will be considered later. Such improvements, together with effective policing, can help to reduce crime levels; if local residents can be convinced that this has happened, they may be more willing to walk or cycle.[18]

The problems caused by greater dispersal of urban activities, which have led to increased distances from home to shops, schools and leisure facilities, can be addressed by planning policy. There are three difficulties here: firstly the trend has been towards larger, more centralised facilities and there would need to be a policy reversal. This may be difficult, as one of the motivating factors behind this trend has been reduction in public expenditure. The second difficulty is that because planning policy can only address new development or change of use of existing stock, and only small amounts of urban fabric are added each year, planning policy is a very slow way of tackling major issues in the built environment. The third difficulty is that many of the facilities are owned and operated by the private sector and the financial interests of companies are likely to be given precedence over the public interest. There has been a trend towards setting up local stores by the large supermarket chains in Britain, partly in response to difficulty in obtaining planning permission to develop out-of-town stores.[19] In theory, this should have increased walking, but often they have replaced existing small shops, and so may not have increased the total stock. In many ways, the 'damage' is already done, with many households taking advantage of the convenience of the car to carry out a large bulk shopping trip. It is hard to see many households switching back to doing all their shopping at the local shops and then carrying it home.

However, just as it has been possible to reduce the pace of development of large, out-of-town superstores, it could be possible to use planning controls to reduce the development of large facilities such as hospitals and schools. As implied above, there would probably be a cost associated with it, but this could, in theory, be offset against the financial saving to the National Health Service from the reduction in illnesses associated with low levels of physical activity. The difficulty would be to establish that there is an increase in the volumes of walking and cycling, and then to put a monetary value on the resulting health improvement.

There is a wider need for research into the financial benefits of health resulting from more physical activity. Transport schemes are appraised (or evaluated) using cost–benefit analysis. This involves putting a monetary value on all the benefits and comparing these with the costs; the scheme chosen is the one where the benefits are greatest relative to the costs. The system now used by the UK Department of Transport for evaluating walking and cycling schemes[20] is based upon research commissioned by the World Health Organisation (WHO),[21] using the Health Economic Assessment Tool (HEAT) for cycling.[22] This involves calculating the number of preventable deaths per person by taking up moderate physical activity through walking and cycling using data from a study in Copenhagen on the reduction in risk of all-cause morbidity by those who cycle for 3 hours a week compared with those who do not commute by bicycle.[23] Until fairly recently, physical activity was not considered at all in the appraisal of road schemes, that is, schemes for providing facilities for cars, which might cause a shift to or from walking and cycling. Nowadays, in appraising road schemes, the relevant key indicator that is used is the number of people achieving 30 minutes a day of moderate activity.[24]

Another approach to reducing the distance people need to travel is to increase residential densities.[25] Densities fell as a result of the suburbanisation process, which led to longer trips; this, in turn, led to some people using cars rather than walking or cycling. It is also more difficult to maintain bus services at low residential densities.[26] Forecasts of significant population growth have led to pressure to build on 'brown-field' sites within existing urban areas. This may cause densities to increase, but will not reduce the distance of existing residents from shops, schools and so on, unless new shops and schools are built to meet the increasing demand, and they are within walking distance of existing residents.

Even if these planning policies of increasing densities and providing local shops and services are implemented further, they will do little or nothing to reduce the problems caused by people who have moved to areas where they can only maintain their lifestyles by using one or more cars for all their trips. Whilst it seems unlikely that many of them are going to return to high density urban living, two points need to be borne in mind. Firstly, if they have moved to pleasant rural or semi-rural environments they may be inclined to indulge in recreational walking and cycling. Secondly, the population is dynamic: new households are being formed all the time, while others dissolve. This means that, whilst the existing households who have moved out of urban areas may not move back, the equivalent households going through the stage in the life cycle when households in the recent past chose to move out might come to a different conclusion and choose a more urbanised lifestyle. The different outcomes to the decision process might result from different states of the housing market and the cost of travel. If this is correct, it suggests that it is important to target households before they move out to lower density rural areas, not after. This process also requires the provision of suitable dwellings to meet these households' needs.

8.5   Policies and measures to increase the volume of active travel

Some of the difficulties of overcoming the barriers to active travel were discussed in the previous section. Despite these difficulties, there is evidence that people are more aware of the benefits of walking and cycling. In a UK survey of attitudes to walking and cycling 97% of the respondents agreed that people should be encouraged to walk to help their health, and 87% agreed the same for cycling.[4] Some negative attitudes to walking and cycling were identified, with 10% of respondents saying that they thought their friends would feel sorry for them if they walked more, with a figure of 13% for cycling. There is potential to shift car drivers out of their cars to active modes. In the survey on short trips by car,[6–8] drivers said that they could shift 31% of their short trips to walk and 7% to cycling.[7] The difficulty is that, for the walkable short trips, 65% would require either personal action or no specific action, while a further 17% would require an improvement in the weather. This means that there is little that government or other agencies can do to shift the majority of trips. For cycling the picture was slightly more positive because, while the respondents indicated that 63% of the trips would require one of the actions cited for walking, they stated that 24% of trips would be transferred if cycling facilities were improved. It should be recognised that there may be a large difference between what people say they would do in a hypothetical situation and what they would actually do.

A number of studies have reviewed schemes to encourage more people to walk and cycle. WHO Europe[27] has identified 13 examples of ways of increasing physical activity from travel across Europe, focusing on children and older people. Davis[28] identified 11 schemes in Great Britain for encouraging active travel. Some examples are as follows:

- Salisbury Doorstep Walks, which are descriptions of 10 local walks for health professionals to give to patients to encourage them to be more active
- Llwynu Primary School Cycling Club, Abergavenny, which is designed to encourage and facilitate cycling by children at the school
- 'Cycling on prescription' at Downfield Surgery in Dundee, which involved the purchase of six bicycles plus a secure shed, helmets, high visibility vests and locks, so that the patients could borrow the bicycles
- Promoting walking and cycling in Stockport, which has involved employing a Project Officer for 22 hours a week to promote active travel

The WHO Europe document[27] includes

- walking programmes for elderly people to promote health and safety in cities in Israel;
- children walking to school in Udine (Italy), which has involved piloting safe routes for walking to school in four primary schools;
- 'Happiness is cycling' in Helsingborg (Sweden), which is a campaign to inform local people about the opportunities available for cycling.

Whilst all these and the other schemes cited in the documents are worthy and may encourage some people to walk or cycle more, none of them have been subjected to a systematic evaluation. Since they all involve expenditure of resources, it is important to see whether the resources have been spent effectively, as they might have been better spent elsewhere. Also, even if some people cycle or walk more when the intervention is initiated, if they all cease very soon after, the scheme is unlikely to have been worthwhile from a physical activity perspective. Similarly, if a scheme simply encourages those who already walk or cycle to walk or cycle more, this is, probably, of much less value than getting people who previously did not walk or cycle to do so. For these reasons, it is important that initiatives are evaluated systematically, as discussed in the next section.

8.6   The effectiveness of policies and measures to increase the volume of active travel

As shown in the previous section, there are a number of initiatives designed to encourage active travel. As implied above, it is important to establish whether they are effective in encouraging more walking and cycling. It is even more useful if they can be shown to be cost effective, that is, deliver increased health benefits that are of greater value than the cost of implementing the initiative, because then the case can be strengthened for similar initiatives.

The evidence on the effectiveness of active travel interventions is not very strong. Ogilvie et al.[29] carried out a systemic review of the literature on initiatives to promote walking and cycling. They initially identified 5606 studies but only 22 met the inclusion criteria. They found a small number of studies that resulted in a shift of about 5% of households' trips from cars to walking and cycling. They reported that volunteers participating in trials experienced short-term improvements in some measures of health or fitness after taking up active commuting. They also found evidence of commuter subsidies and a new railway station encouraging a shift to active travel. However, they concluded that, on balance, most initiatives had not been effective in terms of increasing health benefits. A more recent review[30] suggests that interventions to increase walking which are targeted at the needs of individuals and delivered at this level can be effective, but that the evidence about the effectiveness of interventions at the institution, community or area level is less convincing. Part of the problem is the difficulty of researching into the health effects of transport interventions.[31] Cavill et al.[32] have examined the literature on the economic evaluation of the health effects of walking and cycling interventions and policies and found 17 relevant papers (out of 4264 titles selected for initial inclusion). They identified 16 benefit–cost ratios for walking and cycling schemes; in all cases except one the benefits exceeded the costs.

A review of transport interventions promoting safe cycling and walking[33] published by NICE (National Institute for Health and Clinical Excellence) relied on the evidence in the review by Ogilvie et al.[29] to draw conclusions about the effectiveness of initiatives to promote active travel. NICE examined the potential of four interventions to increase physical activity including pedometers and community-based exercise programmes for walking and cycling.[34] It concluded that there was insufficient evidence to recommend the use of either instrument to promote physical activity other than as part of research studies where effectiveness could be evaluated. More recently, as part of the process of developing NICE guidance on promoting physical activity for children,[35] four interventions to increase physical activity were analysed in terms of cost effectiveness: walking buses, free swimming, dance classes and community sports. Of the four, walking buses (based on evidence by Mackett et al.[36]) were found to be the most effective[37] whilst acknowledging that caution was required in assessing the evidence. One way to encourage walking and cycling is to promote and create suitable built and natural environments. This has been the subject of another NICE Guidance exercise.[38] Again, it was found that there was little sound evidence on the effectiveness of interventions, despite a very wide-ranging review of the literature.

8.7 Conclusions

In this chapter, it has been shown that walking and cycling as forms of travel have been in decline for many years. The main cause of this decline has been the increase in the use of the car. The growth in the availability of the car has been a contributing factor to the decentralisation of urban areas which has, in turn, made it more difficult to walk and cycle to many destinations such as shops and schools. This trend of decentralisation has been exacerbated by policies of concentrating facilities such as hospitals and schools in larger premises while closing down smaller, more local premises.

A number of barriers to active travel have been identified, including lifestyle changes, lack of motivation and difficulties in walking and cycling. The lifestyle changes are linked to a number of factors including the increasing number of mothers who are employed, and parental concerns about allowing children out without adult supervision. A major issue is that many households have chosen residential locations where they depend upon the car for all their trips, which means that it would be very difficult for them to switch to active travel modes. The lack of motivation reflects the relative ease of travel by car for many trips.

To overcome these barriers, major policy initiatives would be required to increase the cost of car ownership and use, reverse the policy of concentrating schools and hospitals in large premises, increase residential densities and ensure the provision of homes in urban areas that meet the aspirations of a wide range of people. Attention also needs to be given to the methods used to appraise schemes for new transport infrastructure to ensure that the health benefits of increased walking and cycling are valued appropriately. There are many smaller scale initiatives that may increase the volumes of active travel. However, there is a lack of evidence of the effectiveness of such interventions and more research is needed into this subject.

Overall, the picture is rather disappointing because of the dominance of the car in everyday mobility. However, given the benefits to health of increased walking and cycling and the fact that a shift from car to active travel offers both travel and health benefits and thus helps to meet the policy agenda of both the national ministries of Health and Transport, and in doing so, saves public expenditure, the potential of intervention is huge. With greater public debate supported by high-quality research into the effectiveness of interventions, it may be possible to implement suitable policies and schemes to help to improve the health of the nation.

References

1. Department for Transport. (2007) Transport Statistics Bulletin: National Travel Survey: 2006, National Statistics, available from http://www.dft.gov.uk/pgr/statistics/datatables publications/personal/mainresults/nts2006/.
2. Department of Health. (2004) At Least Five a Week: Evidence on the Impact of Physical Activity and its Relationship to Health: a report from the Chief Medical Officer, available from http://www.dh.gov.uk/en/Publicationsandstatistics/Publications/PublicationsPolicyAnd Guidance/DH_4080994.
3. Department for Transport. (2007) Towards a Sustainable Transport System: Supporting Economic Growth in a Low Carbon World, available from http://www.dft.gov.uk/about/strategy/ transportstrategy/pdfsustaintranssystem.pdf.
4. Department for Transport. (2002) Attitudes to Walking and cycling, available from http://www.dft.gov.uk/pgr/statistics/datatablespublications/trsnstatsatt/earlierreports/ attitudestowalkingandcycling.
5. Department for Transport. (2007) Transport statistics Great Britain 2007, available from http://www.dft.gov.uk/pgr/statistics/datatablespublications/tsgb/.
6. Mackett, R.L. (2001) Policies to attract drivers out of their cars for short trips. *Transport Policy.* 8:295–306.
7. Mackett, R.L. (2003) Why do people use their cars for short trips? *Transportation.* 30: 329–349.
8. Mackett, R.L., Ahern, A.A. (2000) Potential for mode transfer of short trips: report on the analysis of the survey results. Report to the Department of the Environment, Transport and the Regions. Available on the World Wide Web at http://www2.cege.ucl.ac.uk/cts/shtrp.asp.
9. Holloway, S., Valentine, G. *CyberKids: Children and the Information Age.* London, Falmer Routledge, 2003.
10. National Institute of Child Health and Development. (2000) How do children spend their time? Children's activities, school achievement, and well being. *Research on Today's Issues.* (11), August 2000, Population Reference Bureau for the Demographic and Behavioral Sciences Branch, Center for Population Research, National Institute of Child Health and Human Development, National Institutes of Health, U.S. Department of Education.
11. Mackett, R.L., Lucas, L., Paskins, J., Turbin, J. (2005) The therapeutic value of children's everyday travel. *Transportation Research A.* 39:205–219.
12. Martin, J., Meltzer, H., Elliot, D. *The Prevalence of Disability among Adults. OPCS Surveys of Disability in Great Britain.* Social Surveys Division, Office of Population Censuses and Surveys. London, HMSO, 1988.
13. Ellaway, A., Macintyre, S. (2005) Bonnefoy X: graffiti, greenery, and obesity in adults: Secondary analysis of European cross sectional survey. *British Medical Journal.* 331:611–612. doi 10.1136/bmj.38575.664549.F7.

14. Frank, L.D., Andresen, M.A., Schmid, T.L. (2004) Obesity relationships with community design, physical activity, and time spent in cars. *American Journal of Preventive Medicine.* 27:87–96.
15. Transport for London. *London Travel Report 2007.* London, Mayor of London and Transport for London, 2008.
16. Handy, S. (2006) Questioning assumptions 1: Do New Urbanists walk more? Evaluating new towns from a transportation planner's perspective. *Planning, American Planning Association.* 72 (1):36–37, available from http://www.des.ucdavis.edu/faculty/handy/TTP_seminar/new_urbanism_and_walking.pdf.
17. Transport for London. (2008) Central London congestion charging, impacts monitoring, sixth annual report, July 2008., available from http://www.tfl.gov.uk/assets/downloads/sixth-annual-impacts-monitoring-report-2008-07.pdf.
18. Department for Transport. (1998) Personal security issues in pedestrian journeys., available from http://www.dft.gov.uk/pgr/crime/personalsecurity/personalsecurityissuesinpede3005.
19. Raffaella Sadun. (2008) Does planning regulation protect independent retailers? *Centre Piece, The Magazine of The Centre for Economic Performance, London School of Economics.* 13(2):2–5.
20. Department for Transport. (2007) Guidance on the appraisal of walking and cycling schemes, TAG Unit 3.14.1, Transport Appraisal Guidance, available from http://www.webtag.org.uk/webdocuments/3_Expert/14_Walking_Cycling/3.14.1.htm.
21. World Health Organisation (WHO). (2003) Health and development through physical activity and sport, available from http://whqlibdoc.who.int/hq/2003/WHO_NMH_NPH_PAH_03.2.pdf.
22. Rutter, H., Cavill, N., Dinsdale, H., Kahlmeier, S., Racioppi, F., Oja, P. *Health Economic Assessment Tool for Cycling (HEAT for cycling) user guide.* WHO Regional Office for Europe, Copenhagen, Denmark, Transport, Health and Environment Pan-European Programme, World Health Organization (WHO) Regional Office for Europe, 2007, available from http://www.euro.who.int/Document/E90948.pdf.
23. Andersen, L.B., Schnohr, P., Schroll, M., Hein, H.O. (2000) All-cause mortality associated with physical activity during time, work, sports, and cycling to work. *Archives of Internal Medicine.* 160:1621–1628.
24. Department for Transport. (2009) The Physical Fitness Sub-objective, TAG Unit 3.3.12, Transport Appraisal Guidance, available from http://www.dft.gov.uk/webtag/webdocuments/3_Expert/3_Environment_Objective/3.3.12.htm.
25. Department of Communities and Local Government. (2006) Planning policy statement 3 (PPS3): housing, available from http://www.communities.gov.uk/documents/planning andbuilding/pdf/planningpolicystatement3.pdf.
26. Biddulph, M. *Introduction to Residential Layout.* Oxford, Architectural Press, 2007.
27. Racioppi, F., Dora, C., Krech, R., Von Ehrenstein, O. In: *A Physically Active Life through Everyday Transport with a Special Focus on Children and Older People and Examples and Approaches From Europe* (Ed. Davis, A.) Regional Office for Europe, WHO European Centre for Environment and Health, Rome, Italy, World Health Organization, Regional Office for Europe, 2002, available from http://www.euro.who.int/document/e75662.pdf.
28. Davis, A. *Active Transport: A Guide to the Development of Local Initiatives to Promote Walking and Cycling.* London, Health Education Authority, 1999, available from http://www.nice.org.uk/niceMedia/documents/activetransport.pdf.
29. Ogilvie, D., Egan, M., Hamilton, V., Petticrew, M. (2004) Promoting walking and cycling as an alternative to using cars: systematic review. *British Medical Journal.* 329:763–766.
30. Ogilvie, D., Foster, C., Rothnie, H., Cavill, N., Hamilton, V., Fitzsimons, C., Mutrie, N. (2007) Interventions to promote walking: systematic review. *British Medical Journal.* 334:1204–1213.
31. Ogilvie, D., Mitchell, R., Mutrie, N., Petticrew, M., Platt, S. (2006) Evaluating health effects of transport interventions: methodologic case study. *American Journal of Preventative Medicine.* 31:118–126.

32. Cavill, N., Kahlmeier, S., Rutter, H., Racioppi, F., Oja, P. (2008) Economic analysis of transport infrastructure and policies including health effects related to walking and cycling: a systematic review. *Transport Policy*. 15:291–304.

33. Killoran, A., Doyle, N., Waller, S., Wohlgemuth, C., Crombie, H. *Transport Interventions Promoting Safe Cycling and Walking: Evidence Briefing*. London, National Institute for Health and Clinical Excellence, 2006, available from http://www.nice.org.uk/niceMedia/pdf/Transport_Evidence_Briefing_05-07.pdf.

34. National Institute for Health and Clinical Excellence. (2006) Four commonly used methods to increase physical activity: brief interventions in primary care, exercise referral schemes, pedometers and community-based exercise programmes for walking and cycling. Public Health Intervention Guide number 2, available from http://www.nice.org.uk/PHI002.

35. National Institute for Health and Clinical Excellence. (2008) Guidance on promoting physical activity for children, available from http://www.nice.org.uk/guidance/index.jsp?action=byID&o=11672.

36. Mackett, R.L., Lucas, L., Paskins, J., Turbin, J. *Walking buses in Hertfordshire: Impacts and lessons*, Report, Gower Street, London, Centre for Transport Studies, University College London, 2005, available from http://www2.cege.ucl.ac.uk/cts/research/chcaruse/Walking%20bus%20report%20-%20UCL.pdf.

37. Fordham, R., Barton, G. (2008) A cost-effectiveness scenario analysis of four interventions to increase child and adolescent physical activity: the case of walking buses, free swimming, dance classes and community sports, NICE Programme Guidance on the Promotion of Physical Activity in Children, available from http://www.nice.org.uk/media/C83/74/PromotingPhysicalActivityChildrenCostEffectivenessAnalysis.pdf.

38. National Institute for Health and Clinical Excellence. (2008) Physical activity and the environment: Guidance on the promotion and creation of physical environments that support increased levels of physical activity, available from http://www.nice.org.uk/Guidance/PH8.

9 Greenspace, Obesity and Health: Evidence and Issues

Caroline Brown

9.1 Introduction

As the world's population becomes more and more urbanised, there is increasing attention on the way in which the configuration and quality of the urban environment affects people's health, their well-being and their quality of life. Greenspace is an important element in any urban settlement, and the provision of open space is a particularly significant part of the human habitat. Nature complements, softens and makes liveable the hard infrastructure on which cities depend (buildings, roads, communications networks, etc.), and the term greenspace is used here to denote any and all of the green and open spaces which may be present within a town or city. This can include formal parks and gardens, open spaces such as town squares and cemeteries, the land along rivers, canals and transport corridors, sports pitches, playing fields, golf courses, woodlands, wetlands and sites which are derelict and unused. There are numerous reasons why greenspace is understood to be important for people, and this chapter explores some of those reasons in detail. In particular, this chapter is concerned with examining the relationship between greenspace and obesity.

The chapter begins by considering the link between greenspace, health and the conditions *associated with* obesity, for example, high blood pressure, diabetes and heart disease. Section 9.3 examines greenspace and food, Section 9.4 unpicks the links between greenspace and physical activity, Section 9.5 discusses children and their relationship with greenspace and Section 9.6 reflects on current policy and practice. Although the intention here is to concentrate on the existing research evidence, in some places this is rather patchy. As a result, the chapter includes details of very recent initiatives not yet empirically tested, and provides a commentary on both research and policy gaps.

9.2 Greenspace, health and obesity

The starting point for this chapter is a consideration of the research exploring and demonstrating the effects of nature and greenspace on human health particularly chronic conditions such as cancer and cardiovascular disease, but also mental health problems and general well-being. It is worth considering these here because obesity is associated with a number of chronic conditions including high blood pressure, heart disease, type 2 diabetes, gall bladder disease and osteoarthritis.[1]

The literature includes a number of studies demonstrating the physiological benefits of direct and indirect contact with nature, including the view from a window. The most well-known of these is Ullrich's 1984 study of hospitalised patients and their recovery from surgery.[2] The study demonstrated that all other things being equal, patients with a view of trees required less analgesia and were discharged earlier than patients with a view of a brick wall. Follow-up work has shown that a view of nature and/or greenness reduces levels of stress[3,4] and can reduce both heart rate and blood pressure.[5] This echoes evidence which demonstrates that exercise in a green setting or with views of nature has a greater impact on mood, blood pressure and self-esteem than exercise in a setting with no views or unpleasant views.[6,7] Such research suggests that access to and views of greenspace may not only help to reduce levels of obesity by increasing physical activity, but may also temper the negative health effects of obesity by lowering blood pressure and reducing stress levels. Although the physiological effects of greenspace may be small and temporary, it seems increasingly likely that they play a role in an individual's long-term health, particularly in relation to chronic conditions such as heart disease and cancer.

Linked to this evidence about physiological effects of greenspace is the work which explores the mental health benefits of greenspace. Stress has a psychological as well as a physiological dimension, and it has been observed that views of nature are associated with higher levels of relaxation,[8] improved concentration and self-discipline in young girls[9] and reduced feelings of stress in young adults.[4] Grahn and Stigsdotter's study[10] shows statistically significant links between self-reported levels of stress and use of greenspace, regardless of age, sex and socio-economic status. Frequency and duration of visits both had a positive impact on stress levels, for example, those who visit more often, or spend longer periods in such spaces have lower levels of stress-related illness. Together, this body of work demonstrates that access and exposure to greenspace supports mental health, and in so doing promotes physical health. The link between mental well-being and physical health is widely acknowledged. For example, Burns[11] has stated that the happier a person is, the healthier they are likely to be, the better they will recover from illness and the longer they are likely to live. Other work has shown that low levels of mental well-being are linked to decreased physical well-being, demonstrating a relationship between feelings of hopelessness and mortality.[12]

The cumulative impact of the built environment on health is not yet understood, although we do know a lot about the geography of health inequalities. Public health officials are now considering the possibility that microscopic processes related to stress hormones and cholesterol, for example, may, over a life-course, contribute to, and perhaps explain, the health inequalities that are observed between populations living in good quality neighbourhoods and those living in poor quality neighbourhoods.[13] As we know from the literature, there is now fairly convincing evidence which demonstrates that people who live in greener neighbourhoods suffer from less illness,[14,15] have lower levels of self-reported illness[15,16] and are less likely to die from circulatory diseases or lung cancer.[17] The exact mechanism for these links has not yet been demonstrated, but it seems likely that the effects mentioned above – on blood pressure, heart rate, mood and mental well-being – are likely to play their part in supporting physical health and protecting individuals from chronic health conditions. In this vein, Mitchell and Popham[17] observe that levels of physical activity and response to stress are components of the cause of circulatory diseases. According to their research, one of the possible explanations for the reduced health inequalities among populations living in the greenest neighbourhoods is the influence of greenspace on these factors.

The evidence appears fairly conclusive: greenspace is good for human health, although the relationship with and influence on obesity is not particularly clear. The following sections focus on the links between greenspace and obesity in more detail, beginning with food.

9.3 Greenspace, obesity and food

The balance between energy in (calories consumed) and energy out (physical activity undertaken) lies at the centre of the obesity issue. To date, food and diet has been a major preoccupation of public health initiatives (see Chapter 10). However, it is fair to say that the link between greenspace and food has been largely neglected by policymakers to date, although this is beginning to change.

In modern cities, it is easy to overlook the role of greenspace in providing fresh, local food for urban populations. Supermarkets provide produce from around the world, eroding the link between food consumption, the seasons and the locality, particularly in urban areas where contact with agriculture is at a minimum. Others have written about the link between obesity and diet, highlighting the link with processed, high-fat and high-sugar foods and the absence of fresh, whole food, grown locally.[18] However, there is little emphasis in the current literature on the role of gardens, allotments, community orchards and market gardens in the food environment. Historically, such uses were common in the urban landscape and played an important part in the diets of the working poor. As Ebenezer Howard's garden city model demonstrates, city planning was not only about the provision of housing and industrial land uses but also about food, and his plans were designed to provide urban residents with fresh produce by including market gardens and allotments at the edge of the settlement.[19] Urban allotments have also been an important part of the landscape across many parts of Europe for more than a century. In the 18th and 19th centuries, allotments provided land and space for the poor to grow food, supplementing their diets with fresh food that would otherwise be unaffordable. However, the amount of space given over to food production in urban areas has been dwindling, with an overall decline in the number of allotment sites, urban farms and market gardens in the latter half of the 20th century. In the United Kingdom, figures show that 40% of allotments have been lost since 1970.[20]

From a health and obesity point of view, fresh, whole food grown locally is desirable because it contributes to a seasonally varied diet rich in fresh fruit and vegetables and low in processed, energy intense foods high in fat, sugar and salt. Unfortunately, many poor neighbourhoods not only lack shops selling fresh fruit and vegetables[21] but residents there also lack the opportunity and skills to grow their own fruit and vegetables. For example, work in England has concluded that 'at present, too many areas do not provide access to shops with a wide range of food, particularly fresh food'.[22] This is further borne out by recent government initiatives in both Scotland and England which support local shops to stock fresh fruit and vegetables.[23]

As in the past, many urban dwellers live at high density, and may not have access to an outside space of their own. Even where communal greenspace exists, landscaping and management norms focus on providing spaces which are multifunctional and easy to maintain rather than providing sustenance, fresh food or fuel. The picture may be starting to change. Allotments are increasingly popular across the United Kingdom, and waiting lists for plots are often very long, sometimes more than 10 years – although this is not the case in all parts of the country or across all parts of a city. Anecdotal evidence suggests that much of the new demand for plots is from young professionals, women and families, changing the image of allotments as a working-class, white and male preserve. Despite the demand, allotment sites are still at risk from development projects – and there has been much controversy about the impact of the London Olympic Games on Manor Garden Allotments in Hackney Wick, for example.[24] This site has been relocated to make way for the Olympic Village, however, many allotments sites are lost rather than replaced. The sites which remain in use tend to be on the most marginal land (e.g. sloping steeply, oddly shaped or difficult to access) and in the places where demand for new housing or industrial development is lowest (e.g. in communities which are deprived). This creates the curious situation in which allotments may be close to deprived neighbourhoods where the incidence of obesity is likely to be highest, but they are used less and less by poorer and working-class residents. The reasons for this are twofold: first, as demand grows among professional groups, then it is inevitable that some working-class individuals will have to wait longer to obtain a plot; in addition, demand for allotments among poorer residents tends to be lower. While most allotments are provided by local authorities or allotment societies and managed by a committee of plot holders, some other types of landowner have begun to offer allotments to local residents. The most notable of these is the National Trust – a major landowner in the United Kingdom, known best for its stewardship of historic properties and much of the country's coastline. In early 2009, the Trust announced that it would be creating 1000 allotments.[25] This announcement, along with others, is but a small step towards the vision of Barton et al.,[26] who argue that allotments should be close enough to home to permit easy access by foot. A distance of around 200 m is comfortable for carrying a bucket or pushing a wheelbarrow – although the current reality in most UK cities is that allotment holders may have to travel for several miles to get to their plot. It is important to point out here that the health benefits of allotment gardening extend beyond access to fresh fruit and vegetables: allotment holders also benefit from the physical activity involved in growing their own food and the social and mental health benefits that come from being outdoors and engaging with other plot holders.

While people appear to be more and more interested in growing their own food,[27] allotments are only part of the urban food picture. Setting aside the food grown in domestic gardens, other more radical grass roots projects have recently begun to spring up across the United Kingdom. These projects include the Incredible Edible Todmorden,[28] where activists have been planting public flower beds with vegetables and making the town's greenspaces edible as well as attractive. In Sheffield, activists have been harvesting and distributing fruit from the city's apple, pear and plum trees, giving it out free in and around the city centre,[29] while in Bristol and other cities, local residents are being given help and support to develop their gardening skills.[30,31] Such projects demonstrate that urban greenspaces of all types and sizes can be used to produce fresh food for local residents. However, current planning policy places *no* emphasis on the use of greenspace for food production, or the contribution that allotments and urban food-growing might have for public health and sustainability, particularly in poor communities. CABE Space – government's champion for good quality public space – *does* recognise the role of greenspace for food production, and recommends that local authorities should use their spatial policies to protect and identify land for urban food production.[32] Section 9.6 examines greenspace policy in more detail.

Since the availability of fresh fruit and vegetables influences uptake, then initiatives such at Incredible Edible Todmorden can only have a positive impact on the diet of Todmorden's residents. As yet there is little empirical research which demonstrates the short or long-term impacts of such projects on health, BMI, obesity or diet.

9.4 Greenspace and physical activity

Having looked at the food side of the energy-balance equation, our attention now turns to the issue of physical activity. As various other contributions to this book have demonstrated, the environment in which we live influences our ability and propensity to be physically active (see Chapters 4, 6 and 7). In relation to obesity, physical activity not only helps people reduce and manage their weight but also helps to maintain normal muscle strength and joint function, reduces blood pressure and relieves stress.[1] In line with the rest of this chapter, the focus here is the contribution that greenspace can and might make to tackling obesity.

At its broadest, the research evidence shows strong links between greenspace and levels of physical activity with various studies demonstrating that physical activity rates are higher, and obesity is lower, in neighbourhoods with higher levels of greenery.[33,34] One of these studies demonstrated that people who lived in areas with high levels of greenery were three times more likely to be physically active and 40% less likely to be overweight or obese.[33] Although the causal pathways linking greenspace to health have yet to be isolated, there are two principal relationships worthy of exploration. These are greenspace as a *setting* for exercise and greenspace as a *motivation* for exercise. These areas are discussed in more detail below.

9.4.1 Greenspace as a setting for exercise

One of the most obvious benefits of greenspace is that it provides people with places where they can walk and exercise – often without cost. Many large municipal parks

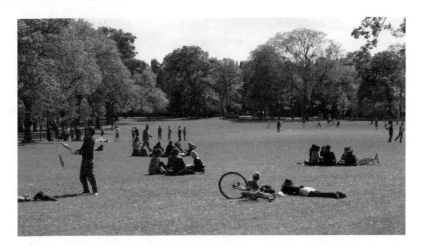

Figure 9.1   Informal activities, The Meadows, Edinburgh.

have open areas where people can sit and play, besides having formal sports facilities such as tennis courts, golf courses and sports pitches. Figure 9.1 illustrates one such space in Edinburgh, Scotland. This park – the Meadows – is not only well used for informal activities (note the juggling practice in the foreground and touch rugby in the background) but also has a number of formal sports functions. These include two cricket squares, tennis courts and a pitch and putt golf course. The Meadows is also used by local primary schools for their sports lessons and weekend football coaching.

The presence or absence of such spaces in a city, and particularly in a neighbourhood, appears to be important in relation to physical activity[33] (see also Chapter 4). As discussed above, the research suggests that the *quantity* of greenspace available is a significant factor. In planning terms, the provision of public parks, playgrounds for children and sports facilities has long been a requirement for neighbourhood planning and new development. This stems from the recognition that having facilities nearby makes it easier for people to access them, and as a result they are more likely to use them. However, we also know that there are disparities between the least deprived and most deprived neighbourhoods in the United Kingdom in terms of the amount of greenspace available,[17] with the least deprived tending to have more greenspace than the most deprived. We also know that regardless of socio-economic factors people are just as likely to use greenspace if access is readily available.[10]

Quantity of greenspace appears to be important for health because it affects the proximity and accessibility of greenspace to local people. Both of these factors have been shown to be important in influencing an individual's ability and desire to engage in exercise[1] and they link to the growing research evidence about the health benefits of walkable neighbourhoods (see also Chapter 3). However, proximity is not the only factor. The health impact assessment of greenspace guide[35] notes that physical activity is influenced by a number of personal factors, and in relation to greenspace the key factors are ease of access, size of greenspace, connectivity to residential/commercial areas, attractiveness (biodiversity, lack of litter) and flexibility. Such observations support the proposition that it is not only the quantity of greenspace that counts in relation to physical activity but also its *quality*. It is well-known that feelings of safety affect use of greenspace, but research in the United States and Australia has also shown that people are more likely to get out and exercise if their neighbourhood is attractive and there is enjoyable scenery.[36] Together such evidence underlines the importance of the *quantity* of greenspace and the *quality* of that space, including its maintenance, accessibility, design and aesthetic value in encouraging and facilitating a physically active population.

In addition to the work which demonstrates the general link between greenspace and physical activity, there is a particular strand which has explored the effects of physical activity in a green setting. This demonstrates, for example, that exercising with a view of green places reduces blood pressure, enhances mood and improves self-esteem to a greater extent than exercising with no views/unpleasant views.[6] Follow-up work examining the effects of exercise in a green setting shows similar benefits, including significant reductions in levels of anger, depression, confusion and tenseness.[7] As discussed earlier, this type of evidence demonstrates the subtle, but very fundamental effects of greenspace on the human body. Not only does *being* in a greenspace help the body cope with stress[10] but *exercising* in a greenspace also appears to offer greater health benefits than exercising indoors.

9.4.2   Greenspace as a motivation for exercise

Besides offering a setting for physical activity, it has been shown that greenspace often provides a *motivation* for individuals to exercise. Getting some fresh air, looking at the view, getting away from things, seeking tranquillity and relaxation – all of these attributes of greenspace appear to give individuals an impetus to be active. These are *additionalities* which cannot be derived from exercising at home, in a gym or another indoor setting, and which are just as important as the activity itself for some people. Evaluations of walking initiatives and Green Gyms have pointed to participants' appreciation of being outside and being with other people in addition to the (health) benefits that they get from being physically active.[37] The result of this is that participants in such programmes were less likely to drop-out than participants in regular gym-based fitness programmes. This suggests that the availability of attractive greenspace thus not only provides an opportunity to be physically active, but in some cases can actually encourage activity that would otherwise not happen at all, or might not be sustained over a longer period.

Another pathway to consider in the built environment–health relationship is that of the neighbourhood effect. This describes the way in which an individual's behaviour is shaped by the behaviour of those around him/her, and is thought to explain why poorer individuals living among better off residents experience less health inequality than poor individuals living in poor neighbourhoods. Put simply, if you live in a place where people are physically active – cycling and walking, jogging, playing informal and formal sports on the local playing fields – then you are more likely to be active yourself.[36] In this sort of neighbourhood being physically active is an accepted norm. Conversely, if you live in a neighbourhood where there are few or no greenspaces or facilities for sport and where cycling is seen as a mark of poverty and not health, it would not be surprising to find low rates of physical activity. A public health professional working in Liverpool in the 1990s, and who did a lot of work promoting cycling in the city, tells a story about attending a community meeting in one of Liverpool's most deprived neighbourhoods. When she arrived at the meeting – on her bike – the local councillor said 'honestly, with all your money and you're still riding a bike . . . ' as if cycling was not something that professionals, or those with cars, would do voluntarily (Ashton, P., per. comm. 1996).[38] In that community cycling was not an accepted behavioural norm, making it much less likely that locals would either own or use a bike to travel around the city. Again, such observations underline how accessible greenspace, which is well used, helps to establish and maintain physical activity – whether that's jogging, cycling, tai chi, football or just an afternoon stroll – as a behavioural norm within that community.

9.5 Greenspace and children's health

Although other chapters in this book deal extensively with the health and physical activity of children and young people (Chapters 6 and 7), it is useful to also discuss them here in the context of greenspace. Because children do not have the same degree of autonomy and choice about their diets, their free-time and their neighbourhoods as adults, then the environment around their homes and schools is particularly important in their physical, mental and social development. Focusing specifically on greenspace, the literature suggests that access to good quality greenspace can have a number of significant health benefits for children. These include promoting normal muscle and bone growth; developing balance and coordination; learning about risk and judgement; promoting feelings of attachment; and assisting with concentration and educational attainment.

In order to develop strong bones, joints and muscles capable of physical activity in adult life, a child needs to be physically active. There is a large body of work devoted to the study of children's play and its relationship with weight and BMI. As might be expected, children who watch more television at age 3 (>8 hours per week) are more likely to be obese at age 7.[21] In addition, a Norwegian study found that outdoor play is more vigorous than indoor play and that children who regularly play in natural areas showed a statistically significant improvement in fitness with better coordination, balance and agility.[38]

Richard Louv has written extensively about the impact of modern society (in the United States) on the development and well-being of children.[39] He coins the term 'nature-deficit disorder' and describes how concerns about safety mean that few children now get to explore their neighbourhoods unsupervised, or scavenge off-cuts of wood from a building site to build themselves dens and treehouses, or learn about judgement and risk taking by climbing trees and fording streams. Louv cites evidence showing that outdoor play in a natural setting is more vigorous, more imaginative, more creative and more egalitarian than play in engineered spaces with asphalt and play structures. In light of such research evidence, policymakers are rethinking their ideas about children's play spaces, moving away from a standard kit, fence and carpet (KFC) approach in which a space is levelled, covered with a 'safety' surface and kitted out with generic play equipment. Wild play and natural play is now being promoted in preference to the KFC approach, emphasising the use of natural materials and natural features to create flexible, dynamic and challenging spaces where children of different ages and physical capabilities can play together. The natural play design movement has been led by professionals in Denmark, Holland and Germany and is now being embraced by policymakers in the United Kingdom.[40]

Besides the benefits derived from active contact with natural spaces, children also benefit from more passive contact with greenspace. Research in the United States has explored educational attainment and concentration in children and the influence of the home setting (e.g. whether it has views of trees and greenery or not).[41] The study found that girls – who, it is theorised, spend more time at home than their male peers – appeared to benefit from a home setting which was green and leafy. In addition, there has been some work which explicitly explores the relationship between neighbourhood greenness and BMI among overweight children.[42] This study looks at the relationships between children's BMI scores over a 2-year period and measures of neighbourhood density and greenness. The results show an inverse relationship between neighbourhood greenness and BMI scores, suggesting that as greenness increases, BMI scores fall. It was also found that children in greener settings were less likely to increase their scores over the 2-year period than children in less-green neighbourhoods. These effects were found to be independent of residential density, age, gender and ethnicity.

Overall, among children and young people access to greenspace provides the same kind of benefits as it does to adults: reducing stress, promoting physical activity and helping to regulate weight. However, it is particularly important for children because of the way in which it influences their future health. Overweight children tend to become overweight adults,[43] and the UK government's obesity strategy places great emphasis on early intervention – from birth – as a means of realising its overall objective of reducing rates of obesity in the general population.[21]

9.6 Greenspace provision and policy

While much of this chapter has concentrated on the evidence linking greenspace and obesity, it is useful to comment on the UK policy which governs the provision, protection and maintenance of urban greenspaces. The simple reason for this is that regardless of the public health evidence about the *value* of greenspace, policy interventions which relate to the location, amount and quality of urban greenspace are the responsibility of numerous government agencies but not public health officials. The discussion, that follows, explores the historic, institutional and policy contexts shaping current UK policy on greenspace.

9.6.1 The historic context

In the United Kingdom, as in many other countries, the provision of public open space in urban areas is shaped to very large part by historical rather than contemporary events. For example, many of London's major greenspaces are the legacy of royal decisions made hundreds of years ago. Hyde Park to give one example was enclosed as a deer park and hunting ground by Henry VIII in the 16th century and is now one of the eight Royal Parks which together cover around 22,000 ha in the capital. In other cities open spaces were laid out as the result of philanthropic activities concerned with alleviating (or at least ameliorating) the squalor of industrial life for the urban poor in the 19th and early 20th centuries. As a result, it is important to understand that much policy effort is directed towards protecting and managing *existing* greenspace rather than providing new spaces. Of course, some new spaces are created within new developments, and the pattern of greenspace provision in more suburban and peripheral urban settings is largely the result of post-war planning policy.

Shockingly, there are no definitive statistics about the number or location of Britain's urban parks and greenspaces, despite various calls for such information to be collated by central government.[44-46] The best estimates currently available suggest that England has more than 23,000 parks and recreational spaces, 300,000 allotments, 400 urban nature reserves and 30,000 sports fields and playgrounds.[20] These figures may seem impressive, but recent research for CABE Space, government's champion for good quality public space, has shown that the quantity of greenspace available to residents varies significantly between regions, between cities and between neighbourhoods.[47] In terms of regional variation, the south-west and south-east of England are among those with the greatest quantity of greenspace per person, while London and some of the northern regions have much lower provision. The most notable variations, however, are seen at the neighbourhood level where the research demonstrated that there was a *fivefold* difference between the quantity of greenspace available to the most affluent and the most deprived neighbourhoods. As discussed earlier, variations in the distribution of greenspace are linked to differential health outcomes, with people living in greener neighbourhoods enjoying better health and lower mortality rates than people living in the least green areas. While disparities in greenspace provision may be the result of historical accident, it is one of the issues which contemporary greenspace and public health policy needs to address.

9.6.2 The institutional context

The multiple links between greenspace and other policy issues mean that responsibility for UK greenspace is divided among a range of bodies. At the national level, the department for Communities and Local Government (CLG) has the main responsibility for greenspace policy, although some activities fall under the remit of the Department for Environment, Food and Rural Affairs (DEFRA). Spatial planning policy is the responsibility of the CLG, and as a result, this department has a considerable influence over the provision and protection of greenspace, particularly in urban areas. Policies related to forestry, nature conservation and agriculture on the other hand fall under the remit of DEFRA. In addition, there are a number of other government agencies with a direct interest in strategies and initiatives for greenspace. Thus, Natural England promotes 'natural' greenspace where nature and ecological processes are allowed to dominate; the Forestry Commission is responsible for protecting and expanding the country's forests and woodlands; English Heritage is interested in parks and gardens with historic value; Sport England is concerned with sports pitches and playing fields; the Audit Commission is interested in local authority spending and management; and, CABE Space has an overall remit to champion high-quality parks and open spaces across urban England. It is noticeable that as yet health bodies do not feature amongst this group of agencies and departments concerned with greenspace issues.

At local authority level responsibility for greenspace is divided slightly differently. While spatial planners are responsible for greenspace strategies and policies about the protection and provision of local greenspace, the management of existing parks and open spaces is usually the responsibility of a different part of the local authority.

The fractured nature of the greenspace sector in the United Kingdom at both national and local government levels has contributed to greenspace being treated as a poor relation in terms of both spending and effort. Recent figures for local authority spending in England[48] show that councils spend *less* on their parks and open spaces per year than they do on their libraries, and libraries are also considered to be very low on the list of political priorities. Concern about this situation has been shaping the sector for a number of years. For example, the creation of CABE Space in 2003 was a direct response to such concerns.[46] Since then CABE Space has been working with others to increase spending and improve the management and planning of greenspace in England's towns and cities.

9.6.3 The policy context

Planning Policy Guidance Note 17 (PPG17)[49] is the principal spatial planning document concerning open space in England. It was published in 2002 following a series of high-level reports and investigations into urban living[50] and urban greenspace[44] which emphasised the economic, social and environmental benefits of high-quality and attractive urban environments. As a national planning document, PPG17 *has* to be taken into account by local authorities and the guidance makes it clear that the provision of open space has numerous benefits, including the health benefits that derive from physical activity and social contact. PPG17 requires local authorities to think strategically about the provision of greenspace in their areas, carrying out an assessment of open space and matching it with an understanding of both current and future needs of the local population for open space of different types (e.g. sports pitches, parks, natural greenspaces, allotments, etc.) setting this out in a distinct open space or greenspace strategy. A companion guide to PPG17[51] gives further guidance to local authorities about the preparation of these strategies. However, monitoring by the CLG[47] shows that there has been relatively slow progress in this regard, and after 5 years only one-quarter of local authorities had a PPG17 style strategy in place, although many others had a strategy in preparation.

As mentioned earlier, one of the key issues which greenspace policy needs to address is the disparity in the provision of greenspace between the least and most deprived neighbourhoods. Perhaps surprisingly, although PPG17 discusses the need to match the provision of open space in an area with the needs of the population for different types of space, it does not set out any national standards for greenspace provision. Because of the variation in greenspace provision between regions, cities and neighbourhoods mentioned above, the UK government has tended to place an emphasis on locally determined standards which are better able to take account of local conditions and needs. Despite this, research in London[52] demonstrates that even local standards are not widely used, partly because such standards do not take into account the quality, accessibility or ecological value of spaces nor do they take account of other types of open space (squares or other paved areas) which also have a part to play in liveable neighbourhoods. Given the evidence about the public health benefits of greenspace this may seem surprising, but the notion of universal quantitative standards has a number of limitations. For example, such standards are essentially arbitrary rather than evidence based and tend to be both rigid and unachievable in many urban settings.[53]

Despite the reticence about such standards, Natural England – the body responsible for nature conservation in England – has developed a set of universal standards for access to natural greenspace. These standards are known as ANGSt (accessible natural greenspace standards) and were first developed in the 1990s. The standards state the following:

- No one should live more than 300 m from a natural greenspace of at least 2 ha.
- There should be at least 1 ha of local nature reserve per thousand population.
- There should be at least one accessible site of 20 ha within 2 km.
- There should be at least one accessible site of 100 ha within 5 km.
- There should be at least one accessible site of 500 ha within 10 km.[53]

The standards are based on the dual benefits provided by natural greenspace within towns and cities, providing both ecological services *and* support for human health and well-being. In relation to the human health benefits of natural greenspace, ANGSt is based on two central ideas: the importance of *everyday* contact with nature, and the notion of a hierarchy of natural spaces in and around our towns and cities. As far as possible ANGSt claims to be evidence based – for example, taking a 300 m straight-line distance from home for the basic measurement since this equates to a 5/6 minute walking threshold beyond which greenspace use declines rapidly.[53]

Alongside ANGSt, there are numerous examples of other greenspace bodies commissioning and publishing research reports about the health benefits of particular types or categories of greenspace.[54] However, while the greenspace sector has been interested in and aware of health concerns for some time, this has not necessarily filtered into local government action. ANGSt, for example, has taken some time to filter into the consciousness, practice and policy of local authorities who have the principal responsibility for managing greenspace. The reasons for this are twofold. The first is that the statutory system of land use planning system has not yet fully rediscovered its long-standing affinity with public health, although the links are becoming stronger and stronger. As a result, local planning authorities are not yet in a position to prioritise public health concerns over and above (or even alongside) other policy goals, for example, economic development or sustainable development. The second problem is that as discussed earlier, the greenspace sector has been rather a poor relation compared to other policy sectors. Ongoing attention to the issue of greenspace by the UK government and its various agencies over the last 10 years has improved the situation enormously. However, greenspace is still underfunded and to some extent undervalued as a policy issue, and a 2006 review of urban greenspace in England noted ongoing concerns about local government management, skills, spending and planning for greenspace.[46]

9.7 Conclusions

This chapter has concentrated on the evidence linking the provision and use of greenspace with obesity. Looking at the links between greenspace and health, physical activity, food environments and children has revealed a rich and varied evidence base which demonstrates that greenspace appears to offer numerous human health benefits. These include reducing stress and its effects on the body; providing a motivation and setting for physical activity; enhancing access to fresh, whole food and influencing play and activity in children. Together, this evidence provides powerful arguments for the provision and protection of greenspaces in and around our towns and cities, and for policy interventions which address the disparities in greenspace provision between neighbourhoods. Unfortunately, while UK policy recognises the health (and other) benefits of greenspace, the historic and institutional context mean that greenspace has been rather undervalued and underfunded as a policy sector for considerable time. The picture is starting to change as evidence of the multiple benefits offered by good quality and accessible greenspace mounts up.

References

1. Frank, L.D., Engelke, P.O., Schmid, T.L. *Health and Community Design: the impact of the built environment on physical activity*. Washington, DC, Island Press, 2003.
2. Ulrich, R.S. (1984) View through a window may influence recovery from surgery. *Science*. 224:420–421.
3. Heerwagen, J.H. The psychological aspects of windows and windowless design. In: *Proceedings of 21st Annual Conference of the Environmental Design Research Association* (Ed. Selby, R.I., *et al.*) EDRA, Edmond, OK, 1990.

4. Hartig, T., Mang, M., Evans, G.W. (1987) Perspectives on wildness: testing the theory of restorative environments. Paper presented at the *Fourth World Wildnerness Congress*, Estes Park, CO.
5. Hartig, T., Evans, G.W., Jammer, L.D., Davis, D.S., Garling, T. (2003) Tracking restoration in natural and urban field settings. *Journal of Environmental Psychology.* 23:109–123.
6. Pretty, J., Peacock, J., Sellens, M., Pretty, C. (2005) The mental and physical health outcomes of green exercise. *International Journal of Environmental Health Research.* 15(5):319–337.
7. Pretty, J., Peacock, J., Hine, R., Sellens, M., South, N., Griffin, M. (2007) Green exercise in the UK countryside: effects on health and psychological well-being, and implications for policy and planning. *Journal of Environmental Planning and Management.* 50(2):211–231.
8. Ulrich, R.S. (1981) Natural versus urban scenes: some psychophysiological effects. *Environment and Behaviour.* 13:523–556.
9. Taylor, A.F., Kuo, F.E., Sulllivan, W.C. (2002) Views of nature and self-discipline: evidence from inner-city children. *Journal of Environmental Pyschology.* 22:49–63.
10. Grahn, P., Stigsdotter, U. (2003) Landscape planning & stress. *Urban Forestry & Urban Greening.* 2:001–018.
11. Burns, G. Naturally happy, naturally healthy: the role of the natural environment in well-being. *The Science of Well-being.* Oxford, Oxford University Press, 2006 pp. 405–431.
12. Everson, S.A., Goldberg, D.E., Kaplan, G.A., *et al.* (1996) Hopelessness and risk of mortality and incidence of myocardial infarction and cancer. *Pyschosomatic Medicine.* 58:113–121.
13. Burns, H., Scotland's Chief Medical Officer. *The Biological Consequences of Living in Adverse Circumstances. Annual Sir Patrick Geddes Lecture.* Edinburgh, RTPI in Scotland, 2008.
14. de Vries, S., Verheij, R., Groenwagen, P., Spreeuwenberg, P. (2003) Natural environments – healthy environments? An exploratory analysis of the relationship between greenspace and health. *Environment and Planning A.* 35:1717–1731.
15. Maas, J., van Dillen, S., Verheij, R., Groenewegen, P. (2009) Social contacts as a possible mechanism behind the relation between green space and health. *Health & Place.* 15:586–595.
16. Maas, J., Verheij, R., Groenewagen, P., de Vries, S., Spreeuwenberg, P. (2005) Greenspace, urbanity and health: how strong is the relation? *Journal of Epidemiological Community Health.* 60:587–592.
17. Mitchell, R., Popham, F. (2008) Effect of exposure to natural environment on health inequalities: an observational population study. *The Lancet.* 372:1655–1660.
18. Norberg-Hodge, H., Merrifield, T., Gorelicke, S. *Bringing the Food Economy Home: Local Alternatives to Global Agribusiness.* London, Zed Books, 2002.
19. Howard, E. The town-country magnet. Reproduced in: *The City Reader* (Eds. LeGates, R.T., Stout, F.) (1996). London, Routledge, 1898.
20. Environment Agency. *The Urban Environment in England and Wales.* Bristol, Environment Agency, 2002.
21. HM Government Obesity Unit. *Healthy Weight, Healthy Lives: One year on.* London, HM Government, 2009.
22. Dowler, E., Blair, A., Donkin, A., Rex, D., Grundy, C. *Measuring Access to Healthy Food in Sandwell.* Sandwell (UK), University of Warwick and Sandwell Health Action Zone, 2001.
23. Department of Health. (2009) Available from http://www.dh.gov.uk/en/News/Recentstories/DH_103380, [cited 2009 01.09.09].
24. Life Island. (2009) Available from http://www.lifeisland.org/, [cited 2009 01.09.09].
25. National Trust. (2009) Available from http://www.nationaltrust.org.uk/main/w-global/w-news/w-latest_news/w-news-growing_spaces.htm, [cited 2009 01/09/09].
26. Barton, H., Grant, M., Guise, R. *Shaping Neighbourhoods: A Guide for Health, Sustainability and Vitality.* London, Spon Press, 2003.
27. The Ecologist. (2009) Ecologist fact April, p. 9.
28. Incredible Edible Todmorden. (2009) Available from www.incredible-edible-todmorden.co.uk, [cited 2009 01.09.09].
29. Grow sheffield. (2009) Available from www.growsheffield.com, [cited 2009 01.09.09].
30. Food Up Front. (2009) Available from www.foodupfront.org, [cited 2009 01.09.09].
31. Grofun. (2009) Available from www.grofun.org.uk, [cited 2009 01.09.09].

32. Sustainable Cities. (2009) Available from http://www.sustainablecities.org.uk/greeninfrastructure/integration/urban-food/, [cited 2009 01.09.09].

33. Ellaway, A., Macintyre, S., Bonnefoy, X. (2005) Graffiti, greenery and obesity in adults: secondary analysis on European cross-sectional survey. *British Medical Journal*. 17:331.

34. Glasgow Centre for Population Health. *Health and the Physical Characteristics of Urban Neighbourhoods: Critical Literature Review*. Briefing Paper No. 2 Concepts Series. Glasgow, GCPH, 2007.

35. Health Scotland, greenspace Scotland, Scottish Natural Heritage & the Institute of Occupational Medicine. *Health Impact Assessment: A Guide*. Stirling, Green space Scotland, 2008.

36. Frumkin, H., Frank, L., Jackson, R. *Urban Sprawl and Public Health, Designing, Planning and Building for Healthy Communities*. Washington, DC, Island Press, 2004.

37. O'Brien, L. *Trees and Woodlands: Nature's Health Service*. Surrey, Forest Research, 2005.

38. Fjortoft, I. (2004) Landscape as playscape: the effect of natural environments on children's play and motor development. *Children, Youth and Environments* 14(2):21–44.

39. Louv, R. *Last Child in the Woods: Saving our Children from Nature-deficit Disorder*. Chapel Hill, NC, Algonquin Books of Chapel Hill, 2005.

40. CABE Space. *Public Space Lessons: Designing and Planning for Play*. London, CABE, 2008.

41. Taylor, A.F., Kuo, F.E., Sullivan, W.C. (2002) Views of nature and self-discipline: evidence from inner-city children. *Journal of Environmental Psychology*. 22:49–63.

42. Bell, J.F., Wilson, J.S., Liu, G.S. (2008) Neighbourhood greenness and 2 years changes in body mass index of children and youth. *American Journal of Preventive Medicine*. 35(6):547–553.

43. Craigie, A.M., Matthews, J.N.S., Rugg-Gunn, A.J., Lake, A.A., Mathers, J.C., Adamson, A.J. (2009) Raised adolescent body mass index predicts the development of adiposity and a central distribution of body fat in adulthood: a longitudinal study. *Obesity Facts*. 2(3):150–156.

44. Department of Transport, Local Government and the Regions (DTLR). *Green Spaces, Better Places: Final Report of the Urban Green Spaces Taskforce*. London, DTLR, 2002.

45. House of Commons. *Committee of Public Accounts: Enhancing Urban Greenspace: Fifty-eighth Report of Session 2005/6*. London, The Stationery Office, 2006.

46. National Audit Office. *'Enhancing Urban Green Space'*. London, The Stationery Office, 2006.

47. Bramley, G., Brown, C., Watkins, D.S. (2009) Not so green and pleasant? Measuring the state of England's urban greenspace. Report to CABE Space: London.

48. Chartered Institute of Public Finance and Accountancy (CIPFA). (2009) Finance & General Statistics 2008/9, www.cipfastats.net.

49. Office of the Deputy Prime Minister (ODPM). *PPG17: Planning for Open Space, Sport and Recreation*. London, ODPM, 2002.

50. Urban Task Force. *Towards an Urban Renaissanace: First Report of the Urban Task Force*. London, Department of Environment, Transport & the Regions, 1999.

51. Office of the Deputy Prime Minister (ODPM). *Assessing Needs and Opportunities: A Companion Guide to PPG17*. London, ODPM, 2002.

52. WS Atkins. *A Review of the Applicability of Standards for Assessing Demand for Open Space in London: Final Report*. London, Unpublished report for London Planning Advisory Committee (LPAC), 2000.

53. English Nature. *Accessible Natural Greenspace Standards in Towns and Cities: A Review and Toolkit for their Implementation*. EN Research Report No. 526. London, English Nature, 2003.

54. O'Brien, L. *Trees and Woodlands: Nature's Health Service*. Surrey, Forest Research, 2005; Health Scotland, Greenspace Scotland, Scottish Natural Heritage & the Institute of Occupational Medicine. *Health Impact Assessment: A Guide*. Stirling, Greenspace Scotland, 2008.

10 Eating Behaviours and the Food Environment

Kylie Ball, David Crawford, Anna Timperio and Jo Salmon

10.1 Introduction

The obesity pandemic has in recent years raised much scientific, political and public interest in the importance of the environment in relation to both eating and physical activity opportunities (the latter are discussed elsewhere in chapters throughout this book). Obesity prevention initiatives in many countries have been characterised by strong calls to modify the environment.[1-3] Such recognition is not new; for example, Rimm and White[4] argued 30 years ago that population obesity was a product of the environment. Despite this, however, there still exists relatively little empirical data from appropriately designed studies investigating associations of environmental factors with individuals' eating behaviours that might impact obesity risk.

This chapter focuses on empirical evidence relating the environment to eating and nutrition-related behaviours relevant to obesity risk in both adults and children. This evidence is interpreted and discussed in light of a number of key conceptual and methodological issues, including the definition of 'neighbourhood environment' and the methods of environmental assessment (subjective vs. objective), the behavioural context and specificity and the application of theoretical conceptual models to further understanding of how environmental factors interact with other determinants to impact eating behaviour and obesity risk. The focus of this chapter is primarily on the influence of physical and economic environmental exposures (principally, food availability, accessibility and affordability) on eating behaviours that might impact obesity risk. However, it is acknowledged that eating behaviours are also influenced by a myriad of factors within the home/family, sociocultural and policy settings.

10.2 Which eating behaviours influence obesity risk?

In order to understand the importance of environmental factors in determining eating behaviours and associated obesity risk, it is important firstly to identify those eating behaviours that are implicated in the development of obesity. Empirical evidence linking specific eating behaviours to adiposity or obesity risk is surprisingly scarce. The limited existing evidence demonstrates that eating behaviours that are most likely associated with increased adiposity include consumption of fast foods, consumption of sugar-sweetened beverages, consumption of foods high in dietary fat (particularly saturated fats), large portion sizes, energy-dense diets and skipping breakfast.[5,6] Conversely, eating behaviours associated with reduced adiposity include consumption of low energy-dense foods including fruits and vegetables, dairy foods (particularly low-fat dairy) and high-fibre foods.

The subsequent review of evidence of environmental determinants of eating behaviours and obesity risk will focus primarily on behaviours associated with adiposity, although given the scarcity of the evidence linking specific eating behaviours to obesity risk, data relating to other eating behaviours will be drawn on where relevant. Clearly, overall energy intakes are a key predictor of obesity risk, but we were unable to identify any studies that examined associations of food availability, accessibility or affordability and overall energy intakes.

10.3   What do we know about the influence of the food environment on eating behaviours?

This section provides an overview of findings from empirical studies examining aspects of the food environment – primarily, food availability, accessibility and affordability – associated with, or predictive of eating behaviours. Data from observational and intervention studies involving both adults and children are presented.

A number of studies have reported on food supply data – that is, data on foods (like fruits or vegetables) available at a national level (e.g. Ref 7). While these studies can tell us about differences or changes in available foods that can be compared with population eating behaviours at an ecological level (e.g. whether countries with greater national availability of fruits and vegetables also have higher proportions of the population meeting fruit and vegetable guidelines), they do not provide strong evidence of associations of the food environment with individuals' consumption of specific foods or the impact of environmental influences on eating behaviours, and hence these studies are not reviewed further here.

10.4   Adults

10.4.1   Observational studies

A limited but growing number of observational studies have examined associations of environmental exposures with specific eating behaviours amongst adults. Two recent systematic reviews have synthesised results of studies examining environmental correlates of consumption of fruit and vegetables[8] and of fat and energy intakes.[9] The review of fruit and vegetable consumption[8] identified that the majority of studies focused on material factors as environmental predictors, generally finding that living in low-income households or neighbourhoods, or being food insecure, was associated with lower fruit and vegetable consumption. Low household income and neighbourhood disadvantage were not, however, strongly associated with energy or fat intakes.[9]

Food accessibility and availability were examined in relatively few studies in both reviews, although these associations have been the focus of a number of studies published more recently. Studies from the US show some evidence for associations of food environmental exposures with diet in adults, although this is far from consistent. For example, having a vegetable garden was associated with higher fruit and vegetable intakes.[10] The presence of a supermarket in the local neighbourhood (US census tract) was positively associated with fruit and vegetable consumption amongst black residents, but not white residents,[11] and the presence of a grocery store, full service restaurant or fast food restaurant was not associated with fruit or vegetable intakes amongst any residents. The presence of grocery stores in the local neighbourhood was negatively associated with saturated fat intakes, but presence of supermarkets, full service or fast food restaurants were not associated with intakes.[11] Proximity to a supermarket was associated with better diet quality amongst pregnant women,[12] and with fruit consumption amongst low-income residents.[13] Greater fresh vegetable availability (assessed by shelf space within stores) within 100 m from home was associated with increased vegetable intake, but not fruit intake, amongst residents in New Orleans. However, in the same study, no associations were found between supermarket access and fruit or vegetable intakes.[14]

Findings from observational studies outside of the United States provide even less evidence to support the notion that food access, availability and affordability impact on dietary intakes. For example, a national study in New Zealand found little evidence of associations of fast food restaurant or supermarket/convenience store access with fruit or vegetable consumption.[15,16] In Melbourne, Australia, density of local fruit and vegetable stores was only weakly correlated with vegetable intakes, but not with fruit intakes, and supermarket density was correlated with neither fruit nor vegetable consumption.[17] A US study showed that the shelf space occupied by healthy foods was negatively correlated with residents' fat intakes,[18] however, in the United Kingdom more recent studies have found no associations between neighbourhood food retail access (e.g. distance to the nearest supermarket, prices of fruits and vegetables) and individual diet (e.g. fruit or vegetable intakes).[19,20]

In summary, findings of observational studies provide some (albeit mixed) evidence of associations of food environmental exposures and eating behaviours predictive of obesity amongst adults in the United States, but very little evidence of such associations in other countries.

10.4.2 Experimental studies

A number of studies have been undertaken to assess effects of environmental intervention strategies on eating behaviours in adults. These have been conducted in both worksites and in the broader community.

In two reviews of environmental interventions targeting eating behaviours, French[21] and Seymour et al.[22] included a review of worksite-based studies, and concluded that results of recent, methodologically sound intervention studies (e.g. Refs 23–27) were modestly positive, indicating that worksite-based nutrition intervention strategies can have beneficial effects on nutrition-related behaviours (primarily fruit and vegetable serves, fat and fibre intakes) amongst worksite populations. However, it is interesting to note that even though these interventions attempted to target broader worksite populations, many still relied primarily on individually based intervention strategies, such as skill building and provision of educational materials. The few that did utilise the capacity for broader environmental change in this setting used strategies such as mass media cafeteria signage, point-of-choice labelling and changes in the food available within worksite cafeterias and vending machines. One difficulty with interpreting results from these studies, however, is the inability to determine which particular component (environmental or educational/individual) was responsible for the behaviour change.

In the broader community, while several large, community-wide interventions targeting healthy eating have been conducted (including the Stanford Three Community Study[28], the Stanford Five-City Project[29], the Minnesota Heart Health Program[30] and the Finnish North Karelia studies[31]), the primary focus of these studies has not been the food environment. Only a relatively small number of methodologically strong, community-based interventions have assessed the effects on diet of modifying aspects of the food environment. Findings from such studies suggest that changes to the availability, accessibility or affordability of healthy foods in the community may result in increased consumption of such foods, although again evidence is mixed. In a review of grocery store interventions,[22] for example, only 5 of the 10 studies identified showed any effects on sales of targeted food items, and those five showed effects for fewer than half of the specific foods targeted. An early study in the United States, for example, found that increasing the amount of allocated space and improving the location of the space for fresh produce in large supermarkets led to increased sales of fruit and vegetable items.[32] An intervention conducted in a grocery store in the Netherlands showed that simply increasing availability of lower fat foods available resulted in reducing energy and percent fat intakes amongst study participants.[33] However, Kristal et al.[34] found that a point-of-purchase intervention in supermarkets had very little impact on fruit and vegetable consumption amongst participants.

Two studies reporting on large-scale food interventions in the United Kingdom also produced mixed findings. In Leeds, reported consumption of fruits and vegetables increased after provision of a large new food retail outlet[35]; however, the uncontrolled, pre–post intervention design of this study does not rule out that such increases may have been due to factors unrelated to the new outlet (such as secular changes in fruit and vegetable intakes generally, in response to increasing messages about the importance of healthy diets). In contrast, a controlled, quasi-experimental study in Glasgow[36] found little evidence for any effect of a new retail outlet on fruit and vegetable consumption.

Finally, price reductions for healthy foods in local markets or supermarkets have been relatively understudied, with the available results suggesting that while such approaches show promise there is insufficient evidence to determine their impact on food purchasing behaviour change.[32,37,38]

A limited number of environmental interventions have been conducted in restaurant settings. These have primarily involved provision of information (such as labelling healthier items on menus). Most of these studies have shown positive effects on purchasing of at least some of the selected items. For example, Albright et al.[39] demonstrated that purchasing of labelled healthier entrée items increased in two of the four restaurants studied. However, other studies found no[40] or inconsistent[41] effects of the restaurant intervention on sales of targeted items.

In summary, findings from existing observational and intervention studies amongst adults provide only limited evidence of an independent role of food promotion, availability, accessibility and affordability on consumption of foods associated with obesity risk, with more consistent evidence arising from methodologically stronger interventions conducted within specific settings (particularly worksites). However, a number of limitations and gaps within the literature remain; these are discussed in more detail in Chapter 13.

10.5   Children and adolescents

10.5.1   Observational studies

A recent review identified 58 papers reporting on observational studies that examined environmental correlates of obesity-related dietary behaviours amongst children and adolescents.[42] That review showed that the majority of the existing studies focused on sociocultural and environmental factors at the household level (e.g. parental education and dietary intakes). However, several papers reported on food availability, accessibility or affordability within the broader environment as correlates of dietary intakes in children or adolescents.

In the school environment, a US study showed that soft drink availability was positively associated with children's soft drink consumption.[43] However, prompts to improve eating at school lunch, and the time that different foods were available at school, were not associated with children's overall energy or total fat intakes.[44] In a study not included in that review, children's fruit intakes did not vary significantly between schools, suggesting little impact of the availability of fresh produce at school on consumption.[45] Amongst adolescents, factors within the school (e.g. an *a la carte* menu, snack and beverage vending machines) were also inconsistently associated with dietary behaviours. Recently studies have begun to objectively examine availability of food outlets surrounding schools. A study in the Netherlands found that availability of supermarkets, fast food outlets, bakeries, small food stores and fruit and vegetable stores within 500 m of school were unrelated to adolescent's snack consumption and snacking behaviour; however, the number of small food stores and the distance from school to the nearest store were inversely associated with adolescent's soft drink consumption.[46] Timperio *et al.*[47] found no associations between children's consumption of takeaway or fast food and the objectively measured presence or number of outlets where these foods could be purchased on the way to school.

In comparison, fewer studies have examined the influence of the objectively assessed features of local neighbourhoods on young people's eating behaviours. In their review, van der Horst *et al.*[42] found no studies examining accessibility, availability or affordability in local neighbourhoods and children's dietary behaviour, and limited and inconsistent evidence of associations between availability of fruit, vegetables and juice in restaurants and grocery stores and dietary behaviours among adolescents. Since that review, several further studies have assessed the associations of environmental factors with children's or adolescents' dietary behaviours. These have generally found support for associations in the expected directions. For instance, relatively consistent negative associations were observed between the objectively assessed availability/accessibility of convenience and fast food restaurants in the local neighbourhood, and children's or adolescents, intakes of fruits and vegetables, in studies in the United States and Australia.[48,49]

10.5.2 Experimental studies

A large number of school-based nutrition interventions targeting a variety of food choices/eating behaviours in both primary and secondary school populations have been conducted (e.g. Child and Adolescent Trial for Cardiovascular Health (CATCH),[50] Pathways,[51] and the 5-A-Day[52] interventions). Overall, these interventions have generally been successful. CATCH and Pathways, for example, modified aspects of the food environment within schools, including reduction in fat in school food service meals, training of food service staff and point-of-purchase promotional signage, in conjunction with classroom curriculum related to healthy eating. Both of these interventions demonstrated healthful changes in student purchasing and eating behaviours, including reductions in fat intakes. It is interesting to note that while a number of studies have shown success in changing eating behaviours in this setting, relatively few have succeeded in impacting body weight amongst school populations. Nonetheless, the evidence suggests that implementing environmental changes within-school settings may represent an effective component of school-based nutrition interventions aimed at modifying eating behaviours.

As with the worksite interventions, the majority of school-based interventions have tended to be multifaceted, and hence it is not possible to evaluate the importance of environmental components as opposed to other intervention components. However, several school-based interventions have focused exclusively on environmental changes. The CHIPS study,[53] based in 12 high schools and 12 worksites in the United States, found that lowering the prices of lower fat snacks increased the purchase of these snacks, with increases in direct proportion to the price reductions. Promotional signage at the point of sale also had a small independent effect on increasing sales. Similarly, several studies[54–56] have shown that increasing the availability of healthful food choices in school cafeterias increased sales of these food items. Collectively these studies provide evidence that the environmental exposures, food pricing and availability have strong influences on food purchasing choices in school settings, and food promotion may also have an independent effect.

10.6   Summary of evidence

Evidence on associations of environmental exposures with obesity-related eating behaviours, while increasing, remains limited and findings inconsistent. Observational studies, particularly outside of the United States, do not provide strong support that environments impact eating behaviours predictive of obesity, but should be viewed in light of a number of research gaps/limitations. There have, in general, been relatively few replicated observational studies investigating associations of food accessibility, availability and affordability and eating behaviours amongst children or adults. Results from intervention studies provide somewhat stronger evidence supporting the importance of environmental influences on eating behaviours, although results are equivocal. Currently, the evidence base regarding the contribution and importance of environmental factors in influencing eating behaviours related to obesity risk is insufficient to justify well-informed public health programs or policies. The following section provides an overview of the key implications of the existing evidence for future research and practice.

10.7   How should we interpret existing evidence?

While research into the influence of food access, availability and affordability is still in its infancy, the mixed findings that have emerged from the studies that have been conducted to date raise a number of issues that warrant further exploration. These relate to the importance of the behavioural context, whether subjective or objective environments should be considered and whether current conceptual models are adequate and appropriate. Given there is presently a stronger body of empirical evidence on the role of the environment in influencing physical activity behaviours than there is for eating behaviours, the discussion below will draw on that literature where appropriate.

10.8   Defining the neighbourhood environment

Within much of the research reviewed in Section 10.3 and in emerging research, there is a strong focus on the neighbourhood environment and as such, this is an important issue to consider when interpreting the existing evidence of the relation between the environment and eating. However, applying a definition of a local neighbourhood for individuals is difficult and this has consequently varied greatly across studies. In addition, evidence suggests substantial between-person variation in perceptions of what constitutes a 'neighbourhood'. For example, a qualitative study of mainly Latina or Hispanic women living in the United States found that those living in lower income areas perceived their neighbourhood to have much smaller boundaries (one-quarter the size) compared with women from higher income areas.[57] In a recent review of literature on environmental influences on eating and physical activity behaviours, we highlighted a number of factors that may account for the inconsistent results that have emerged.[58] Amongst these factors were the use of different administrative definitions of neighbourhoods, the use of different size buffers around study participants' home addresses, a lack of agreement about whether to assess subjective or objective features of the neighbourhood environment, and a lack of consensus about which environmental exposures to assess (these latter two points will be discussed in Sections 10.8.1 and 10.8.2, respectively).

10.8.1   Should we assess subjective or objective food environments?

The majority of the research which has been reviewed in this chapter has incorporated objective measures of the food environment, but to date, descriptive research into the relation between the environment and eating behaviours has also relied on subjective perceptions of environmental characteristics.[59,60] What is more important, the actual food environment to which a person is exposed, or their perceptions of that environment? Does it matter whether or not a fresh fruit and vegetable store is actually present in a person's neighbourhood, or is this only important if they are aware of it?

Surprisingly, little research has examined the concordance between perceived and actual measures of the environment. In a study of the mismatch between perceptions of the availability of recreational facilities for physical activity and objective audits of those facilities, we found that a substantial portion of the community were unaware of such facilities in their neighbourhood and that this varied according to age, income, self-efficacy for physical activity and physical activity levels.[61] These findings are important since they highlight that studies of environment–behaviour relations that rely only on perceptions should be interpreted with caution. Studies that use measures of the perceived environment as a proxy for assessing the actual environment may incorrectly identify an association where none exists or vice versa. It may be argued that the most important type of measure to use is the one that best predicts or explains behaviour. In physical activity research, some studies have found objective measures[62] to be more predictive, and others have shown subjective measures[63] to be more strongly associated with behaviour. In one of the few studies to assess objectively measured and perceived environmental correlates of food-related behaviours, Giskes et al.[64] reported that perceived availability and prices of recommended foods in supermarkets were associated with the purchase of these foods, whereas objectively assessed availability and prices were not. Clearly, further research is necessary to determine the most appropriate means of assessing environmental exposures that impact on food purchasing and eating behaviours.

10.8.2   The importance of understanding the behavioural context

In their seminal review of research designed to promote nutrition-related behaviours, Baranowski et al.[65] argued that nutrition promotion interventions are more likely to be successful when they focus on a specific behavioural outcome (e.g. reducing soft drink consumption, as opposed to reducing total sugar intake). Similarly, research into the relation between environment and diet is likely to yield more interpretable results when it is focused on understanding specific eating behaviours. For example, a consideration of the environmental influences on total sugar intake may be less likely to yield meaningful results than a study that focuses on soft drink intake because we have greater capacity to assess the environmental influences on soft drink intake (i.e. because total sugar intake is determined by multiple eating behaviours and therefore will involve multiple environmental exposures).

It is also important to recognise that people live their lives in multiple settings or contexts[66] and all these may potentially have some impact on eating behaviours. For example, for many adults the foods that are available at work (e.g. cafeterias and vending machines) and around their place of work (local food outlets, such as cafes, restaurants and fast food stores) may also be important. They may also purchase food or be exposed to food advertising on billboards and at food outlets on their way to and from work, particularly if they use public transport to commute to work. The foods available in the neighbourhoods where an adult lives and works, or where children live and where they study, will, therefore, potentially influence eating behaviours, but, with few exceptions,[47,67] such multiple settings have not been considered simultaneously in examinations of environmental influences on eating behaviours.

The behavioural context of food and eating is also likely to vary across the population. The settings that children are exposed to will be different from those of adults, where the school and after-school care settings will feature. This is also likely to differ between young children and teenagers, who have more independence and discretionary funds. However, even among a particular population group the importance of different settings will vary. For example, amongst adults of high socio-economic position (SEP), the availability of supermarkets and other food outlets, like fruit and vegetable stores, in their local neighbourhood may be less important than for low SEP groups, who may not have ready access to private transport and rely on public transport or walking to shop for food. The same may also be true for those older adults who have lost the capacity to drive. It is therefore possible that the same food environment may have quite different impacts on eating behaviours amongst two people who live in close proximity but have different socio-demographic characteristics (e.g. a working parent and a frail retired person living alone).

10.8.3   Are existing conceptual models adequate and appropriate?

It has been argued that 'nothing is more practical than a good theory', and it is well recognised that the application of behavioural theory is critically important in order to gain a comprehensive knowledge of the determinants of complex phenomena such as eating behaviours. However, to date many of the theoretical models that have been used to assist with understanding and influencing people's eating behaviours have focused primarily on individual cognitions (e.g. attitudes, intentions, preference, self-efficacy) and to a lesser extent proximal social factors such as the influence of family, friends or work colleagues (e.g. Ref 68). More recently, social ecological models that emphasise the influence of a broad range of environmental aspects have been favoured.[66,69] These models posit that there are multiple levels of influence on behaviour that interact across the individual, sociocultural, physical and policy environments within and across different settings and population groups. For example, factors that may influence what a child eats for morning recess in a school setting could include presence of a school canteen, the school's healthy canteen policy, snack options available, whether parents provided food or money for morning recess, the cost of the items, what the child's friends have to eat, the time taken to queue at the canteen and what the child would prefer to eat. As this simple example illustrates, the influences on eating behaviours can occur at multiple levels and can vary by context, setting and population group.

Few studies to date have been designed to comprehensively examine such multiple levels of influence on people's eating behaviours. Perhaps this is because such research is methodologically challenging, usually requiring large population-based samples and reliable and valid measures of these influences. While it is unlikely that behavioural science will ever manage to explain all of the variance in people's eating behaviours, the benefit of such studies is able to examine the *relative* levels of influence and therefore identify the key factors that should be targeted in intervention studies. There is also a need for more sophisticated theoretical models that better explain how determinants at different levels (i.e. individual vs. environmental) interact to explain eating behaviours, and the mediators (mechanisms) and moderators (effect modifiers) of change in people's eating behaviours over time and resulting from interventions.

Many of the studies of environmental influences on eating behaviour have been atheoretical in nature. Whether existing theoretical models are most appropriate for explaining and influencing adults' and children's eating behaviours is an issue requiring further consideration. Most of the current theories used in health behaviour research have been developed for use with adults. While developmental theories have been used to understand how children learn behaviour (e.g. social learning theory), the role of the family and broader neighbourhood environments is not well enunciated in such theories. It has been argued that the most successful and efficacious behavioural interventions are those that have utilised a theoretical framework[70]; therefore, it is important that future research on the role of the environment in children's and adults' eating behaviours applies relevant and informative behavioural theories.

10.9 Conclusions and future research directions

While there is emerging evidence of the influence of the environment on people's eating behaviours, as reviewed in this chapter, there are some obvious gaps in evidence and future research needs. For example, careful conceptualisation and measurement of environmental exposures likely to influence eating behaviours is paramount. This should be determined by the specific study aims and informed by appropriate theoretical frameworks. There is a need for the development and validation of measures of food environmental characteristics that are feasible for large epidemiological studies and across a variety of locations and contexts. Consideration should also be given to the multiple contexts in which people live, work, study and play, and research is required to investigate the relative importance of environments across such contexts in impacting eating behaviours. Given the discrepancies in findings from observational studies across different countries (primarily between the United States and other parts of the developed world), research enabling direct comparisons across localities would be of value.

Further evidence based on studies employing appropriate methodologically strong study designs, such as multilevel studies, prospective and longitudinal research, and intervention studies is also required. Given the practical difficulties in conducting appropriately controlled randomised interventions of environmental strategies, particularly on a large scale, the use of quasi-experimental research designs including capitalising on 'natural experiments' is warranted. There is also a need for intervention designs which allow for identification of the efficacy of various intervention elements, for example, education versus increasing availability versus promotion versus pricing.

Very few studies have examined the influence of culture or policy. Culture is an understudied concept, often naively operationalised as ethnicity. Cultural factors, however, encompass much more than one's ethnic group, and incorporate shared values, beliefs and practices that are likely to pose a strong influence on eating behaviours, yet for which little empirical evidence exists. Policies in relation to people's eating behaviours have also been infrequently studied, and rarely has the full complement of various types of policy been applied in a single study. Policies may be formal written codes or laws legislated at the national, organisational or local government level, written standards that guide choices, or unwritten social norms. For example, in some places, such as Sweden and Quebec in Canada, the government has implemented a policy banning food advertising during children's television viewing times. Further research investigating the influence of the cultural and policy environments on people's eating behaviours is required.

Finally, decades of research establishing the importance to healthy eating of individual factors (such as taste and preferences, perceptions of convenience and self-efficacy) should not be overlooked in the recent enthusiasm of researchers and policymakers to identify environmental determinants of eating behaviours. Theoretically, grounded research incorporating appropriate multilevel study designs and tests of cross-level interactions will be of great value in further understanding of the relative importance of individual and environmental determinants of eating behaviours and obesity risk.

References

1. Australian National Obesity Taskforce. Healthy Weight 2008: *Australia's Future*. 2008 [cited 2008 June 8], available from: http://www.healthyactive.gov.au/publications.htm.

2. Hill, J.O., Peters, J.C. (1998) Environmental contributions to the obesity epidemic. *Science.* 280:1371–1374.
3. Katz, D.L., O'Connell, M., Yeh, M.C., Nawaz, H., Njike, V., Anderson, L.M., Cory, S., Dietz, W. (2005) Public health strategies for preventing and controlling overweight and obesity in school and worksite settings: a report on recommendations of the Task Force on Community Preventive Services. *MMWR Recommendations and Reports.* 54(RR-10):1–12.
4. Rimm, A.A., White, P.L. Obesity: its risks and hazards. In: *Obesity in America: A Conference.* (Ed. Bray, G.A.) 1st Edition, NIH Publication No 80-359 U.S. Department of Health, Education, and Welfare, Public Health Service, National Institutes of Health, Bethesda, MD, 1979. pp. 103–124.
5. Greenwood, J., Stanford, J. (2008) Preventing or improving obesity by addressing specific eating patterns. *Journal of the American Board of Family Medicine.* 21:135–140.
6. Newby, P.K. (2007) Are dietary intakes and eating behaviors related to childhood obesity? A comprehensive review of the evidence. *The Journal of Law, Medicine and Ethics.* 35(1):35–60
7. Naska, A., Vasdekis, V.G.S., Trichopoulou, A., Friel, S., Leonhauser, I.U., Moreiras, O., Nelson, M., Remaut, A.M., Schmitt, A., Sekula, W., Trvgg, K.U., Zajkás, G. (2000) Fruit and vegetable availability among 10 European countries - how does it compare with the 'five a day' recommendation. *British Journal of Nutrition.* 84(4):549–556.
8. Kamphuis, C.B., Giskes, K., de Bruijn, G.J., Wendel-Vos, W., Brug, J., van Lenthe, F.J. (2006) Environmental determinants of fruit and vegetable consumption among adults: a systematic review. *British Journal of Nutrition.* 96(4):620–635.
9. Giskes, K., Kamphuis, C.B.M., Lenthe, F.J.V., Kremers, S., Droomers, M., Brug, J. (2007) A systematic review of associations between environmental factors, energy and fat intakes among adults: is there evidence for environments that encourage obesogenic dietary intakes? *Public Health Nutrition.* 10(10):1005.
10. Devine, C.M., Wolfe, W.S., Frongillo, E.A.J., Bisogni, C.A. (1999) Life course events and experiences: association with fruit and vegetable consumption in 3 ethnic groups. *Journal of the American Dietetic Association.* 99:309–314.
11. Morland, K., Wing, S., Diez Roux, A. (2002) The contextual effect of the local food environment on residents' diets: the atherosclerosis risk in communities study. *American Journal of Public Health.* 92(11):1761–1767.
12. Laraia, B.A., Siega-Riz, A.M., Kaufman, J.S., Jones, S.J. (2004) Proximity of supermarkets is positively associated with diet quality index for pregnancy. *Preventive Medicine.* 39(5):869–875.
13. Rose, D., Richards, R. (2004) Food store access and household fruit and vegetable use among participants in the US Food Stamp Program. *Public Health Nutrition.* 7(8):1081–1088.
14. Bodor, J.N., Rose, D., Farley, T.A., Swalm, C., Scott, S.K. (1997) Neighbourhood fruit and vegetable availability and consumption: the role of small food stores in an urban environment. *Public Health Nutrition.* 11(4):413–420.
15. Pearce, J., Hiscock, R., Blakely, T., Witten, K. (2008) The contextual effects of neighbourhood access to supermarkets and convenience stores on individual fruit and vegetable consumption. *Journal of Epidemiology and Community Health.* 62:198–201.
16. Pearce, J., Hiscock, R., Blakely, T., Witten, K. (2008) A national study of the association between neighbourhood access to fast-food outlets and the diet and weight of local residents. *Health and Place.* doi: 10.1016/jhealthplace.2008.04.003.
17. Ball, K., Crawford, D., Mishra, G. (2006) Socio-economic inequalities in women's fruit and vegetable intakes: a multilevel study of individual, social and environmental mediators. *Public Health Nutrition.* 9(5):623–630.
18. Cheadle, A., Psaty, B.M., Curry, S., Wagner, E., Diehr, P., Koepsell, T., Kristal, A. (1991) Community-level comparisons between the grocery store environment and individual dietary practices. *Preventive Medicine.* 20(2):250–261.
19. Pearson, T., Russell, J., Campbell, M.J., Barker, M.E. (2005) Do 'food deserts' influence fruit and vegetable consumption?--a cross-sectional study. *Appetite.* 45(2):195–197.
20. White, M., Buntin, J., Raybould, S., Adamson, A., Williams, L., Mathers, J. Do Food Deserts Exist? A multi-level, geographical analysis of the relationship between retail food access,

socio-economic position and dietary intake. Final report to the Food Standards Agency, 2004.

21. French, S.A. Population approaches to promote healthful eating behaviors. In: *Obesity Prevention and Public Health*. (Eds. Crawford, D., Jeffery, R.W.). Oxford, Oxford University Press, 2005. pp. 101–127.

22. Seymour, J.D., Yaroch, A.L., Serdula, M., Blanck, H.M., Khan, L.K. (2004) Impact of nutrition environmental interventions on point of purchase behavior in adults: a review. *Preventive Medicine*. 39(Suppl. 2):S108–S136.

23. Beresford, S.A., Thompson, B., Feng, Z., Christianson, A., McLerran, D., Patrick, D.L. (2001) Seattle 5 a day worksite program to increase fruit and vegetable consumption. *Preventive Medicine*. 32:230–238.

24. Buller, D., Morrill, C., Taren, D., Aickin, M., Sennott-Miller, L., Buller, M.K., Larkey, L., Alatorre, C., Wentzel, T.M. (1999) Randomized trial testing the effect of peer education at increasing fruit and vegetable intake. *Journal of the National Cancer Institute*. 91:1491–1500.

25. Jeffery, R., French, S., Raether, C., Baxter, J.E. (1994) An environmental intervention to increase fruit and salad purchases in a cafeteria. *Preventive Medicine*. 23:788–792.

26. Sorenson, G., Thompson, B., Glanz, K., Feng, Z., Kinne, S., DiClemente, C., Emmons, K., Heimendinger, J., Probart, C., Lichtenstein, E. (1996) Work site-based cancer prevention: primary results from the Working Well Trial. *American Journal of Public Health*. 86: 939–947.

27. Tilley, B., Glanz, K., Kristal, A., Hirst, K., Li, S., Vernon, S., Myers, R. (1999) Nutrition intervention for high-risk auto workers: results of the Next Step Trial. *Preventive Medicine*. 28(3):284–292.

28. Fortmann, S., Williams, P., Hulley, S., Haskell, W., Farquhar, J.W. (1981) Effect of health education on dietary behavior: the Stanford three community study. *American Journal of Clinical Nutrition*. 34:2030–2038.

29. Farquhar, J., Fortmann, S., Maccoby, N., Haskell, W.L., Williams, P.T., Flora, J.A., Taylor, C.B., Brown, B.W. Jr, Solomon, D.S., Hulley, S.B. (1985) The Stanford Five-City Project: design and methods. *American Journal of Epidemiology*. 122:323–334.

30. Luepker, R., Murray, D., Jacobs, D., *et al.* (1994) Community education for cardiovascular disease prevention: risk factor changes in the Minnesota Heart Health Program. *American Journal of Public Health*. 84:1383–1393.

31. Puska, P., Salonen, J., Nissinen, A., Tuomilehto, J., Vartiainen, E., Korhonen, H., Tanskanen, A., Rönnqvist, P., Koskela, K., Huttunen, J. (1983) Change in risk factors for coronary heart disease during 10 years of a community intervention programme (North Karelia project). *British Medical Journal*. 287:1840–1844.

32. Curhan, R.C. (1974) The effects of merchandising and temporary promotional activities on the sales of fresh fruits and vegetables in supermarkets. *Journal of Marketing Research*. 11:286–294.

33. Westrate, J., van het Hof, K., van den Berg, H., Velthuis-te-Wierik, E.J., de Graaf, C., Zimmermanns, N.J., Westerterp, K.R., Westerterp-Plantenga, M.S., Verboeket-van de Venne, W.P. (1998) A comparison of the effect of free access to reduced fat products or their full fat equivalents on food intake, body weight, blood lipids and fat-soluble antioxidants levels and haemostasis variables. *European Journal of Clinical Nutrition*. 52:389–395.

34. Kristal, A., Goldenhar, L., Muldoon, J., Morton, R. (1994) Evaluation of a supermarket intervention to increase consumption of fruits and vegetables. *American Journal of Health Promotion*. 11 422–425.

35. Wrigley, N., Warm, D., Margetts, B., Whelan, A. (2002) Assessing the impact of improved retail access on diet in a 'food desert': a preliminary report. *Urban Studies*. 39(11):2061–2082.

36. Cummins, S., Petticrew, M., Sparks, L., Findlay, A. (2005) Large scale food retail interventions and diet. *British Medical Journal*. 330(7493):683–684.

37. Anliker, J., Winne, M., Drake, L. (1992) An evaluation of the Connecticut Farmers' market coupon program. *Journal of Nutrition Education*. 24:185–191.

38. Balsam, A., Webber, D., Oehlke, B. (1994) The Farmers' Market Coupon Program for low-income elders. *Journal of Nutrition for the Elderly*. 13:35–42.

39. Albright, C., Flora, J., Fortmann, S. (1990) Restaurant menu labeling: impact of nutrition information on entree sales and patron attitudes. *Health Education Quarterly*. 17:157–167.
40. Scott, L., Foreyt, J., Manis, E., O'Malley, M., Grotto, A. Jr. (1979) A low-cholesterol menu in a steak restaurant. *Journal of the American Dietetic Association*. 74:54–56.
41. Dubbert, P., Johnson, W., Schlundt, D., Montague, N. (1984) The influence of caloric information on cafeteria food choices. *Journal of Applied Behavior Analysis*. 17:85–92.
42. van der Horst, K., Oenema, A., Ferreira, I., Wendel-Vos, W., Giskes, K., van Lenthe, F., Brug, J. (2007) A systematic review of environmental correlates of obesity-related dietary behaviors in youth. *Health Education Research*. Jul 21:203–226.
43. Grimm, G., Harnack, L., Story, M. (2004) Factors associated with soft drink consumption in school-aged children. *Journal of the American Dietetic Association*. 104:1244–1249.
44. Zive, M., Frank-Spohrer, G.C., Sallis, J., McKenzie, T.L., Elder, J.P., Berry, C.C., Broyles, S.L., Nader, P.R. (1998) Determinants of dietary intake in a sample of white and Mexican-American children. *Journal of the American Dietetic Association*. 98:1282–1289.
45. Vereecken, C., Bobelijn, K., Maes, L. (2005) School food policy at primary and secondary schools in Belgium-Flanders: does it influence young people's food habits. *European Journal of Clinical Nutrition*. 59:271–277.
46. van der Horst, K., Timperio, A., Crawford, D., Roberts, R., Brug, J., Oenema, A. (2008) The school food environment: associations with adolescent soft drink and snack consumption. *American Journal of Preventive Medicine*. 35(3):217–223.
47. Timperio, A., Ball, K., Roberts, R., Andrianopoulos, N., Crawford, D. (2009) Children's fast food intake and availability of food outlets near home and on the way to school. *Public Health Nutrition*. 12:1960–1964.
48. Jago, R., Baranowski, T., Baranowski, J.C. (2006) Observed, GIS, and self-reported environmental features and adolescent physical activity. *American Journal of Health Promotion*. 20(6):422–428.
49. Timperio, A., Ball, K., Roberts, R., Campbell, K., Andrianopoulos, N., Crawford, D. (2008) Children's fruit and vegetable intake: associations with the neighbourhood food environment. *Preventive Medicine*. 46:331–335
50. Leupker, R., Perry, C., McKinlay, S., *et al.* (1996) Outcomes of a field trial to improve children's dietary patterns and physical activity: the Child and Adolescent Trial for Cardiovascular Health (CATCH). *JAMA*. 275:768–776.
51. Caballero, B., Clay, T., Davis, S.M., Ethelbah, B., Rock, B.H., Lohman, T., Norman, J., Story, M., Stone, E.J., Stephenson, L., Stevens, J., Pathways Study Research Group (2003) Pathways: a school-based, randomized controlled trial for the prevention of obesity in American Indian schoolchildren. *American Journal of Clinical Nutrition*. 78:1030–1038.
52. Foerster, S., Gregson, J., Beall, D.L., Hudes, M., Magnuson, H., Livingston, S., Davis, M.A., Joy, A.B., Garbolino, T. (1998) The California children's 5-a-Day Power Play! Campaign: evaluation of a large-scale social marketing initiative. *Family and Community Health*. 21:46–64.
53. French, S.A., Jeffery, R.W., Story, M., Breitlow, K.K., Baxter, J.S., Hannan, P., Snyder, M.P. (2001) Pricing and promotion effects of low-fat vending snack purchases: the CHIPS study. *American Journal of Public Health*. 91:112–117.
54. French, S.A., Story, M., Fulkerson, J.A., Hannan, P. (2004) An environmental intervention to promote lower-fat food choices in secondary schools: outcomes of the TACOS Study. *American Journal of Public Health*. 94(9):1507–1512.
55. Perry, C.L., Bishop, D.B., Taylor, G.L., Davis, M., Story, M., Gracy, C., Bishop, S.C., Mays, R.A., Lytle, L.A., Harnack, L. (2004) A randomized school trial of environmental strategies to encourage fruit and vegetable consumption among children. *Health Education and Behavior*. 31:65–76.
56. Whitaker, R., Wright, J., Finch, A., Psaty, B.M. An environmental intervention to reduce dietary fat in school lunches. (1993) *Pediatrics*. 91:1107–1111.
57. Yen, I.H., Scherzer, T., Cubbin, C., Gonzalez, A., Winkleby, M.A. (2007) Women's perceptions of neighborhood resources and hazards related to diet, physical activity, and smoking: focus group results from economically distinct neighborhoods in a mid-sized U.S. City. *American Journal of Health Promotion*. 22:98–106.

58. Ball, K., Timperio, A.F., Crawford, D.A. (2006) Understanding environmental influences on nutrition and physical activity behaviors: where should we look and what should we count? *The International Journal of Behavioral Nutrition and Physical Activity*. 3:33.

59. Inglis, V., Ball, K., Crawford, D. (2008) Socioeconomic variations in women's diets: What is the role of perceptions of the local food environment? *Journal of Epidemiology and Community Health*. 62(3):191–197.

60. Veugelers, P., Sithole, F., Zhang, S., Muhajarine, N. (2008) Neighborhood characteristics in relation to diet, physical activity and overweight of Canadian children. *International Journal of Pediatric Obesity*. 3:152–159.

61. Ball, K., Jeffery, R.J., Crawford, D.A., Roberts, R.J., Salmon, J., Timperio, A.F. (2008) Mismatch between perceived and objective measures of physical activity environments. *Preventive Medicine*. 47:294–298.

62. Sallis, J.F., Hovell, M.F., Hofstetter, C.R., Elder, J.P., Hackley, M., Caspersen, C.J., Powell, K.E. (1990) Distance between homes and exercise facilities related to frequency of exercise among San Diego residents. *Public Health Reports*. 105:179–185

63. Hoehner, C.M., Brennan Ramirez, L.K., Elliott, M.B., Handy, S.L., Brownson, R.C. (2005) Perceived and objective environmental measures and physical activity among urban adults. *American Journal of Preventive Medicine*. 28(2, Suppl. 2):105–116.

64. Giskes, K., Van Lenthe, F.J., Brug, J., Mackenbach, J.P., Turrell, G. (2007) Socioeconomic inequalities in food purchasing: the contribution of respondent-perceived and actual (objectively measured) price and availability of foods. *Preventive Medicine*. 45(1):41–48.

65. Baranowski, T., Weber, K., Cullen, W., Baranowski, J. (1999) Psychosocial correlates of dietary intake: advancing dietary intervention. *Annual Review of Nutrition*. 19:17–40.

66. Stokols, D. (2000) Social ecology and behavioural medicine: implications for training, practice and policy. *Behavioral Medicine*. 26:129–138.

67. Jeffery, R.W., Baxter, J., McGuire, M., Linde, J. (2006) Are fast food restaurants an environmental risk factor for obesity? *The International Journal of Behavioral Nutrition and Physical Activity*. 3:2.

68. Ajzen, I. From intentions to actions: a theory of planned behavior. In: *Action-control: From Cognition to Behavior*. (Eds. Kuhl, J., Beckman, J.) Heidelbert, Germany, Springer, 1985. pp. 11–39.

69. Bronfenbrenner, U. (1977) Toward an experimental ecology of human development. *American Psychologist*. 32:513–531.

70. Cliska, D., Miles, E., O'Brien, M.A., Turl, C., Tomasik, H.H., Donovan, U., Bevers, J. (2000) Effectiveness of community-based interventions to increase fruit and vegetable consumption. *Journal of Nutrition Education*. 32:241–252.

11 Food Policy and Food Governance – Changing Behaviours

Amelia A. Lake and Jane L. Midgley

11.1 Introduction

In 1944 Boudreau stated, 'Food policy is a social and political weapon of no mean importance today'[1] (p. 215). In the present era, food and food policy remain an emotive topic; issues around food, health and food safety are seldom out of the news.[2] Food policy and food governance (the relationship between stakeholders and government) have an important role defining and understanding why we eat what we eat. Food choice is a complex amalgamation and interrelationship between both sociocultural and biological factors.[2] While food is physiologically essential for the body to function, it is well accepted that sociocultural and environmental determinants can have a strong role in deciding which foods are consumed. Interest in the food environment and its role in promoting obesity has gained recent prominence,[3] however, this exploration of the food environment as a component of the obesogenic environment is a relatively new field of research.[4]

The obesogenic environment has been defined as 'the sum of influences that the surroundings, opportunities, or conditions of life have on promoting obesity in individuals or populations.' (p. 564).[5] These 'obesogenic environments' are considered to be one of the driving forces behind today's escalating obesity crisis.[5] The ANGELO (analysis grid for environments linked to obesity) framework[5] can be used to define the obesogenic environment. In this framework, the environment is divided into two levels 'micro-environments' and 'macro-environments'; the former includes schools, workplaces, home environment, retailers, community groups and neighbourhoods; the latter includes policy, education systems, the media, transportation systems and health systems. Within the ANGELO framework there are four categories of environment: physical ('what is available'), political (which broadly includes policy), sociocultural ('attitudes and beliefs') and the economic environment.[6] Policy and governance relating to food can be seen to cut across all of the four categories of the environment.

Eating habits can be described as one of the most complex of human behaviours.[2] Food habits and food choices are a negotiated set of behaviours within a social setting which are open to a wide variety of influences,[2,7] one of which is the broader food environment. The food environment can be defined as any opportunity to obtain food.[8] This definition of the food environment can include physical, sociocultural, economic and policy factors at both micro- and macro-level.[8] It includes food availability and accessibility in addition to food advertising and marketing.[9]

Micro-level studies have focused on schools and workplaces. Recent policy changes in England and research have enforced the fact that schools are recognised as an important environment that can shape and influence the health-related habits of young people.[10,11] Prior to the new English school food guidelines, research in secondary schools reported that a large variety of unhealthy options made it difficult for young people to choose a healthy diet.[10] Since May 2006, changes in English school food policy have sought to dramatically modify the food environment in schools and have an impact upon young people's eating behaviours.[12] The ongoing evolution and evaluation of these interventions will be of interest to numerous stakeholders. What foods are available *outside* the school grounds is an environment of interest to both researchers and policymakers. In the United States, a study found a clustering of fast food restaurants around schools.[13] In England, there has been interest in the school fringe (shops that surround secondary schools – pupils aged 11–18 years). A pilot study of two secondary schools in the south-east of England[14] found that pupils obtained food from the shops that surrounded their secondary school, rather than their school canteen. The research observed that the nutritional quality of these fringe purchases was low, in particular the overconsumption of sugar by girls. This research suggested that the current focus on school food be expanded to include the foods available on the school fringe.

In terms of the macro-food environment, messages about food reach individuals in numerous ways including educational materials, information about food products and information from food retailers.[15] Sophisticated advertising and marketing campaigns are used to promote food products. It is reported for every $1 spent by the World Health Organisation (WHO) to improve nutrition, $500 is spent by the food industry on processed foods.[16] In the United Kingdom, advertising of fruit and vegetables is considerably lower than other foods. Figures from the 2003 Advertising Statistics Yearbook[17] report £15.2 million being spent on total confectionery advertising in 2002, compared with £2.8 million on fresh fruit and £1.2 million on fresh vegetables. However, since 2007 the OFCOM, an independent organisation which regulates the UK's broadcasting, telecommunications and wireless communications sectors, restrictions on TV advertising to children (under 16 years old) are likely to have influenced these figures.

A number of studies have explored the food environment at a macro-level and have looked at fast food outlets and their geographical position in relation to socio-economic status (see also Chapter 12 by Pearce and Day). Cummins *et al.*[18] reported that greater the level of neighbourhood deprivation in Scotland and England, the more likely the neighbourhoods were exposed to McDonalds restaurants. Conversely, work in Glasgow found no association between area of deprivation and access to takeaway outlets.[19] In New Zealand[20], travel distance to outlets selling fast food was found to be twice as much for the least socially deprived neighbourhoods as compared with the most deprived neighbourhoods.

This distance 'pattern' was also observed in outlets where healthy food could be purchased such as supermarkets and smaller food outlets. As a result of this work, Pearce et al.[20] emphasise the need to explore all aspects of the food environment, not just the fast food environment (see Chapter 12).

The macro-environment is constantly changing. The food environment or the 'foodscape' in the United Kingdom has changed rapidly over the last 20 years;[21] accompanying this change have been increases in rates of overweight and obesity. Using historical Yellow Pages data from 1980 and 2000 while focusing on an area within the North East England, Burgoine et al.[21] reported dramatic rise in the total number of food outlets between 1980 and 2000 (79%). There were modest increases in food retail outlets (16%); however, the overall number of outlets to obtain 'foods for consumption away from home' increased by 259% from 27 in 1980 to 97 in 2000.[21]

Addressing the economic environment, the cost of food is a critical factor in food choice. Our environment provides vast amounts of cheap food.[22] US economic analysis[23] has pointed to the inverse relationship between the energy density of food (kJ/g) and the energy cost ($/MJ). The least healthy foods high in added sugar and fat are more affordable than the recommended healthy alternatives of lean meats, wholegrains, fresh fruit and vegetables.[23] The lower cost of food as a proportion of household expenditure is seen as an indicator of economic progress and improving health.[24] While the amount spent by households in the United Kingdom on food supplies has reduced to 10%, lower income households spend more than 23% of household income and higher income households spend less than 15% of their income on food.[22]

Eating has been described as more of a 'public' rather than 'private' phenomenon now, compared with the past.[25] Eating out, particularly the increase in quick meals outside the home,[26] has been 'embedded' in our culture.[27] This increase in consuming food outside of the home requires a better understanding of what drives the decisions of the food industry.[28] In a series of interviews with senior menu development and marketing executives at chain restaurants in the United States, Glanz et al.[28] reported that economic drivers and consumer demand determine whether or not healthier options are available in restaurants.

The 2003 WHO report entitled *Diet, Nutrition and the Prevention of Chronic Disease*[29] reflects how shifts in the world food economy are mirrored in global dietary patterns. In the introductory chapter, James et al. describe the historical context of the obesity epidemic and the huge imbalance in the energy requirements available to us compared with our current energy expenditure. Food and Nutrition Policy has a significant role in the world food economy and global food markets. Policy determines what foods are grown through to which foods are present in the retail outlets in which the consumers make their food choices.

This chapter addresses the complex relationship between policies which influence food (in terms of agricultural, planning and health policies), the food environment and individual food intake. The chapter looks specifically, but not exclusively, at England and the United Kingdom. Chapter 10 by Ball et al. has explored eating behaviours in relation to the food environments and has highlighted the relationship between the environment and nutrition-related behaviours, relevant to obesity risk, both in adults and children.

11.2   Dietary guidelines and recommendations with reference to obesity prevention

Unhealthy diets are linked to a number of chronic diseases, including obesity. It is well established that dietary habits in early life influence the risk of developing several chronic diseases.[30] Food and nutrition are central themes in global and national health policies.[29,31] In the United Kingdom, 'healthy eating' has been an integral aspect of successive health policies.[31–34]

While nutrition is a relatively young science which only began to be systematically studied at the beginning of the 20th century,[35] dietary guidelines and dietary advice have been remarkably stable. Current UK Dietary Reference Values (DRVs) were published in 1991.[36] In the United Kingdom, food-based healthy eating guidelines using the Eatwell Plate[37,38] focus on increasing fruit and vegetables and fibre and decreasing foods high in salt, sugar and fat. Dietary advice, with regard to prevention of overweight and obesity, is based around the simple physiological concept of energy balance. In order to maintain a healthy weight, energy balance (i.e. energy in and energy out) must be maintained.

Despite contradictory and confusing messages in the media about health and nutrition,[39] the British public do appear to be increasingly aware of, and interested in, the relationship between the foods they consume and their health.[40] The message to consume more fruit and vegetables is probably one of the most consistent dietary messages over recent years.[40] Fat reduction messages, associated with the reduction of cardiovascular disease, have had an impact nationally, where daily intake of fat has decreased by >30 g over the last 20 years and saturated fatty acids have fallen by >20 g.[41] Where intakes of fat have fallen nationally, intakes of sodium have shown very little movement (excluding sodium in table salt, 2.6 g/day since 1985[41]). Recently the Food Standards Agency (FSA)'s focus on salt has targeted both the individual consumer as well as the food industry to reduce levels of salt in foods.[42]

Following the publication of the Foresight Obesity Report in Autumn 2007,[24] the English policy response to the obesity epidemic has resulted in the publication of the cross-government strategy *Healthy Weight, Healthy Lives*.[43] This document sets out the ambition to be the 'first major nation to reverse the rising tide of obesity and overweight in the population . . .' (p. v).[43]

11.3   Individual versus the environment

The 2008 Healthy Weight, Healthy Lives strategy[43] suggests policies which extend from the individual to their environment with a strong focus on the environment (see Chapter 2). However, in the Foreword, Prime Minister Gordon Brown clearly states that the responsibility of maintaining a health weight lies with the individual: 'There should be no doubt that maintaining a healthy weight must be the responsibility

Table 11.1   Healthy Weight, Healthy Lives – five areas for tackling excess weight.

1. Children	Healthy growth and healthy weight – early prevention of weight problems to avoid the 'conveyor-belt' effect into adulthood
2. Promoting healthier food choices	Reducing the consumption of foods that are high in fat, sugar and salt and increasing the consumption of fruit and vegetables
3. Building physical activity into our lives	Getting people moving as a normal part of their day
4. Creating incentives for better health	Increasing the understanding and value people place on the long-term impact of decisions
5. Personalised advice and support	Complementing preventative care with treatment for those who already have weight problems

Source: Adapted from Healthy Weight Healthy Lives.[43]

of individuals first – it is not the role of Government to tell people how to live their lives and nor would this work.' (p. iii).[43] The Prime Minster's next sentence is sensible, yet it fails to acknowledge that environments which are supportive are also important in supporting changes in lifestyle: 'Sustainable change will only come from individuals seeing the link between a healthy weight and a healthy life and so wanting to make changes to the way that they and their families live.' (p. iii).[43]

Described as 'multifaceted and complex' (p. 5),[43] reversing the tide of obesity is well recognised as requiring societal ownership and effort from individuals, communities, industry and government (see Chapter 2). Guidance in Healthy Weight, Healthy Lives focuses on five areas for tackling excess weight[43] (see Table 11.1). The second point specifically promotes healthier food choices with a focus (unsurprisingly) on reducing the intake of foods high in fat, salt and sugar and increasing the intake of fruit and vegetables. The approach to achieving this goal places much emphasis on government, industry and food advertising and marketing as it does on the individual.

11.4   Food policy

This section focuses on the United Kingdom and specifically England; the food policy landscape in the United Kingdom is complex for two main reasons. First, food is an issue that cuts across a number of policy areas. Second, food policy is multilevel in its governance with international agreements and standards flowing down and being implemented and supported by additional regional (European) and national policies; the flow of the policy framework and decisions are 'top-down' (p. 279).[44] Regarding the multilevel nature of food governance, an additional layer of complexity is added by the governance arrangements of the United Kingdom as most food-related policy is devolved from the United Kingdom to the governments of Scotland, Wales and Northern Ireland, with subtle differences appearing since 1999 when devolution became effective. This means that to make our way through the complex situation we have ordered the discussion by a general review of food policy framework in England and then by specific policy areas (health, agriculture and planning). In this way, the policy and governance issues of the food environment that impact directly on the individual are highlighted. The discussion is based on English policy which is made by the UK Government, and it is the UK Government that retains membership of regional and international organisations such as the UN, Codex Alimentarius Commission and the European Community and also has power to act on food-related issues that were 'reserved' in the devolution settlement such as international development and trade.

11.4.1   The overarching food policy landscape

Within England, the Department for Environment, Food and Rural Affairs (Defra) is the lead department for food policy, although admittedly neither England nor the United Kingdom possesses a discrete 'food policy'. For decades, policy concerning food has been developed in a rather piecemeal way with each department attending to its own food-related priorities in isolation; so, for example, Defra (and its predecessor the Ministry of Agriculture, Fisheries and Food, MAFF) focused on agriculture and fisheries policy primarily in response to European Commission (EC), Common Agricultural Policy (CAP) and Common Fisheries Policy, while the Department of Health focused on nutritional health. However, in July 2008 the Cabinet Office (which supports the Prime Minister and aims to improve the coherence, quality and delivery of policy for the UK Government) published its report *Food Matters*.[45] This report recommended four strategic policy objectives as the basis for food policy in England, these were to ensure 'Fair prices, choice, access to food and food security through open and competitive markets; continuous improvement in the safety of food; a further transition to healthier diets; and a more environmentally sustainable food chain' (p. iii).[45] The report argued that the objectives and recommendations could have relevance to the rest of the United Kingdom, the EC and other countries globally. The responsibility for leading food policy developments across the UK Government fell on Defra. However, each government department is responsible for ensuring that the objectives have been adopted; the Department of Health and the FSA have developed strategic objectives that support food safety and healthy diets. The strategic overview to developing a secure and sustainable food system is the context for English (and United Kingdom) food-related policy actions which the following sections discuss in more detail.

A more detailed strategy for 'a secure and sustainable food system' will be published by the UK Government during 2009–2010 following public consultation.[46] By gaining public comments on the key aims the emergent policy should, in theory at least, be developed by engaging with individuals and supporting them to change their behaviour to meet policy objectives which through consultation may reflect their own objectives. For example, amongst the questions the consultation poses for reducing diet-related chronic disease are 'Who is responsible for ensuring we eat healthily? What should the balance of freedom of choice versus restricting choices that are not in our best interests? Do you think consumers have enough information to be able to make healthy food choices?'[47]

11.4.2 Public health

Food-related public health policy in England as the foregoing sections have discussed has focused on changing food behaviour (to make healthy food choices and follow a healthy and nutritionally balanced diet) as well as food safety. A number of nutritional health interventions through the Department of Health are aimed at children (such as fruit in schools programme) and particularly those from the poorest backgrounds. The latter includes the Healthy Start scheme (vouchers given to pregnant and new mothers, children under four years of age from low-income households, i.e. receiving support from the state welfare system, and all pregnant mothers under 18 years with vouchers able to be spent on milk, fruit and vegetables) and encouraging children and young people from low-income households to claim free school meals that they are entitled to.[48]

Policy relating to food safety has perhaps done the most to change the food environment of the individual. The FSA leads on food safety. The FSA is a non-departmental public body that was created in 2000 as a result of the James Report[49] on the public confidence in the safety of British food following a number of high-level food scares. The report identified that under the then existing system of food controls there was 'the potential for conflicts of interest within MAFF arising from its dual responsibility for protecting public health and for sponsoring the agriculture and food industries' (para 1.11)[50] to which the government agreed that a separation of interests was needed. To resolve this conflict of interest and to 'put an end to the climate of confusion and suspicion which has resulted from the way food safety and standards issues have been handled in the past' (para 1.10)[50] the policy responsibilities for agriculture were separated from the responsibility for food safety standards along the food chain and the protection of public health by the creation of the FSA.

The FSA's remit was to develop policies or to provide advice, information or assistance on matters that related to food safety or other consumer food interests. Today the FSA is directly responsible for the safety of the food available to United Kingdom consumers (through its inspection services and guidance given to local authorities in inspecting food businesses) but also through public information campaigns and encouraging changes to the nutrient balance in processed foods; where we eat and what we eat. For example, the FSA is introducing a national scheme called 'Scores on the doors', where the scores given by local authority food hygiene inspectors are published (displayed in the business or online) so that consumers can use this information to make informed choices about where they buy food from. In the case of what we eat, the FSA has also supported the mandatory (compulsory) fortification of folic acid to either bread or flour, and encouraged through a continuing campaign regarding reduced salt use by consumers as discussed earlier and by the food industry in processed foods.

11.4.3 Agriculture

The EC's CAP exerts the strongest policy influence affecting the production of food in Europe today and in recent decades. The CAP was created 50 years ago as Article 33 of the 1957 Treaty of Rome, from which time it has been an integral part and legacy of community policy. The five objectives of the CAP under Article 33(1) were as follows:

(i)   To increase agricultural productivity by promoting technical progress and by ensuring the rational development of agricultural production and the optimum utilisation of the factors of production, in particular labour
(ii) To ensure that a fair standard of living for the agricultural community, in particular, by raising the individual earnings of those employed in agriculture
(iii) To stabilise markets
(iv) To assure the availability of supplies
(v)   To ensure that supplies reach consumers at reasonable prices.

As such, the supply of food products reaching the market and their affordability were key objectives, but the policy was one which at its core supported the agricultural industry and rural communities dependent on the industry.

In simplified terms, the policy functioned by giving financial support directly to farmers based on their levels of production. This had the outcome that while productivity was raised, production decisions were made irrespective of market conditions. Therefore, after the excesses of grain mountains and milk lakes of the 1980s and 1990s, reforms were introduced to counter the over-production and intensive agricultural production methods encouraged by the system to reduce the level of direct support so that food production decisions were more attuned to the market. The reforms were known as Agenda 2000 with further reforms occurring at the mid-term review in 2003. Consequently, support continued to be provided to producers recognising agriculture's 'multifunctional' role in supporting the wider social, economic and environmental conditions of the places where agriculture occurs (i.e. crediting actions and public benefits provided rather than how much was produced or farmed). As such, direct agricultural support levels have reduced and receipt of payment has become linked to wider public good provision such as meeting animal health and welfare standards and environmental standards (soil health, water management, etc.). The rationale behind this has been to increase agriculture's responsiveness to market and consumer demands and becoming more entrepreneurial rather than production decisions being made based on the support received.[51,52] The balance of funding support has shifted ('modulated') to improve agricultural efficiency, the social and economic development and diversification of rural areas (which can include activities such as food marketing) and environmental improvements.

The continued focus of English (and UK Government) policy regarding agriculture and food is on production and productivity, especially with respect to environmental and sustainable production as well as ensuring that the industry improves its economic position without reliance on public supports.[53–56] In the past, there has been a consistent lack of emphasis on the relationship between agriculture, its output – food – and the nutritional health of consumers, although food safety was recognised and is incorporated in the support system. One noticeable exception being that one stated principle for sustainable farming and food in England should be to 'Produce **safe, healthy products** in response to market demands, and ensure that all consumers have access to nutritious food, and to accurate information about food products' (p. 12 emphasis in original).[54]

It is only recently that the UK Government, through the Council of Food Policy Advisers set up following the Food Matters report, has begun to explore linkages between healthy eating and production; 'There is, for example, no reason why we can't grow more fruit and vegetables in the UK – and we should aim to do so... We will be looking at any barriers to increasing both production and consumption of fruit and vegetables in England, and agreeing what needs to be done to overcome them' (p. 10).[56] Indeed a recent House of Commons Environment, Food and Rural Affairs select committee report noted that more could be done to improve fruit and vegetable production in the United Kingdom as the government's '5-a-day' campaign had raised demand for fruit but only 10% of the fruit consumed in the United Kingdom by value was grown in the United Kingdom.[57]

It may be that the connection between food production and the health of consumers is beginning to be taken into consideration in agricultural policy although it remains to be seen to what extent. The connection is something that has been seen elsewhere for sometime; the specific cost of CAP to public health in Sweden[58] and the relation was highlighted by the Welsh Assembly Government[59] as well as policy attempts to improve the link between healthy food production and consumption in the Scottish Diet Action Plan[60] albeit unsuccessfully.[61]

11.4.4 Planning policy

Planning is a place-shaping activity – managing space and the quality of social, economic and environmental changes that occur – and local planning authorities (LPAs) co-produce the food environment mainly through the planning application decision-making process (these may be changes to land and building use such as building on greenfield sites and reducing the availability of agricultural/horticultural land, permitting food processing activities or the building of supermarkets and other food retail outlets). It is in shaping the food environment that significant policy overlaps occur and affect the food environment of the individual although these may not be directly recognised.[62] For example, Petticrew et al. noted that new supermarket openings may improve local diets, local employment opportunities, community self-esteem and attract housing and regeneration investment into the area, and that these may consequently raise social capital, feelings of well-being and improve general health.[63] A direct causal relationship is hard to prove as major regeneration schemes may often involve attracting supermarkets/major food retailers and so overlapping policies may lead to similar outcomes.[63] Results from a survey of LPAs for the Competition Commission (CC) inquiry into grocery retailing supported the existence of the positive externalities through policy interrelationships; 37% of respondents felt that major supermarkets brought benefits to their residents, 56% agreed that major supermarkets make an area more attractive to other businesses and 82% noted that they can be an important anchor to a new development or regeneration scheme.[64]

The UK's planning system is 'plan-led', with a hierarchical (top-down) structure of plans and guidance. In England, the planning framework comprises of Regional Spatial Strategies (RSS, prepared by regional planning bodies, generally Regional Development Agencies) and the Local Development Framework (through a series of Local Development Documents (LDDs), which local authorities as LPAs are responsible for). This is supplemented by central government planning policy statements (PPSs), gradually replacing planning policy guidance notes (PPGs) on particular topics; indirectly these split into issues concerning food retail and production as part of overarching PPSs as there is no overarching food planning guidance.

Most food retail policy in local planning documents mainly relates to fast food outlets and restaurants, rather than food grocery retail according to LPAs.[64] This is in contrast to the planning guidance on town centres (PPS 6) which focuses more on food grocery retail: the importance of street and covered markets (including farmers markets) are stressed, with LPAs required to ensure that markets remain attractive and competitive as they offer local choice, add to the diversity and vitality of town centres and contribute to the rural economy.[65] In market towns and villages advice is given that the development should be appropriate in scale to the needs and size of the settlement, with a more positive perspective given to development in deprived areas. This approach, encouraging retail development in existing town centres, rather than out-of-town centres, is known as the 'sequential approach'. This was brought about following concerns over the increase in supermarket numbers (from 457 in 1986 to 1102 in 1997) and its association to their share of grocery spend (rising from 29.9 to 53.7% over the same period) as large retailers focused on smaller settlements to increase their market share during the 1990s.[66] This was a response to the era of massive superstore building of the 1980s to early 1990s following property recession and the focus on smaller stores and the new competition from low-cost food retailers in high streets and town centres.[67] The argument for sequential citing being that small towns had small customer catchment areas which meant that there was a limited food retail market so new stores should be positioned in the town centre to retain its vitality. While it was recognised that new stores would affect existing food retailers the policy argument was that these would be marginal businesses.[66] Consequently, the approach has meant that supermarkets have to show the need for a new food store (such as measures of population to food retail outlet ratios, economic investment and leakages). The survey of LPAs for the CC inquiry found the existing policy criteria – conformity with the development plan, establishment of need and the sequential approach – provided a good framework for considering planning applications from major grocery retailers.[64]

The planning system is less clear on land used for food production; even though the Sustainable Food and Farming Strategy argued that the key objective should be to maintain land in food production[54] the most recent demands by policymakers to raise production has not contemplated land use.[56] PPS7 (sustainable development in rural areas) emphasises that the 'best and most versatile agricultural land', land graded as having the greatest agricultural productivity potential, should be taken into account alongside other sustainability considerations, with development, such as house building, occurring on poorer quality land wherever possible.[68] Moreover, LPAs may 'include policies in their LDDs to protect specific areas of best and most versatile agricultural land from speculative development' (p. 16).[68]

Of course, food is produced in more domestic settings such as gardens and in more urban sites such as allotments, community gardens and city farms. This latter group are classed as 'open space' by PPG17 (open space, sport and recreation)[69] (see also Chapter 9). In this guidance note the government recognises the value of allotments for health and argues that the value of open space to local communities and areas should be recognised and given protection through local standards and policies by LPAs against development, even if such sites appear underused.

11.5   Food provision and food access

While national policymakers are beginning to orientate themselves to the issues posed by food, it is on a more local level that the individual balances aspects of food access and food provision. Indeed, even at the local level (community or neighbourhood), the individual is still faced with a food environment that is a combination of local decision-making and food retailing, which in turn impacts on the food decisions and health of the individual.

Local authorities in their role as local food authorities undertake important responsibilities in the enforcement and delivery of food-related policies. This covers an array of responsibilities: inspections of animal health and welfare, environmental health and food hygiene standards in food businesses, health and safety, planning decisions on the food environment and the requirement (as Local Education Authorities) to provide and increase the take-up of free school meals to eligible pupils. Local authorities are beginning to become involved in developing food strategies. For example, the Mayor of London published a food strategy for the region (which comprises a number of local authorities).[70] The strategy aimed to encourage London residents, visitors and organisations to 'take responsibility for the impacts of their food choices' to recognise the integration between food and farming and through the actions promoted would ensure that 'all Londoners have ready access to a healthy, affordable and culturally appropriate diet' (p. 11).[70] In relation to encouraging consumer engagement to engender positive behaviour change, the London food strategy developed a number of action points from healthy eating campaigns, reward cards for healthy and sustainable food choices and expand opportunities for small-scale food production through allotments, gardens and other initiatives and alternative food networks. This would be complemented by other actions including those to ensure the commercial vibrancy of London which also looked to the planning system to provide support to different retailers to meet the strategy's aims.[70] However, as Steel has commented without the involvement of major retailers in developing the strategy in reality the strategy's ability to achieve its objectives would be 'negligible' as it 'cannot tackle the real forces shaping the city's food systems' (p. 149).[71] This may be a rather disheartening view given what was and still may be very forward policy thinking on food and local/regional food systems within the United Kingdom, but it emphasises the critical reality that for most individuals what you eat is dependent on food retailers.

Evidence continues to be presented regarding retail provision and food access and the negative impacts of this on individual health in a range of localities and socio-economic groups, mainly deprived areas and poorer households.[72–75] This is due to a combination of available income (or lack of it), cost and ease of travel to food retailers and returning with heavy bags as well as availability of culturally appropriate foods (with the associated food, health and cooking knowledges). In turn, there appears to be a case that policymakers (often planners, regardless of level) do not take into account the view of low-income consumers, and in turn by consequence poor related health outcomes and inequalities that may result.[73,75] It is only recently that the Government has considered the benefits of working with retailers to promote healthy choices such as supporting small retailers (convenience stores/corner shops) to stock fruit and vegetables which in pilots led to 40% more sales of fruit and vegetables.[76] However, we cannot infer from these statistics that the rise in sales led to a rise in fruit and vegetable consumption.

Yet what is actually eaten – the qualities required in its production, its appearance, taste, safety and possibly nutrition – is dominated by the major food retailers. As Marsden comments consumer groups 'are increasingly marginalized in what is an increasingly privately regulated food governance system dominated by retail capital' (p. 27).[77] This occurs as the major retailers gain international influence through private sector organisations such as EurepGAP (a producer and retailer organisation) which sets private production standards on fruit and vegetables, which are often in excess of public standard requirements. Through the global food sourcing practices of multinational food retailers, the private standards become an informal or quasi-global standard and lead to the standards governing the food system becoming more international.[78] As these standards are set by the retailers, it means that the qualities of what products are purchased and eaten by individuals are increasingly determined by the retailers themselves. This is particularly the case in recent years where governments worldwide have faced budget cuts and incorporated private standards into their own inspection regimes.[78] For example, in 2007 a new inspection system based on the Red Tractor scheme was launched in the United Kingdom.[79] Under the scheme, British producers pay membership which involves inspection to be accredited with meeting animal and environmental health and food safety standards and marketed with a publicly recognised logo. The new system incorporated the scheme's inspection information into government inspection databases, so state inspectors can highlight sectors with a higher food safety risk or individual producers with low safety standards. As such the power of the retailer remains a powerful force.

11.6   Future for food policy

Before taking a future perspective, it may be useful to reflect on the past. Diet is dynamic and evolving, changes in diet can be traced alongside changes in society and policy. An example of this is during the years of the World War II where there was strict control over food intake with rationing and a limited range of foods available. At this point in history, the UK government was in control of the nation's diet.[80] The introduction of food rationing around the time of World War II was a dietary equaliser. Rationing continued until 1954 after which the intake of meat, sugar, fats and sweets increased accompanied by a decrease in bread, potatoes and vegetables.[81] From the 1960s dietary change, such as increased convenience food, accompanied social changes including many more women working outside the home, increased affluence and travel abroad.[82] Immigrants from Asia and from Italy opened restaurants, which were popular with the British public and influenced consumption patterns through to the 1980s.[82]

At the beginning of the 1990s, Murcott[81] (p. 1) described Britons as being 'more food conscious than at any previous point in the nation's history'. Interest in eating and food was seen at all levels of society from policymakers to the media and cook books had a large share of the non-fiction market.[81] This change in food and eating awareness may have been a reflection of the way the eating patterns and habits of the British society were changing alongside other wider social changes. A survey conducted in 1996 on cooking and eating habits in Great Britain by Mintel Marketing Intelligence Special[83] reported that although 40% of respondents believed they followed a traditional diet, 49% reported eating pasta as part of their normal diet. Cultural rules for food patterns and habits exist enforced by convention and social interaction, while social and economic factors facilitate dietary change.[82]

Changing the patterns of dietary behaviour within the general population would help policymakers achieve nutritional targets. A review of the literature suggests that dietary changes are more likely to occur if food composition, price and marketing are changed (components of the food environment), rather than trying to change individual behaviour.[84] Individual's dietary behaviours do change, but the reasons for this have yet to be fully examined and understood.[85]

UK food policy and governance largely still focuses on individual food choices and food policy environment rather than appreciating that the individual makes their food choices within the food environment *and* food policy environment. Perhaps we could hypothesise that this effect is because the intervening issue between food policy and the individual's food choices is the retailer. Ultimately the retailer holds considerable power.

This chapter has explored how the simple act of eating, one of the most basic and yet most complex of human behaviours, is determined through a series of policy- and governance-driven decisions. As food policies and food strategies are being developed within the United Kingdom and elsewhere, there remain a number of problems and questions that require resolution. First, as more policy areas are linked together (e.g. sustainability and health) how are these balanced? Should and can they be equal or should different aspects be prioritised? For example, prioritising affordable food over health outcomes or health outcomes over sustainable production? In turn, how are sub-components of different policy areas prioritised and incorporated into responses (e.g. obesity vs. malnutrition)?

Second, can a food policy whether developed at the highest or lowest policy levels fully incorporate all the complex, varied and often competing interests that are present? In Western economies foods are global commodities where international political and economic factors are frequently the main drivers which determine our food environment (in addition to the underlying physical environmental conditions, e.g. soil type). Often those with the ability to campaign and lobby, as well as those with the larger resources have the greatest influence on food-related decisions. To support individual food choices, provide healthy food environments and reduce health inequalities, can communities improve their food environment? While momentum is building for more local level initiatives, how different interests will be brought together is still unclear. Moreover, from a practitioner perspective can the different policy guidance sufficiently inform decisions and work in practice?

Third, how dynamic can a food policy be? Can an overarching policy really allow rapid responses to new challenges as they emerge? Perhaps it is here that greater consideration of the individual's behaviours within their food environment is required. A policy and governance framework that can take into account the different influences acting upon the individual (retail power, planning decisions, etc.) needs to be developed. This is required to generate a more coherent response to counter the overwhelming obesogenic food environment that surrounds individuals. In order to address the current obesity epidemic there needs to be a seismic shift in how policy at every level approaches the food environment in relation to individual behaviours.

References

1. Boudreau, F.G. (1944) Food and nutrition policy here and abroad. *American Journal of Public Health and the Nations Health.* 34(3):215–218.
2. Lake, A.A., Hyland, R.M., Rugg-Gunn, A., Mathers, J.C., Adamson, A.J. (2009) Combining social and nutritional perspectives: from adolescence to adulthood (The ASH30 Study). *British Food Journal.* 111(11):1200–1211.
3. Jones, A., Bentham, G., Foster, C., Hillsdon, M., Panter, J. *Obesogenic Environments Evidence Review: Foresight Tackling Obesities: Future Choices Project.* London, Government Office for Science, 2007.
4. McKinnon, R.A., Reedy, J., Morrissette, M.A., Lytle, L.A., Yaroch, A.L. (2009) Measures of the food environment: a compilation of the literature, 1990–2007. *American Journal of Preventive Medicine.* 36(4, Suppl. 1):S124–S133.
5. Swinburn, B., Egger, G., Raza, F. (1999) Dissecting obesogenic environments: the development and application of a framework for identifying and prioritizing environmental interventions for obesity*1. *Preventive Medicine.* 29(6):563–570.
6. Swinburn, B., Egger, G. (2002) Preventive strategies against weight gain and obesity. *Obesity Reviews.* 3(4):289–301.

7. Lake, A.A., Hyland, R.M., Rugg-Gunn, A.J., Wood, C.E., Mathers, J.C., Adamson, A.J. (2007) Healthy eating: perceptions and practice (The ASH30 study). *Appetite*. 48(2):176–182.
8. Townshend, T., Lake, A.A. (2009) Obesogenic urban form: theory, policy and practice. *Health & Place*. 15(4):909–916.
9. Lake, A., Townshend, T. (2006) Obesogenic environments: exploring the built and food environments. *The Journal of the Royal Society for the Promotion of Health*. 126(6):262–267.
10. Ludvigsen, A., Sharma, N. (2004) Burger boy and sporty girl: children and young people's attitudes towards food in school, available from http://www.barnardos.org.uk/ burger_boy_report_1.pdf, [cited 2003 September 18].
11. Brug, J., van Lenthe, F. Chapter 14. Conclusions and Recommendations. *Environmental determinants and interventions for physical activity, nutrition and smoking: A Review*. Zoetermeer, Speed-Print, 2005.
12. Department for Education and Schools. (2006) Nutritional standards for school lunches and other school food. The final decisions on the report of the school meals review panel on school lunches and the advice of the School Food Trust on other school food. London.
13. Austin, S.B., Melly, S.J., Sanchez, B.N., Patel, A., Buka, S., Gortmaker, S.L. (2005) Clustering of fast-food restaurants around schools: a novel application of spatial statistics to the study of food environments. *American Journal of Public Health*. 95(9):1575–1581.
14. Sinclair, S., Winkler, J. *The School Fringe: What Pupils Buy and Eat from Shops Surrounding Secondary Schools*. London, Nutrition Policy Unit. London Metropolitan University, 2008.
15. Harrabin, R., Coote, A., Allen, J. (2003) Health in the News. Risk, reporting and media influence. Summary. 2003, available from www.kingsfund.org, [cited 2003 18.09.03].
16. Millstone, E., Lang, T., eds. *The Atlas of Food*, London: Earthscan; 2003.
17. The Advertising Association. *Advertising Statistics Yearbook 2003*. London: The Advertising Association and WARC; 2003.
18. Cummins, S.C.J., McKay, L., MacIntyre, S. (2005) McDonald's restaurants and neighborhood deprivation in Scotland and England. *American Journal of Preventive Medicine*. 29(4):308–310.
19. Macintyre, S., McKay, L., Cummins, S., Burns, C. (2005) Out-of-home food outlets and area deprivation: case study in Glasgow, UK. *International Journal of Behavioral Nutrition and Physical Activity*. 2(1):16.
20. Pearce, J., Blakely, T., Witten, K., Bartie, P. (2007) Neighborhood deprivation and access to fast-food retailing: a national study. *American Journal of Preventive Medicine*. 32(5):375–382.
21. Burgoine, T., Lake, A.A., Stamp, E., Alvanides, S., Mathers, J.C., Adamson, A.J. (2009) Changing foodscapes 1980–2000, using the ASH30 study. *Appetite*. 53(2):157–165.
22. Lobstein, T., Jackson Leach, R. *Tackling Obesities: Future Choices – International Comparisons of Obesity Trends*, Determinants and Responses – Evidence Review: Foresight, 2007.
23. Drewnowski, A., Darmon, N. (2005) Food choices and diet costs: an economic analysis. *The Journal of Nutrition*. 135(4):900–904.
24. Foresight. *Tackling obesities: future choices – project report*. London, Government Office for Science, 2007.
25. The Strategy Unit Cabinet Office. (2008) Food: an analysis of the issues, available from http://www.cabinetoffice.gov.uk/media/cabinetoffice/strategy/assets/food/food_analysis.pdf.
26. Cheng, S.-L., Olsen, W., Southerton, D., Warde, A. (2007) The changing practice of eating: evidence from UK time diaries, 1975 and 2001. *The British Journal of Sociology*. 58(1):39–61.
27. Riley, M. (1994) Marketing eating out: the influence of social culture and innovation. *British Food Journal*. 96(10):15–18.
28. Glanz, K., Resnicow, K., Seymour, J., Hoy, K., Stewart, H., Lyons, M., *et al.* (2007) How major restaurant chains plan their menus. *American Journal of Preventive Medicine*. 32(5):383–388.
29. World Health Organisation. *Diet, Nutrition and the Prevention of Chronic Disease*. Technical Report Series 916. Geneva, WHO/ FAO Expert Consultation, 2003.

30. Kleinman, R.E. (2000) Complementary feeding and later health. *Paediatrics*. 106(5):1287.
31. Department of Health. *Choosing Health? Choosing a Better Diet: A Consultation on Priorities for a Food and Health Action Plan*. London: Department of Health, 2004.
32. Department of Health. *The Health of the Nation: A Strategy for Health in England*. London, HMSO, 1992.
33. Department of Health. *Eat Well II: A Progress Report from the Nutrition Task Force on the Action Plan to Achieve the Health of the Nation Targets on Diet and Nutrition*. London, Department of Health, 1996.
34. Department of Health. *Saving Lives: Our Healthier Nation*. White Paper Cm 4386. London, The Stationery Office, 1999.
35. Bender, A. Food and nutrition: principles of nutrition and some current controversies in Western Countries. In: *The Food Consumer*. (Eds. Ritson, C., Gofton, L., McKenzie, J.) John Wiley & Sons, Inc., Chichester, 1986 pp. 37–58.
36. Department of Health. *Report on Health and Social Subjects: 41. Dietary Reference Values for Food Energy and Nutrients for the United Kingdom*. London, HMSO, 1991.
37. Food Standards Agency. (2007) Eatwell plate, available from http://www.eatwell.gov.uk/healthydiet/eatwellplate/.
38. Food Standards Agency. (2005) 8 tips for eating well, available from http://www.eatwell.gov.uk/healthydiet/eighttipssection/8tips/.
39. Buttriss, J. (2003) Scene setting: who is the voice of nutrition in Britain? *Proceedings of the Nutrition Society*. 62:573–575.
40. Kelly, C.N.M., Stanner, S.A. (2003) Diet and cardiovascular disease in the UK: are the messages getting across? *Proceedings of the Nutrition Society*. 62:583–589.
41. Department for Environment, Food and Rural Affairs & National Statistics. *National Food Survey 2000: Annual Report on Food Expenditure, Consumption and Nutrient Intakes*. London, The Stationery Office, 2001.
42. Food Standards Agency. (2009) Salt, available from http://www.salt.gov.uk/, [cited 2009 27/08/09].
43. Cross-Government Obesity Unit, Department of Health & Department for Children, Schools and Families. *Healthy Weight, Healthy Lives: A Cross-government Strategy for England*. London, 2008.
44. Lang, T., Heaseman, M. *Food Wars: The Global Battle for Mouths, Minds and Markets*. London, Earthscan, 2004.
45. Cabinet Office. *Food Matters, Towards a Strategy for the 21st Century*. London, Cabinet Office, 2008.
46. Defra. *Food Matters: One Year On*. London, Defra, 2009a.
47. Defra. (2009b) Food 2030 Defra online discussion, Diet-related chronic disease. Available at http://sandbox.defra.gov.uk/food2030/2009/08/reducing-diet-related-chronic-disease/.
48. HM Treasury. *PSA Delivery Agreement 12: Improve the Health and Wellbeing of Children and Young People*. London, TSO, 2007.
49. James, P. (1997) *Food Standards Agency Report – An Interim Proposal by Professor Philip James 30 April 1997*, London, MAFF/Department of Health Scottish Executive. Available at http://archive.food.gov.uk/maff/archive/food/james/cont.htm.
50. MAFF. *The Food Standards Agency: A Force for Change: (Cm3830)*. London, TSO, 1998.
51. EC. *The EU Rural Development Policy 2007–2013, Fact Sheet*. Luxembourg, EC, 2006.
52. EC. *Simplification of the Common Agricultural Policy, Fact Sheet*. Luxembourg, EC, 2006.
53. HM Treasury and Defra. (2005) A Vision for the Common Agricultural Policy. Available at http://www.defra.gov.uk/farm/policy/capreform/pdf/vision-for-cap.pdf.
54. Defra. *The Strategy for Sustainable Food and Farming: Facing the Future*. London, Defra, 2002.
55. Defra. *Sustainable Farming and Food Strategy: Forward Look*. London, Defra, 2006.
56. Defra. *The Future of our Farming*. London, Defra, 2009. Available at http://www.defra.gov.uk/farm/policy/pdf/farm-future-leaflet090709.pdf.
57. House of Commons Environment, Food and Rural Affairs Committee. *Securing Food Supplies Up to 2050: The Challenges Faced by the UK, HC213-1*. London, TSO, 2009.

58. Elinder, L.S., Joossens, L., Raw, M., Andreasson, S., Lang, T. *Public Health Aspects of the EU Common Agricultural Policy*. Stockholm, Sweden, National Institute for Public Health, 2003.

59. Welsh Assembly Government. (2007) *Quality of Food Strategy*. Task and Finish Group report. Available at http://wales.gov.uk/consultation/dphhp/qualityoffood?lang=en.

60. Scottish Office. *Eating for Health: A Diet Action Plan for Scotland*. Edinburgh, Scottish Office, 1996. Available at: www.scotland.gov.uk/library/documents/diet-00.htm.

61. Lang, T., Dowler, L., Hunter, D.L. *Review of the Scottish Diet Action Plan: Progress and Impacts 1996–2005*. Edinburgh, Health Scotland, 2006.

62. Midgley, J. (2007) The food state: public policy and its relationship to the food we eat. Unpublished working paper for the Institute of Public Policy Research, London.

63. Petticrew, M., Cummins, S., Ferrell, C., Findlay, A., Huggins, C., Hoy, C., Kearns, A., Sparks, L. (2005) Natural experiments: an underused tool for public health? *Public Health*. 119(9):751–757.

64. Competition Commission. (2007) Working paper on planning issues. Available at: www.competition-commission.org.uk/inquiries/ref2006/grocery/emerging_thinking_working_papers.htm.

65. Communities and Local Government (CLG). *Planning Policy Statement 6: Planning for Town Centres*. London, TSO, 2005.

66. Communities and Local Government (CLG). (1998) *Impact of Large Foodstores on Market Towns and District Centres*. Available at: http://www.communities.gov.uk/archived/publications/planningandbuilding/impactlarge.

67. Wrigley, N. (1998) PPG6 and the contemporary UK food store development dynamic. *British Food Journal*. 100(3):154–161.

68. CLG. *Planning Policy Statement 7: Sustainable Development in Rural Areas*. London, TSO, 2004.

69. CLG. (2002) *Planning Policy Guidance 17: Planning for Open Space, Sport and Recreation*. Available at www.communities.gov.uk/publications/planningandbuilding/planningpolicyguidance17.

70. London Development Agency. *Healthy and Sustainable Food for London: The Mayors Food Strategy*. London, London Development Agency, 2006.

71. Steel, C. *Hungry City: How Food Shapes Our Lives*. London, Vintage, 2009.

72. Ellaway, A., Macintyre, S. (2000) Shopping for food in socially contrasting localities. *British Food Journal*. 102(1):52–59.

73. Robinson, N., Caraher, M., Lang, T. (2000) Access to shops: the views of low-income shoppers. *Health Education Journal*. 59:121–136.

74. Holmes, B. (2007) 'Food security', Vol 3 Chapter 20 unpaginated, in *Low income diet and nutrition survey*. A survey carried out on behalf of the Food Standards Agency by Natcen, Kings College London and University College London. Available at: www.food.gov.uk/science/dietarysurveys/lidnsbranch/.

75. Bowyer, S., Caraher, M., Eilbert, K., Carr-Hill, R. (2009) Shopping for food: lessons from a London borough. *British Food Journal*. 111(5):452–474.

76. Department of Health. (2009) Change4Life corner shops to open across the country, national news release 28 July. Available at http://nds.coi.gov.uk/Content/Detail.aspx?NewsAreaId=2&ReleaseID=405312&SubjectId=2.

77. Marsden, T. (2002) Food matters and the matter of food: toward a new food governance? *Sociologia Ruralis*. 40(1):20–29.

78. Fulponi, L. (2006) Private voluntary standards in the food system: the perspective of major food retailers in OECD countries. *Food Policy*. 31(1):1–13.

79. FSA. (2007) 'Farming industry and local authorities set to reap the benefits of new inspection scene says FSA', press release 04 June. Available at www.food.gov.uk/news/newsarchive/2007/jun/farminginspect.

80. McKenzie, J. An integrated approach – with special reference to the study of changing food habits in the UK. In: *The Food Consumer*. (Eds. Ritson, C., Gofton, L, McKenzie, J.M.) Chichester, John Wiley & Son, Inc., 1986, 155–167.

81. Murcott, A. (1998) Hungry for change. Available at: http://www.timeshighereducation.co.uk/story.asp?storyCode=106842&sectioncode=26.
82. Mitchell, J. (1999) The British main meal in the 1990s: has it changed its identity? *British Food Journal.* 101(11):871–883.
83. *Mintel Marketing Intelligence Special Report. Cooking and eating habits.* London, Mintel International Group, 1996.
84. Mela, D.J. (1999) Food choice and intake: the human factor. *Proceedings of the Nutrition Society.* 58(3):513–521.
85. Satia, J.A., Kristal, A.R., Curry, S., Trudeau, E. (2001) Motivations for healthful dietary change. *Public Health Nutrition.* 4(5):953–959.

12 Neighbourhood Histories and Health: Social Deprivation and Food Retailing in Christchurch, New Zealand, 1966–2005

Jamie Pearce and Peter Day

12.1 Introduction

There is considerable international evidence for strong social and ethnic disparities in a range of health outcomes including life expectancy, childhood mortality, various types of morbidity such as cancer incidence and health-related behaviours including alcohol consumption.[1] Using a range of metrics, the overwhelming majority of the evidence has found that socially and materially disadvantaged groups tend to have poorer health status. Importantly, the 'health gap' is not limited to differences between the 'rich' and the 'poor' but rather there remains a gradient in health across *all* social groups.[2] Furthermore, in most rich nations there has been a sharp rise in health inequalities over the past 20–30 years.[3,4] This time period has coincided with the implementation of market-oriented economic and social policies which have widened inequalities in accessing health-determining resources such as wealth, education, employment and health care.[5] In addition to a widening gradient in health status across various social and ethnic groups, it is increasingly recognised that there are enduring health inequalities between areas of differing socio-economic circumstances. Geographical inequalities in health have been noted in most Organisation for Economic Co-operation and Development (OECD) countries.[6–9] Research has consistently established that more socially deprived areas tend to have worse health than less deprived areas, and that this spatial divide is widening.[10] For example, in the United Kingdom life expectancy has continued to increase in the most socially advantaged areas at a greater pace than in the most disadvantaged areas. Inequalities in health between rich and poor areas of the country have continued to widen significantly since the early 1980s.[8]

New Zealand is no exception to these international trends in health inequalities. Relative inequalities in health between social and ethnic groups rose sharply during the 1980s and 1990s,[11] a period where the adoption of a neoliberal social and economic agenda resulted in considerable structural change in New Zealand society.[12] For instance, during the late 1980s and early 1990s levels of income inequality in New Zealand rose more sharply than any other rich nation.[13] Similarly, spatial inequalities in health in New Zealand have risen markedly over the past two decades.[14-16] When regions across the country are ranked by deprivation, inequalities in life expectancy grew during the 1980s and 1990s by approximately 50%.[17] Other New Zealand research has noted that alternative measures of health and health-related behaviours are spatially patterned in a similar way. For example, obesity rates are twice as high in the most deprived quintile of neighbourhoods in New Zealand compared to the least deprived quintile.[18] However, whilst there is considerable evidence documenting spatial inequalities in health in New Zealand and elsewhere, the reasons for the growing spatial divide remain elusive.

The explanations for rising inequalities in health status are likely to be multi-faceted. In recent years, there has been a resurgence of interest among geographers, epidemiologists and public health researchers in 'contextual' or 'neighbourhood' influences on health outcomes, and health inequalities.[19-21] This body of research seeks to establish whether various characteristics of the places in which people live (contextual argument) have an effect on assorted health outcomes that are independent of the combined characteristics of the people living in those areas (compositional argument). Methodological developments in techniques such as multilevel modelling and Geographical Information Systems (GISs) have significantly advanced the neighbourhoods and health research agenda, and it is widely accepted that neighbourhoods tend to exert an influence on many individual-level health outcomes.[22] In New Zealand, a broad array of potential neighbourhood characteristics with a plausible health effect have been appraised,[23] including neighbourhood social capital,[24] regional inequality,[25] access to primary health care resources[26] and neighbourhood provision of gambling outlets on individual-level gambling and problem gambling behaviour.[27]

One theme in the recent neighbourhoods and health literature that has received substantial attention is the notion that locational access to 'everyday' health-related features within neighbourhoods may partially explain neighbourhood variations in health.[28] For example, the salutary health effects of neighbourhood resources such as recreational opportunities, parks and greenspace and food retail provision have been noted. In one European study, high levels of greenery and low levels of graffiti and litter in residential environments were associated with individual-level physical activity and not being overweight.[29] Similarly, the increased recognition of the public health burden of the emerging 'obesity epidemic' has prompted researchers to try and elucidate the potential contextual drivers of diet and nutrition, as well as their social distribution. The growing focus on the *contextual* drivers of obesity is a response to the limited impact that individual-level interventions have had in reducing the prevalence of this health outcome. Therefore, it has been suggested that more attention needs to be paid to furthering our understanding of how 'obesogenic environments' are related to diet-related health outcomes.[30]

Neighbourhood access to opportunities to procure 'healthy' (e.g. fruits and vegetables) and 'unhealthy' (e.g. fast food) food has been suggested as a key driver of social inequalities in dietary intake and associated health outcomes such as heart disease, hypertension, various types of cancer and type 2 diabetes.[31,32] Studies in a number of countries have found that access to food retail outlets often varies by measures of neighbourhood socio-economic status (e.g. mean income, percentage minority ethnic group). Findings in the United States have overwhelmingly demonstrated that more socio-economically disadvantaged neighbourhoods are inclined to have poorer access to larger supermarkets. These areas also tend to have higher numbers of smaller convenience stores where the range of food choice tends to be lower, and the cost of food higher.[33–37] The preponderance of evidence in United States also suggests that residing in a neighbourhood with poor locational access to a food store has a detrimental impact on the quality of diet and diet-related health outcomes of local residents.[31,38]

Outside the United States, the evidence for poorer access to food retailing in more deprived neighbourhoods or what has been termed a 'food desert' is more mixed.[39] Research in the United Kingdom is equivocal with some studies supporting the presence of food deserts[40–42] or beneficial health effects of the opening of a new supermarket,[43,44] and others finding a small[45] or no[46] effect. Studies in Canada[47] and Australia[48] have not supported the presence of food deserts. In New Zealand, at the national-level, locational access to supermarkets and convenience stores was better in *more* deprived neighbourhoods,[49] and the health effects associated with neighbourhood access were not consistent.[50] With regard to fast food outlets, the weight of evidence from the international literature suggests that outlets are also more prevalent in lower socio-economic neighbourhoods. Results from the United States,[36,51] the United Kingdom[52,53] and Australia[54] concur. Similarly, in New Zealand, locational access to fast food outlets (both multinational chains and locally operated outlets) was patterned in a similar way,[55] although the health effects of geographical access on local residents were equivocal.[56] An international review of the influence of the food environment on individual-level nutrition and weight is provided elsewhere.[57]

To summarise the New Zealand findings, at the national-level, food retailing is preferentially located in more deprived neighbourhoods,[49,55,57] and this relationship is consistent in the majority of regions across the country, including Christchurch.[58] In the current study, we extend the previous New Zealand work by including a temporal dimension to the analyses, and consider whether the contemporary picture of the social distribution of food retailing has persisted over time. To our knowledge, all previous studies in New Zealand and elsewhere that have evaluated the association between neighbourhood access to food retailing and the socio-economic circumstances of the neighbourhood have been cross-sectional, and only considered a single point in time. Therefore, no prior work has examined whether the geographical distribution of food retailing has become more socially polarised over time. This omission is perhaps surprising given that causal inference cannot be determined from studies of this type.[59] Further, there is increasing evidence that to fully evaluate neighbourhood effects on health, neighbourhood exposure over the whole life-course must be accounted for.[60] For instance, it has been suggested that neighbourhood exposures (e.g. to social deprivation) earlier in life may subsequently have important health effects.[61] Therefore, evaluating individual-level exposure to aspects of the food environment at different points through the life-course is an important conceptual advance. The current study extends previous work by examining the social distribution of food retail outlets in the Christchurch urban area over the past 40 years. Using a repeated cross-sectional study design, we consider whether the geography of food retailing in Christchurch has become more socially polarised since the mid-1960s.

12.1.1   Data and methods

Data on the location of all food retail outlets located within the Christchurch City Territorial Authority area were extracted from the Yellow Pages business telephone directories at approximate 10-year intervals between 1966 and 2005. Data were obtained for 1966, 1976, 1985 (the telephone directory in 1986 could not be located), 1996 and 2005 (the most recent edition at the time of data collection). All outlets were geocoded to provide a geographic coordinate of an outlet's location, which enabled the identification of the 2001 Census Area Unit (CAU) in which it was located. In 2001, there were 106 CAUs across the city, with a median population of 2949 (range 246–5931). Each food outlet was allocated to one of the following categories: bakery, butchery, dairy, delicatessen, fast food outlet, fruit and vegetable shop, grocery store, supermarket, restaurant or tea room/coffee shop. The retail food mix of some categories has changed markedly over the study period. For example, in the 1960s fast food outlets consisted of mainly traditional fish-retailer and 'fish'n'chip' shops but in later years include chicken shops, pizza outlets, Asian and Indian food takeaway shops and multinational fast food chain stores such as McDonalds, Burger King and Kentucky Fried Chicken (KFC). Several categories reflect the relative scale of business and the range of retail food available. 'Dairies' comprise of small convenience stores while the grocery store category comprises of medium-sized food retail outlets selling a wider variety of foodstuffs. Supermarkets tend to be larger stores selling a greater range of food. Supermarkets have also evolved over time from smaller 'superettes' that were common in the 1970s and 1980s to larger chain stores such as 'Woolworths', 'New World', 'Countdown', 'Pak'n'Save' and 'Fresh Choice'. The restaurant category comprises of licensed and non-licensed food establishments listed in the Yellow Pages under restaurants, and includes businesses with on-premise dining and a primary activity of providing restaurant food. Tea rooms/coffee shop category comprises of outlets listed under the tea room/café/coffee shop classification where these terms were often included in the business name.

To consider whether the prevalence of food retailing varied between neighbourhoods of differing levels of social deprivation, each CAU was categorised into a quintile of deprivation using the 1991 New Zealand Deprivation Index (NZDep91). The NZDep91 is calculated from census data on 10 socio-economic characteristics (e.g. family composition, tenure and benefit receipt).[62] Ideally, an equivalent neighbourhood measure of social deprivation would have been used for each of the 5 years considered, but a comparable index was not available prior to 1991. Therefore, the NZDep91 index was used as the indicator of area social deprivation for each year. This approach was considered satisfactory given: (1) its mid-way

Table 12.1 Correlation between proportion of the population in a 'professional and technical' occupation and the 1991 New Zealand Deprivation score.

	Year					
	1966	1976	1985	1991	1996	2005
Correlation coefficient*	−0.50	−0.50	−0.54	−0.58	−0.57	−0.53

*Significant at $p < 0.01$

proximity in the period under study and (2) its consistently high correlation with occupational class in each year when compared with quintiles of the proportions of professional/technical workers residing in each CAU (Table 12.1). The high correlation between occupational class in each year and NZDep91 suggested that areas which were deprived in 1991 were deprived in 1966 and in each subsequent year of the analyses.

The index was used to categorise all CAUs (using 2001 boundaries) across the city into quintiles of low to high deprivation. For each quintile, the total number of food outlets per 10,000 population were calculated using the corresponding census as the denominator population (usual resident population). Additional analysis stratified the results by the type of food retailing (supermarkets, fruit and vegetable shops, etc.) and compared CAUs in the highest deprivation quintile with CAUs in the lowest deprivation quintile. Due to the large number of outlets in the central business district that would have heavily skewed the results and the relatively few people living in this area of Christchurch, the city centre CAU (Cathedral Square) was excluded from all analyses of the social distribution of food retailing.

12.2 Results

Over the study period, the total number of food retail outlets in Christchurch increased from 902 in 1996 to 1138 in 2005 (Table 12.2). The retail types showing the largest increases were tea rooms/coffee shops, which rose more than eightfold in number; restaurants more than sevenfold; fast food outlets and bakeries more than fivefold; and the number of supermarkets more than doubled between 1976 and 2005 (there were no supermarkets in 1966). Conversely, the number of grocery stores decreased from 378 in 1966 to 78 in 2005 (a 93% reduction), fruit and vegetable shops from 102 to 16 (84% reduction) and butchers 179 to 36 outlets (80% reduction). Although the total number of outlets rose by 26%, the population of the city increased by almost 40%, and hence there was a small reduction in the total number of outlets per population from 35.9 per 10,000 in 1966 to 32.4 per 10,000 in 2005.

Maps of the geographical distribution of retail food outlets in Christchurch at the beginning and end of the study period (1966 and 2005) illustrate these trends (Figures 12.1–12.3). For example, in 1966 there were a large number of grocery stores spread across Christchurch with most suburbs having a number of outlets, but by 2005 there was a sparse scattering of (probably larger) grocery stores and

Table 12.2   Total number of food outlets in Christchurch (1966–2005) by retail type.

Retail type	Year				
	1966	1976	1985	1996	2005
Bakery	18	19	50	114	99
Butchery	179	174	167	58	36
Dairy	83	119	156	130	104
Delicatessen	14	17	25	12	7
Fast food outlet	65	57	247	272	325
Fruit and vegetable shop	102	47	48	34	16
Grocery store	378	158	92	34	28
Supermarket	–	16	32	28	34
Restaurant	46	80	148	245	350
Tea rooms/coffee shop	17	18	18	98	139
Total count	902	705	983	1025	1138
Total population	251,348	286,472	286,521	313,905	351,507
Rate per 10,000 population	35.9	24.6	34.3	32.7	32.4

particularly supermarkets across the city (Figure 12.1). On the other hand, the small number of fast food outlets, restaurants and tea room/coffee shops that were concentrated in the central city in 1966 had by 2005 spread across most of the urban area, although a significant proportion remained in the central city area (Figure 12.2). In 1966, there was a high density of bakeries, butchers, delicatessens and fruit and vegetable shops across the city, particularly in eastern suburbs, but by 2005 the pattern of these outlets was considerably less dense and more evenly distributed across the city (Figure 12.3).

The relationship between the number of food retail outlets per 10,000 population and social deprivation (NZDep91) for CAUs across Christchurch demonstrated a consistent social gradient for each year examined (Figure 12.4). The number of food retail outlets per 10,000 population generally increased across neighbourhoods stratified into quintiles from low to high deprivation with a consistently higher prevalence of retail food outlets in more deprived areas over the 40-year period. For example, in 1966 the number of outlets per 10,000 population in quintile 1 (low deprivation) was 21.8 compared to 38.0 in quintile 5 (high deprivation). The corresponding figures in 2005 were 13.3 and 37.8. The consistency of this relationship is shown when the ratio of the number of food outlets per 10,000 in the CAUs with the highest compared to lowest deprivation quintile stratified by retail type are examined (Table 12.3). A ratio of greater than 1.0 demonstrated that there were higher rates of retail outlets in the most deprived quintile of neighbourhoods

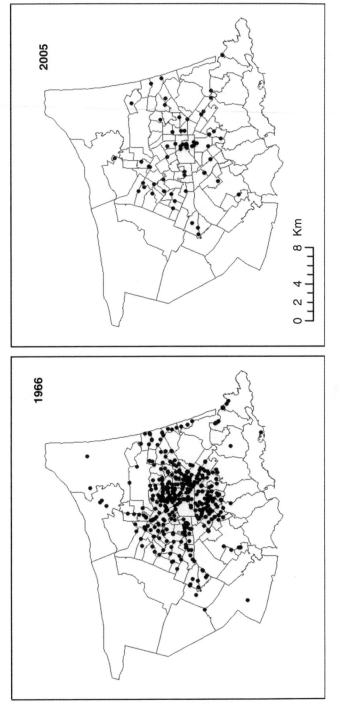

Figure 12.1 Distribution of grocery stores and supermarkets across Christchurch (1966 and 2005).

189

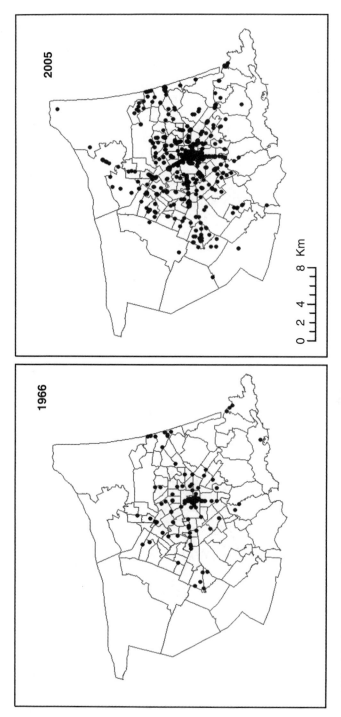

Figure 12.2 Distribution of fast food outlets, restaurants and tea rooms/coffee shops across Christchurch (1966 and 2005).

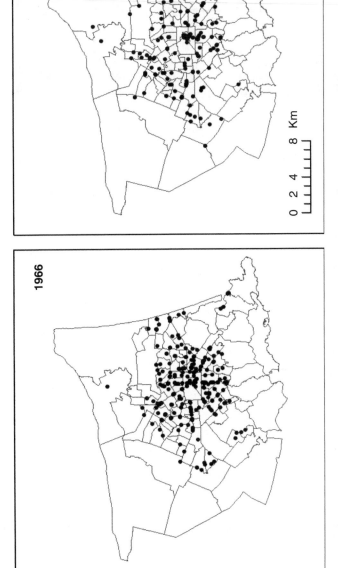

Figure 12.3 Distribution of bakeries, butcheries, delicatessens and fruit and vegetable shops across Christchurch (1966 and 2005).

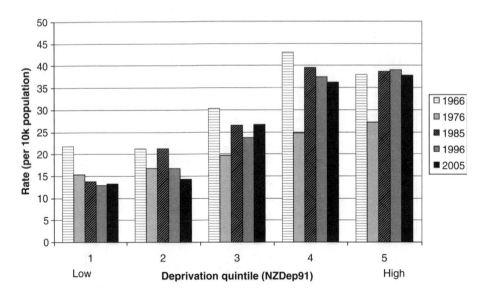

Figure 12.4   Retail food outlets per 10,000 population by deprivation quintile, 1966–2005.

Table 12.3   Ratio of the number of food outlets per 10,000 population in the most deprived quintile of areas compared with least deprived quintile, 1966–2005.

Retail type	Year				
	1966	**1976**	**1985**	**1996**	**2005**
Bakery	3.7	2.5	5.0	4.2	4.0
Butchery	1.5	1.5	1.8	1.4	1.6
Dairy	1.1	1.3	2.4	2.4	2.0
Delicatessen	–	5.9	1.5	2.1	–
Fast food outlet	8.1	3.4	9.0	4.8	4.4
Fruit and vegetable shop	2.0	9.3	10.1	3.1	4.1
Grocery store	1.8	1.2	0.9	0.8	2.1
Supermarket	–	1.3	1.8	0.8	1.5
Restaurant	2.5	–	5.2	3.8	2.4
Tea rooms/coffee shop	–	0.4	2.7	2.8	2.6
Total	1.7	1.8	2.8	3.0	2.8

compared to the least deprived quintile. If the ratio was less than 1.0 then the opposite was the case. The ratio for all outlets increased from 1.7 in 1966 to 2.8 in 1985 and remained fairly constant in 1996 and 2005. For most types of retail the ratios were generally greater than 1.0 across all years with bakeries, fast food outlets, dairies, fruit and vegetable shops, restaurants and tea rooms/coffee shops consistently having ratios greater than 2.0.

12.3 Discussion

Previous studies in New Zealand that have considered the cross-sectional association between food/alcohol retailing and neighbourhood deprivation have shown that opportunities to procure food,[49,57,58] fast food[55] and alcohol[57] are more frequent in socially deprived neighbourhoods. The findings of the current Christchurch study are consistent with the earlier national-level findings. Our research adds to the earlier body of evidence by demonstrating that the social gradient in the distribution of food and alcohol retailing remained consistent over the 40-year study period. These results in Christchurch conflict with much of the international evidence, particularly in the United States, where locational access to food retailing tends to favour less deprived, high income or low ethnic minority communities.[35–37,40] However, for fast food outlets, the Christchurch results concur with those in most other countries including the United States,[51] the United Kingdom[52,53] and Australia.[54]

What explains the different findings in New Zealand compared to most other countries? Many explanations are possible but include factors such as differences in residential segregation, and the consequent ability of local communities to influence decision-making and land use planning. In the United States, it is likely that various characteristics of urban neighbourhoods will exert a greater influence on the health and well-being of local residents due to the higher degree of residential segregation in most US cities. Selective migration streams over a long period of time have seen higher income and white residents shift into the suburbs of many metropolitan centres in the United States, leaving low-income and black residents to remain in the urban centres, a process known as 'white flight'.[63] The growing concentration of low-income and black residents in spatially confined parts of US cities is likely to exacerbate neighbourhood health effects in the United States including the concentration of particular demographic groups who are the target market of particular food retailers in specific localities (e.g. supermarkets targeting wealthier neighbourhoods and not low-income areas). Further, residential segregation is likely to exacerbate differentials in land use planning strategies and political empowerment between high- and low-income neighbourhoods, and hence influence local decision-making with regard to locating various types of food retailing.[64]

The results of this study have some potentially important implications for policy development in New Zealand. Enhancing our understanding of the environmental mechanisms that influence residential health provides numerous opportunities for policy interventions. If characteristics of the local physical infrastructure (including food retailing) are important in shaping health outcomes, health-related behaviours or well-being, then there is considerable scope to develop area-based initiatives to improve health and reduce health inequalities. This assumption is integral to various policy initiatives such as the WHO Healthy Cities program,[65,66] and the current UK (Labour) Government's New Deal for Communities initiative.[67] An improved understanding of the local food environment offers the potential to improve inequalities in diet-related health outcomes. In a number of settings, improving locational access to shops selling healthy food (e.g. supermarkets) and restricting access to outlets selling unhealthy food (e.g. fast food restaurants) has been advocated as a strategy to improve the diets of residents living in deprived neighbourhoods.[68] However, our findings suggest that in Christchurch, inequalities in access to food outlets are unlikely to mediate the well-established relationship between neighbourhood deprivation and poor health. Our findings add evidence to earlier research by demonstrating that the relationship between neighbourhood access to food retailing and social deprivation has been established for over four decades. Nonetheless, it would be valuable if future work could use detailed longitudinal information to examine whether inequalities in diet and diet-related health outcome at the individual-level can be explained by neighbourhood access to food outlets early in the life-course.

The limitations of this study need to be considered. First, because the retail outlet data prior to 2005 were historical it was not possible to verify the accuracy and completion of the data. However, the data for 2005 were informally 'ground truthed' by checking the validity of the data in neighbourhoods well known to the authors and there was a high degree of correspondence. Second, features other than locational access are also likely to influence whether local residents will use the retail opportunities in their neighbourhood. Factors such as neighbourhood variations in the price of goods, shopping preferences, daily mobility patterns such as the journey to work may influence shopping habits and result in the procurement of food outside of the *residential* neighbourhood. Third, there are numerous potential methodological approaches for capturing key characteristics of the local food environment. In this study, we have simply used the census boundaries in which each food outlet is located and associated the corresponding measure of social deprivation. It could be argued that more sophisticated, and possibly more accurate, measures of neighbourhood access, such as using GIS representations[69] (see also Chapter 5 by Edwards), may influence the associations that were observed between access and area deprivation. Future work could usefully examine the sensitivity of the results in studies such as the current one to the measures used to capture the food environment.

12.4 Conclusion

In this study in Christchurch, New Zealand, we used a repeated cross-sectional study design at 10-yearly intervals to evaluate the social distribution of neighbourhood access to food retailing, and considered whether this geography has changed over the past 40 years. We found that opportunities to procure food in Christchurch are patterned by neighbourhood deprivation. Across the city, more deprived neighbourhoods tend to have better access to all types of food provision, a trend that has been apparent throughout the study period. Since the mid-1960s, more socially deprived neighbourhoods in Christchurch have persistently had better geographical access to both 'healthy' (e.g. supermarkets and grocers) and 'unhealthy' (e.g. fast food) retailing. Given the strength and consistency of these findings over time, it seems unlikely that neighbourhood access to food retailing is a key driver of the observed social and spatial inequalities in diet and nutrition-related health outcomes in New Zealand. Improving nutrition and reducing inequalities in diet remain key research and policy priorities in New Zealand. Therefore, it is important that researchers in New Zealand investigate the potential of alternative area level drivers for inequalities in diet such as neighbourhood differences in the cost of food (e.g. fruits and vegetables), national and local advertising of healthy and unhealthy food or community transport options.

The international evidence evaluating the role of the local food retail environment in shaping nutrition-related health outcomes and behaviours is incongruent, and distinct variations have been noted between nations, also discussed in Chapter 10 by Ball *et al*. However, all previous studies have been cross-sectional and considered only a single point in time, and this approach has been a significant impediment to the field of research because it is increasingly recognised that neighbourhood exposures to health promoting and damaging characteristics operate throughout the life-course. Given the global increase in obesity levels in recent years, we encourage researchers to examine the changing socio-spatial distribution of food retailing in their own countries.

12.5 Acknowledgement

The authors thank Rowan Haigh (University of Canterbury) for collecting the food retail data.

References

1. WHO Commission on Social Determinants of Health. *Closing the Gap in a Generation: Health Equity Through Action on the Social Determinants of Health*. Final report of the Commission on Social Determinants of Health. Geneva, WHO, 2008.
2. Davey Smith, G. *Health Inequalities: Lifecourse Approaches*. Bristol, Policy Press, 2003.
3. Mackenbach, J.P., Bos, V., Andersen, O., Cardano, M., Costa, G., Harding, S., Reid, A., Hemstrom, O., Valkonen, T., Kunst, A.E. (2003) Widening socioeconomic inequalities in mortality in six Western European countries. *International Journal of Epidemiology.* 32:830–837.
4. Mackenbach, J.P., Stirbu, I., Roskam, A.J., Schaap, M.M., Menvielle, G., Leinsalu, M., Kunst, A.E. (2008) Socioeconomic inequalities in health in 22 European countries. *New England Journal of Medicine.* 358:2468–2481.
5. Pearce, J., Dorling, D. (2009) Tackling global health inequalities: closing the health gap in a generation. *Environment and Planning A.* 41:1–6.
6. Davey Smith, G., Dorling, D., Mitchell, R., Shaw, M. (2002) Health inequalities in Britain: continuing increases up to the end of the 20th century. *Journal of Epidemiology and Community Health.* 56:434–435.
7. Hayes, L., Quine, S., Taylor, R., Berry, G. (2002) Socio-economic mortality differentials in Sydney over a quarter of a century, 1970–94. *Australian and New Zealand Journal of Public Health.* 26:311–317.
8. Shaw, M., Davey Smith, G., Dorling, D. (2005) Health inequalities and New Labour: how the promises compare with real progress. *BMJ.* 330:1016–1021.
9. Singh, G.K., Siahpush, M. (2006) Widening socioeconomic inequalities in US life expectancy, 1980–2000. *International Journal of Epidemiology.* 35:969–979.
10. Shaw, M., Dorling, D., Gordon, D., Davey Smith, G. *The Widening Gap: Health Inequalities and Policy in Britain*. Bristol, Policy Press, 1999.

11. Blakely, T., Fawcett, J., Atkinson, J., Tobias, M., Cheung, J. *Decades of disparity II: Socioeconomic Mortality Trends in New Zealand, 1981–1999*. Wellington, Ministry of Health, 2005.

12. Le Heron, R.B., Pawson, E. *Changing Places: New Zealand in the Nineties*. Auckland, NZ, Longman Paul Ltd, 1996.

13. Atkinson, A. Income Inequality in OECD Countries: Data and Explanations. *CESifo Working Paper Series No. 881*, 2003.

14. Pearce, J., Barnett, R., Collings, S., Jones, I. (2007) Did geographical inequalities in suicide among men aged 15–44 in New Zealand increase during the period 1980–2001? *Australian and New Zealand Journal of Psychiatry*. 41:359–365.

15. Pearce, J., Dorling, D., Wheeler, B., Barnett, R., Rigby, J. (2006) Geographical inequalities in health in New Zealand, 1980–2001: the gap widens. *Australian and New Zealand Journal of Public Health*. 30:461–466.

16. Pearce, J., Tisch, C., Barnett, R. (2008) Have geographical inequalities in cause-specific mortality in New Zealand increased during the period 1980–2001? *New Zealand Medical Journal*. 121:15–27.

17. Pearce, J., Dorling, D. (2006) Increasing geographical inequalities in health in New Zealand, 1980–2001. *International Journal of Epidemiology*. 35:597–603.

18. Ministry of Health. *A Portrait of Health: Key Results of the 2002/03 New Zealand Health Survey*. Wellington, Ministry of Health, 2004.

19. Macintyre, S., Ellaway, A., Cummins, S. (2002) Place effects on health: how can we conceptualise, operationalise and measure them? *Social Science and Medicine*. 55:125–139.

20. Diez Roux, A.V. (2001) Investigating neighborhood and area effects on health. *American Journal of Public Health*. 91:1783–1789.

21. Diez-Roux, A.V. (1998) Bringing context back into epidemiology: variables and fallacies in multilevel analysis. *American Journal of Public Health*. 88:216–222.

22. Pickett, K., Pearl, M. (2001) Multilevel analyses of neighbourhood socioeconomic context and health outcomes: a critical review. *Journal of Epidemiology and Community Health*. 55:111–122.

23. Stevenson, A., Pearce, J., Blakely, T., Ivory, V., Witten, K. (2009) Neighbourhoods and health: a review of the New Zealand literature. *New Zealand Geographer*. 65:211–221.

24. Blakely, T., Atkinson, J., Ivory, V., Collings, S., Wilton, J., Howden-Chapman, P. (2006) No association of neighbourhood volunteerism with mortality in New Zealand: a national multilevel cohort study. *International Journal of Epidemiology*. 35:981–989.

25. Barnett, R., Pearce, J., Moon, G. (2005) Does social inequality matter? Assessing the effects of changing ethnic socio-economic disparities on Maori smoking in New Zealand, 1981–96. *Social Science and Medicine*. 60:1515–1526.

26. Hiscock, R., Pearce, J., Blakely, T., Witten, K. (2008) Is neighbourhood access to health care provision associated with individual-level utilisation and satisfaction? *Health Services Research*. 43:2183–2200.

27. Pearce, J., Mason, K., Hiscock, R., Day, P. (2008) A national study of neighbourhood access to gambling opportunities and individual gambling behaviour. *Journal of Epidemiology and Community Health*. 62:862–868.

28. Macintyre, S., Ellaway, A. Neighbourhoods and health: an overview. In: *Neighbourhoods and Health*. (Eds. Kawachi, I., Berkman, L.) Oxford, Oxford University Press, 2003.

29. Ellaway, A., Macintyre, S., Bonnefoy, X. (2005) Graffiti, greenery, and obesity in adults: secondary analysis of European cross sectional survey. *British Medical Journal*. 331:611–612.

30. Egger, G., Swinburn, B. (1997) An "ecological" approach to the obesity pandemic. *British Medical Journal*. 315:477–480.

31. Laraia, B.A., Siega-Riz, A.M., Kaufman, J.S., Jones, S.J. (2004) Proximity of supermarkets is positively associated with diet quality index for pregnancy. *Preventive Medicine*. 39:869–875.

32. Morland, K., Wing, S., Diex-Roux, A. (2002) The contextual effect of the local food environment on residents' diet: the atherosclerosis risk in communities study. *American Journal of Public Health*. 92:1761–1767.

33. Alwitt, L., Donley, T. Retail stores in poor urban neighborhoods. (1997) *Journal of Consumer Affairs*. 31:139–164.

34. Chung, C., Myers, S. (1999) Do the poor pay more for food? An analysis of grocery store availability and food price disparities. *Journal of Consumer Affairs*. 33:276–296.

35. Moore, L.V., Diez Roux, A.V. (2006) Associations of neighborhood characteristics with the location and type of food stores. *American Journal of Public Health*. 96:325–331.

36. Morland, K., Wing, S., Diez Roux, A., Poole, C. (2002) Neighborhood characteristics associated with the location of food stores and food service places. *American Journal of Preventive Medicine*. 22:23–29.

37. Zenk, S.N., Schulz, A.J., Israel, B.A., James, S.A., Bao, S.M., Wilson, M.L. (2005) Neighborhood racial composition, neighborhood poverty, and the spatial accessibility of supermarkets in metropolitan Detroit. *American Journal of Public Health*. 95:660–667.

38. Zenk, S.N., Schulz, A.J., Hollis-Neely, T., Campbell, R.T., Holmes, N., Watkins, G., Nwankwo, R., Odoms-Young, A. (2005) Fruit and vegetable intake in African Americans – income and store characteristics. *American Journal of Preventive Medicine*. 29:1–9.

39. Cummins, S., Macintyre, S. (2006) Food environments and obesity – neighbourhood or nation? *International Journal of Epidemiology*. 35:100–104.

40. Clarke, G., Eyre, H., Guy, C. (2002) Deriving indicators of access to food retail provision in British cities: studies of Cardiff, Leeds and Bradford. *Urban Studies*. 39:2041–2060.

41. Ellaway, A., Macintyre, S. (2000) Shopping for food in socially contrasting localities. *British Food Journal*. 102:52–59.

42. Whelan, A., Wrigley, N., Warm, D., Cannings, E. (2002) Life in a 'food desert'. *Urban Studies*. 39:2083–2100.

43. Wrigley, N., Warm, D., Margetts, B. (2003) Deprivation, diet, and food-retail access: findings from the Leeds 'food deserts' study. *Environment and Planning A*. 35:151–188.

44. Wrigley, N., Warm, D., Margetts, B., Whelan, A. (2002) Assessing the impact of improved retail access on diet in a 'food desert': a preliminary report. *Urban Studies*. 39:2061–2082.

45. Cummins, S., Petticrew, M., Higgins, C., Findlay, A., Sparks, L. (2005) Large scale food retailing as an intervention for diet and health: quasi-experimental evaluation of a natural experiment. *Journal of Epidemiology and Community Health*. 59:1035–1040.

46. Pearson, T., Russell, J., Campbell, M.J., Barker, M.E. (2005) Do 'food deserts' influence fruit and vegetable consumption? – a cross-sectional study. *Appetite*. 45:195–197.

47. Smoyer-Tomic, K., Spence, J., Amrhein, C. (2006) Food deserts in the prairies? Supermarket accessibility and neighborhood need in Edmonton, Canada. *Professional Geographer*. 58:307–326.

48. Winkler, E., Turrell, G., Patterson, C. (2006) Does living in a disadvantaged area mean fewer opportunities to purchase fresh fruit and vegetables in the area? Findings from the Brisbane food study. *Health and Place*. 12:306–319.

49. Pearce, J., Witten, K., Hiscock, R., Blakely, T. (2007) Are socially disadvantaged neighbourhoods deprived of health-related community resources? *International Journal of Epidemiology*. 36:348–355.

50. Pearce, J., Hiscock, R., Blakely, T., Witten, K. (2008) The contextual effects of neighbourhood access to supermarkets and convenience stores on individual fruit and vegetable consumption. *Journal of Epidemiology Community Health*. 62:198–201.

51. Block, J.P., Scribner, R.A., Desalvo, K.B. (2004) Fast food, race/ethnicity, and income: a geographic analysis. *American Journal of Preventive Medicine*. 27:211–217.

52. Cummins, S.C.J., Mckay, L., Macintyre, S. (2005) McDonald's restaurants and neighborhood deprivation in Scotland and England. *American Journal of Preventive Medicine*. 29:308–310.

53. Macdonald, L., Cummins, S., Macintyre, S. (2007) Neighbourhood fast food environment and area deprivation–substitution or concentration? *Appetite*. 49:251–254.

54. Reidpath, D.D., Burns, C., Garrard, J., Mahoney, M., Townsend, M. (2002) An ecological study of the relationship between social and environmental determinants of obesity. *Health and Place*. 8:141–145.

55. Pearce, J., Blakely, T., Witten, K., Bartie, P. (2007) Neighborhood deprivation and access to fast food retailing: a national study. *American Journal of Preventive Medicine*. 32:375–382.
56. Pearce, J., Hiscock, R., Blakely, T., Witten, K. (2009) A national study of the association between neighbourhood access to fast food outlets and the diet and weight of local residents. *Health and Place*. 15:193–197.
57. Pearce, J., Day, P., Witten, K. (2008) Neighbourhood provision of food and alcohol retailing and social deprivation in urban New Zealand. *Urban Policy and Research*. 26:213–227.
58. Pearce, J., Witten, K., Hiscock, R., Blakely, T. (2008) Regional and urban–rural variations in the association of neighbourhood deprivation with community resource access: a national study. *Environment and Planning A*. 40:2469–2489.
59. Diez Roux, A.V. (2004) Estimating neighborhood health effects: the challenges of causal inference in a complex world. *Social Science and Medicine*. 58:1953–1960.
60. Naess, O., Claussen, B., Thelle, D.S., Davey Smith, G. (2004) Cumulative deprivation and cause specific mortality. A census based study of life course influences over three decades. *Journal of Epidemiology and Community Health*. 58:599–603.
61. Naess, O., Leyland, A.H., Davey Smith, G., Claussen, B. (2005) Contextual effect on mortality of neighbourhood level education explained by earlier life deprivation. *Journal of Epidemiology and Community Health*. 59:1058–1059.
62. Crampton, P., Salmond, C., Sutton, F. *NZDep91 Index of Deprivation Instruction Book*. Wellington, Health Services Research Centre, 1997.
63. Massey, D., Denton, N. *American Apartheid: Segregation and the Making of the Underclass*. Cambridge, MA, Harvard University Press, 2003.
64. Kwate, N.O. (2008) Fried chicken and fresh apples: racial segregation as a fundamental cause of fast food density in black neighborhoods. *Health and Place*. 14:32–44.
65. Blackman, T. *Placing Health: Neighbourhood Renewal, Health Improvement and Complexity*. Bristol, Policy Press, 2006.
66. Davies, J.K., Kelly, M.P. *Healthy Cities: Research and Practice*. London; New York, Routledge, 1993.
67. Stafford, M., Nazroo, J., Popay, J.M., Whitehead, M. (2008) Tackling inequalities in health: evaluating the New Deal for Communities initiative. *Journal of Epidemiology and Community Health*. 62:298–304.
68. Cummins, S., Macintyre, S. (2002) "Food deserts" – evidence and assumption in health policy making. *British Medical Journal*. 325:436–438.
69. Pearce, J., Witten, K., Bartie, P. (2006) Neighbourhoods and health: a GIS approach to measuring community resource accessibility. *Journal of Epidemiology and Community Health*. 60:389–395.

13 Environmental Correlates of Nutrition and Physical Activity: Moving Beyond the Promise

Frank J. van Lenthe
and Johnannes Brug

13.1 Introduction

According to the principles of a planned approach to promote population health, the development of effective interventions and policies aimed at curbing the obesity epidemic requires a proper understanding of its determinants. Obesity is the result of a lasting positive imbalance between energy intake and energy expenditure. Energy intake can be modified by changes in nutrition. Energy expenditure can mainly be modified by increasing physical activity, which raises the question of what the determinants of these behaviours are.

Research on the determinants of nutrition and physical activity behaviours has, in recent decades, mostly been rooted in social-cognitive theories, and was mainly focused on identifying individual-level, cognitive or belief-based behavioural determinants. However, in the past decade attention shifted towards environmental determinants of such energy-balance behaviours. This change followed and further instigated a paradigm shift from a health education 'planned learning experiences to facilitate voluntary change in behaviour'[1] to a health promotion 'the combination of educational and environmental supports for actions and conditions of living conducive to health'[2] approach in encouraging prevention of unnecessary weight gain. Further, it coincided with the development of socio-ecological models of health behaviours[2] as well as methodological developments, in particular the introduction of multilevel analysis in public health research.[3] As is clear in previous chapters, many studies are nowadays conducted to explore the association between environmental factors on the one hand, and physical activity and nutrition behaviour on the other.

13.2 Environmental correlates of physical activity and diet: underlying reasons for promising findings

Research on the determinants of energy-balance behaviours has long been focused on identifying individual cognitions. Studies applied well-known theories, such as the Theory of Planned Behaviour[4] and the Social-Cognitive Theory[5] to measure cognitions and to relate them to physical activity. The aim of these studies is to predict individual behaviour and explore individual-level, primarily cognitive potential determinants. The available evidence suggests that approximately 20–40% of variance in energy-balance behaviours can be explained by these social-cognitive potential determinants.[6] The interest in the role of the environment for physical activity and diet is perhaps to some extent due to this finding, that is, that a major part of these behaviours remain 'unexplained'. There are, however, more compelling reasons to search for environmental correlates of physical activity and diet. Firstly, the rise in obesity started in the early 1980s and in the last 25 years the prevalence of obesity has increased dramatically. While this happened in the United States initially, many countries have been or are experiencing similar trends. In order to understand the dramatic increase in obesity in many countries in the world, there is a need to focus on determinants that have changed *populations* in all these countries.

Although factors such as those described in social-cognitive models can, of course, change over time, it is a legitimate question to ask why they would have changed in themselves in such a short period of time for so many people. It seems reasonable to assume that there are underlying structural 'upstream' changes that have occurred in our societies and that may have resulted in the substantial increase in obesity at the population level in so many countries. Along with other changes, urbanisation may be one such structural change. Secondly, studies have reported that obesity is not randomly distributed within countries. A consistent finding in many western countries is the higher prevalence of obesity in lower as compared to higher socio-economic groups.[7] If physical activity and/or an unhealthy dietary intake were primarily the result of individual cognitions, the consistency of the socio-economic gradient in obesity would be rather coincidental. It is more likely that underlying exposures shared by socio-economic groups result in lower levels of physical activity and/or a higher dietary energy intake, leading to higher obesity rates. It may well be that such environmental influences are mediated by changes in cognitions and beliefs, but population changes in obesity do suggest that there are common, structural upstream or more 'ultimate' determinants at work. Thirdly, after the introduction of multilevel analytical techniques in public health research, studies have shown neighbourhood inequalities in obesity. Residents from more deprived neighbourhoods have an increased risk of obesity, compared to residents of more affluent neighbourhoods, and these inequalities can only to some extent be explained by the composition of the neighbourhoods.[8]

Following these lines of reasoning, the identification of environmental correlates of physical activity and diet emerged as a promising field. In the past 10 years, a first generation of studies has been published; the following sections explore what can be concluded.

13.3 Environmental correlates of physical activity

The expectation of promising findings is reflected by the large number of studies conducted in the past 10 years. There is now a considerable number of review papers, and even some review of reviews. One of the first studies summarising the links between the physical environment and physical activity, published in an urban planning journal, suggested that 'environmental barriers to physical activity are still poorly understood' (p. 209).[9] A first systematic review in a public health journal appeared in 2002 and identified 19 studies in which physical environmental characteristics were linked to physical activity.[10] The majority of studies measured a variety of perceptions of the environment. Most studies in the review did find associations between perceptions of the environmental and physical activity, but there were only few consistent associations; though overall, the results were described as 'promising'.[10] On the more specific issue of environmental correlates of walking – a type of physical activity that most people can engage in, similar conclusions were drawn from other review studies. Owen et al. showed a 'modest but consistent' body of evidence of relationships between the physical environment and walking.[11] Trost et al. reviewed studies linking the physical environment to physical activity and showed that the strength of the associations varied from study to study. They concluded that there was 'sufficient evidence to identify several new environmental correlates of physical activity' (p. 1999).[12] Saelens et al. reviewed the transportation literature and concluded that evidence suggested that residents from communities with higher population density, greater connectivity and more land use mix reported higher rates of walking/cycling for utilitarian purposes.[13] Cunningham and Michael reviewed the literature on aspects of the built environment for physical activity and older adults, and identified six studies in older adults.[14] In this review inconsistent results were found, this was attributed to problems of measuring the built environment.

With these conclusions in mind, we conducted a systematic review on environmental determinants of physical activity in 2004.[15] The study included a substantially larger number of studies ($n = 47$) and the results could be classified in more detail. Environmental characteristics were classified using the analysis grid for environments linked to obesity (ANGELO) framework[16] (which distinguishes the physical, social–cultural, economic and political environment), and studies were classified by types of physical activity (such as total physical activity, moderate physical activity, commuting activity, walking and bicycling). If in more than half of the investigated samples in the included studies significant associations were found, we concluded that there was 'convincing evidence'; a possible association was found if 40–50% of the associations were statistically significant in at least three studies. The review showed that particularly in the field of the physical environmental characteristics, only 'possible' associations were found. A possible positive association was found for convenience of recreational facilities in relation to sports/vigorous physical activity. Connectivity of trails was convincingly associated with commuting activities. A possible association was found between the availability of sidewalks and walking and (in men only) between environmental aesthetics and walking. These mixed findings were also reported in a more recent review on the associations between parks and recreation settings and physical activity.[17] Studies linking the built environment to walking and cycling for leisure time showed that only few measures were correlated to physical activity.[18] Panter et al. reviewed environmental determinants of active travel in youth and also reported mixed results, perhaps with the exception of route length.[19]

To conclude, there has been a substantial increase in studies linking (predominantly physical) environmental characteristics to elements of physical activity. Initially, results were seen as promising, but currently, there is lack of consistent evidence for specific associations, perhaps with the exception of environmental correlates of recreational walking and walking and cycling for transport.[20] Can we thus conclude that the environment is not so important for physical activity as was initially proposed? We argue that the reviews briefly reviewed in this chapter are based on a 'first generation' of studies that can merely explore the issue, but that, in general, are too weak to draw firmer conclusions. There is a clear need to improve the research in this field.

13.4   Environmental correlates of diet

In research exploring environmental correlates of dietary intakes, physical environmental characteristics have been regarded as promising possible determinants for many years. For example, studies in socio-economically contrasting neighbourhoods suggested that a poorer dietary intake of residents of deprived, as compared to residents of more affluent neighbourhoods, could be ascribed to lower accessibility and to higher prices of healthy foods.[21] Two studies summarising the evidence of the association between environmental correlations of fruits and vegetables, fat and energy intake, however, showed that the evidence linking the physical environment and dietary intake is still far from consistent and convincing.[22,23] The reviews made clear that a great diversity of environmental factors was studied, but also that the number of replicated studies for each determinant was limited, or that replications were lacking completely. Thus, it appeared to be premature to conclude that environmental factors were related to these dietary outcomes. The studies also found more consistent evidence of environmental correlates at the household level than at the neighbourhood level.

Food patterns of children, particularly in children aged 12 years and younger, are to a large extent determined by their parents. Not surprisingly therefore, the majority of studies on environmental correlates of children's diets have concentrated on parental and home environmental factors. Indeed, van der Horst *et al.*, who systematically searched for all studies on the association between environmental determinants and total energy intake, fat intake, fruit and vegetable intake, snacks/fast food, soft drinks until the end of 2004, showed that a majority of studies explored household (parental) characteristics. Only some studies were focused on schools-environmental factors, and little information was available about physical environmental factors.[24] This review thus also shows that there is no clear and consistent evidence about the link between physical environmental factors and nutrition behaviours.

13.5   Moving beyond the promise: a research agenda

We started this chapter by providing some arguments for a shift in emphasis in behavioural nutrition and physical activity research from personal-level factors towards environmental determinants of physical activity and nutrition. There are good reasons to think in terms of a promising field of research; yet, the current state of research shows inconsistent results and thus unclear patterns. This may of course be because the role of environmental characteristics is not as important as we initially believed it was. On the other hand, it has been called 'actually surprising' that associations have been found, given that it concerns distal factors that are often crudely or even poorly measured.[25] Indeed, given the infancy of this complex field of research, more and better research can and should help to interpret the strength of the association between environmental characteristics and physical activity and diet. We provide eight recommendations for further research.

13.5.1 Providing robust answers to the right questions

With perhaps a few exceptions, studies on the association between environmental characteristics and behavioural nutrition, and physical activity and obesity, have used cross-sectional study designs. These studies provide an answer to the question whether environmental characteristics are associated with these outcomes. They contribute to understanding the correlates of present behaviours and health states, that is, correlates of the obesity epidemic, *as it currently is*. It is at least equally important to further understand what may have caused the rising trend in unfavourable physical activity and nutrition patterns, overweight and obesity, that is, to identify correlates, predictors and determinants of the observed change over time. Prevalence rates in, for example, the United States have doubled or even tripled in the past two decades, and in many other countries steeply rising trends are observed at present. To curb the increase in the prevalence, we need to identify the predictors and possible determinants of these increases. These may very well be different from the correlates or determinants of the current prevalence, as can be illustrated for the association between fast food outlets and dietary intake.

Fast food consumption is one of the usual suspects for the obesity epidemic. Different studies have shown that people who eat fast food more, or more frequently, have a higher risk to become overweight or obese.[26] It has been argued that the easy availability and accessibility of fast food outlets makes people eat more and increases their risk for unnecessary weight gain. Several studies have focused on the association between the proximity to fast food outlets and the consumption of fast food, both in adults and in children. Contrary to what would be expected, studies linking the neighbourhood density or proximity of fast food outlets to snack consumption or obesity did not find a positive association[27,28]; in fact, one study reported that living closer to fast food outlets was associated with a lower body mass index (BMI).[27] However, in order to interpret such results appropriately, information about overall accessibility and variation in accessibility may be important. In the United States, for example, one-third of all schools have at least one fast food outlet or convenience store within 800 m from the school.[29] In the city of Glasgow, United Kingdom, more than two food premises (restaurants, cafes, takeaways and fast food restaurants) per 1000 residents were identified in 2003.[30] Thus, in contemporary societies large segments of the population have good access to fast food outlets, and therefore relevant variation in access to outlets may be limited. If we do take into account that most individuals will also have good fast food accessibility in other environments than their home neighbourhood (e.g. where they work or go to school) the variation is likely to be even smaller than observed when only the home environment is taken into account. It may, therefore, not be too surprising that at present no associations between proximity to fast food outlets, fast food consumption and obesity may be found.

In studying the role of fast food outlet density in the obesity epidemic, it may be more important to investigate if the rise in number of fast food outlets, and the growing proximity over the years, that is, before almost everyone has easy access to such outlets, preceded and predicted changes in behavioural nutrition and weight status. Studies in the United States have shown a dramatic increase in the number of fast food restaurants. The proportion of fast food restaurants from the total number of restaurants has almost doubled between 1997 and 2007,[31] that is, in a period in which obesity rates in children and adults have also steeply increased. To our knowledge, there are no studies available directly linking this increase in fast food outlets to the increase in childhood obesity with an appropriate design, but this longitudinal association deserves to be further investigated. To summarise, a lack of consistency in associations between present-day potential obesogenic environmental factors on the one hand and present-day behaviours or weight status on the other do not tell us much about the role such environmental factors may have played in shaping the obesity epidemic and obesogenic behaviours. Studies are needed in which associations between the development of environmental characteristics and behavioural nutrition and physical activity, as well as obesity, are investigated.

13.5.2 Development and application of a true socio-ecological theory

The increased recognition of the need to understand health behaviours in their (environmental) context has resulted in socio-ecological health promotion frameworks which differentiate between elements of the environment,[16,32] and link environmental characteristics to health behaviours, sometimes mediated by individual characteristics.[33,34] These frameworks are very helpful, but can be enriched by analysing and benefitting from insights from disciplines that have a much longer tradition in studying environments that may be relevant for behavioural nutrition and physical activity research; disciplines such as urban geography, sociology and economics.

A crucial feature of good socio-ecological theory for behavioural nutrition and physical activity is that it increases our understanding of the dynamics of the living environment in relation to relevant behaviours. It allows the formulation of appropriate hypotheses, and helps to design and conduct studies to test these hypotheses. This is well illustrated in studies in which the proximity to facilities is related to (un)healthy diet, physical activity or obesity. In such studies, an important question concerns the role of area deprivation, often measured by, for example, the mean neighbourhood income or the percentage of unemployment. Arguably, deprivation is a confounder: in deprived neighbourhoods there may be fewer shops to buy, for example, fruits and vegetables, the number of fast food outlets is higher, and people may eat less fruits and vegetables and consume more fast food. From this perspective, is it appropriate to statistically adjust for neighbourhood deprivation in analyses linking proximity to outlets to consumption? Good theory, however, would better support the strategy for analyses. Gentrification results in a change in neighbourhood deprivation, for example, a change in mean neighbourhood income because wealthier residents move out of neighbourhoods to new neighbourhoods and financially less well off people move in. Based on theory, this may result in a migration of fruit shops out of deprived neighbourhoods.[35] Thus, the change in neighbourhood deprivation would cause a change in the availability of fruit shops and in this situation, one should not adjust for neighbourhood deprivation. Studies have shown that adjustment for neighbourhood deprivation can make a substantial difference in the association between accessibility of outlets and health-related behaviours.[36] Improved socio-ecological theory describing how different environmental factors are related to each other avoids such problems.

13.5.3 Integrating different elements of the environment

To help guide research into environment and health behaviour, the environment can be seen as everything outside the individual. This is, of course, a very broad and general formulation. In studies investigating the obesogenic environment, most attention has been paid to physical environmental factors, that is, availability and accessibility opportunities to eat too much and move too little. The ANGELO framework, however, identifies different categories of the environment: the physical, social-cultural, economic and political environment.[16] Our review, in which environmental characteristics were classified according to this framework indeed showed that the majority of associations studied concerned the physical living environment.[15] The same study, however, reported a much more consistent association for the social environment with physical activity and nutrition, than for the physical environment. Social support was a social-environmental factor that appeared to be important for physical activity, while modelling or social learning appeared to be of particular relevance for nutrition, especially for children and adolescents. These reviews indicate that we should look beyond the physical environment to gain better insights into obesogenic environments, and the social environment is a promising research avenue to explore.

Our review showed that especially more proximal social-environmental factors have been studied in relation to behavioural nutrition and physical activity, such as subjective norms, perceived social support and example behaviour (descriptive norms), of important others. There is an increasing interest in the more distal aspects of the social–cultural environment, for example, factors that may shape the conditions for receiving social support. This concerns, in particular, social cohesion and related concepts (social capital, social disorganisation) and social networks. There is a general concern that modern societies have resulted in a decline in social cohesion in western societies. A majority of studies tend to support the hypothesis that social cohesion enhances health, but there is still little empirical research linking social cohesion to physical activity and diet.[37] Moreover, recent research suggests that health-related behaviours and obesity spread through social networks.[38] If indeed this is the case, and to the extent that social cohesion reduces social networks and social support for health-related behaviour, a decline in social cohesion may have contributed to declining levels of physical activity. Further research on the importance of this broader social environment is therefore warranted.

Relatively little knowledge is available on aspects of the cultural environment, such as shared norms and values with respect to healthy eating and physical activity. Based on ideas from the French sociologist Pierre Bourdieu, Roskam and Mackenbach[39] hypothesised that the adoption of healthier lifestyles in a time where unhealthy choices are available everywhere can be seen as a way of 'distinction' from others. This could be one of the mechanisms through which socio-economic inequalities in physical activity and a healthy diet can be explained. Some studies have linked (class-related) cultural resources ('cultural capital') to health, but still little is known on the link to physical activity and a healthy diet.[40,41]

Finally, in relation to this theme, what is the role of economic characteristics? Within affluent countries, there is little evidence that food prices differ geographically, exposing certain groups in societies to higher prices. Arguably, however, some healthy foods are more expensive than unhealthy food and sports facilities can be expensive, and as such there can be an association between the economic environment and these behaviours. Drewnowski and Darmon have argued that refined grains, added sugar and added fats are among the least expensive sources of energy.[42] But it is unclear if people use a price/calorie ratio as an important motivation for food choice and other current studies including prices of healthy food have produced findings that are difficult to understand. Giskes et al. showed that perceptions of prices did not match with objective prices,[43] and also that residents who perceived fruits and vegetables as expensive were more likely to consume them.[44] Current research has strongly focused on identifying 'single' environmental correlates. Future research, however, should integrate elements of different environments and should develop hypotheses based on this integration.

13.5.4 Improving the measurement of (physical) environmental characteristics

Integrating methods to measure objective environmental characteristics

An important critical comment about much research currently conducted concerns the measurement of environmental characteristics. In this early phase of research, we often still depend on non-validated, self-report measures, or on more objective assessments of environmental characteristics based on measures that were not designed to study possible determinants of behavioural nutrition and physical activity. More recent research specifically designed to explore the role of the environment for physical activity and diet introduced other techniques, such as geographic information systems for measuring density and distance to characteristics. A series of audit instruments have been developed to measure particularly those characteristics that could not be captured by routinely available databases.[45,46] It is now widely accepted that in many situations distances to facilities 'on their own' are weakly or unrelated to diet and physical activity; reality is more complex. There is a need to integrate different aspects of the physical environment, such as distances to parks, in combination with their quality and safety. Indicators capturing different aspects of the physical environmental characteristics may provide stronger associations with physical activity and diet.[47]

Understanding the relation between objectively measured characteristics and individual perceptions of the environment

In addition to collecting information about objective environmental characteristics through methods described above, assessment of how people perceive their environment remains important. Perceptions of the environment capture how residents view their environment; people see, hear, smell and otherwise experience their environment, and this information is cognitively processed leading to perceptions. It is likely that different people perceive the same environment differently, based on, for example, their motivations, past behaviours, values and preferences. Perceptions of the environment are, therefore, more proximal potential determinants of behaviour than the 'real', objective measures of the environment. Various studies indeed indicate that perceptions of the environment are more strongly associated with physical activity and nutrition behaviours than objective measures of environments. However, these results are mostly based on cross-sectional studies, and these stronger associations may not be indications of causality. It may very well be that self-reported 'perceptions' of the environment are rather justifications of their present behaviour: if asked to (dis)agree with statements like 'There are sufficient sports facilities in my area' it is likely that inactive persons will agree, as an 'excuse' for their lack of activity. Physically inactive persons may also be less knowledgeable about available sports facilities in their living environment than active persons, since they have less experience in using these facilities. Moreover, in cross-sectional studies, asking the same residents to provide information about their behaviour and potential environmental correlates of these behaviours may easily result in 'same source bias': personality characteristics may result in a tendency to answer questions on both behaviours and the environment in the same (positive or negative) direction, which results in spurious correlations.

The legitimacy of objectively measured characteristics is rooted in the fact that this is the environment that can be changed through policy, so that many persons are reached, and such real changes would be expected to also influence what people perceive. Instead of arguing whether one way of measurement is superior to the other, research should preferably include both, should focus on further understanding the differences and take these differences and unique contributions into account in the interpretation of study findings. For example, Kamphuis recently found that socio-economic inequalities in perceptions of the environment were partly explained by objectively measured environmental characteristics, and also by psychosocial factors of individuals.[48]

13.5.5   Exploring environmental–individual interactions

Although integration of different environmental characteristics may result in stronger associations between 'the environment' and physical activity and diet, it is not likely that a combination of environmental characteristics will completely explain these behaviours. For both physical activity and diet, individual cognitions and personality characteristics are important. One of the key challenges in future research is to integrate both individual and environmental characteristics. Initially, studies often statistically adjusted for cognitions in research aimed at identifying the independent association between environmental correlates and physical activity and diet. It has been argued that environmental characteristics are partly related to the behaviours via these cognitions, and that statistical adjustment of the mediators takes away part of the effect of the environment. Therefore, mediation analysis, with all its complexities in itself, is now an important area of research.[49] In addition, an improved understanding of moderation, that is, the extent to which environmental characteristics have stronger, or weaker, associations with physical activity and diet in combination with individual characteristics, has been emphasised.[50] Thus far, this mainly concerned socio-demographic and personality characteristics. Adopting a life-course perspective, in which attitudes may develop in youth (e.g. prior to the choice of the living environment), it can be hypothesised that the environment moderates the association between attitudes and these behaviours. There is still little attention for this type of moderation.[34] Research needs to further elucidate the (complex) interaction between environmental determinants and individual-level correlates of physical activity and diet.

13.5.6   Improving statistical methods: beyond multilevel modelling

To date, the available studies on the environment-behaviour associations are mostly based on studies using secondary analyses. This means that environmental characteristics are most often based on indicators from available databases, and these databases are mostly available at aggregated area levels, such as the neighbourhood level. This concerns, for example, indicators for the availability of shops and sport facilities, the density of fast food outlets, and also indicators for social cohesion. Using this approach, all residents within an administrative boundary are thus regarded as 'equally exposed', and residents outside the area are regarded as 'not exposed' to the environmental characteristics of the adjacent neighbourhoods. Of course, this may not match with reality. Residents living 'at the edge' of a neighbourhood may live closer to facilities just outside their neighbourhood than to similar facilities in their own neighbourhood. A traditional multilevel model provides information about the variation within neighbourhoods, but does not model the correlation between neighbourhoods (spatial autocorrelation). Geostatistical models provide information about clustering within neighbourhoods and also about the correlation between neighbourhoods. There is some evidence that such an approach results in stronger associations between contextual determinants and health outcomes.[51] A related problem is that the appropriate scale for environmental characteristics and for specific behaviours does not match with traditional or statistical boundaries. Geostatistical models incorporate a notion of the appropriate space into statistical analyses and, therefore, provide important additional information. Similarly, the use of ego-centred boundaries of an individual's living environment, including both objective and selective boundaries, will further enhance our understanding of associations.[52]

13.5.7   Improving causality

Applying new methods in observational research

The studies described in the overview in previous paragraphs report on associations, which may be the result from confounding (a third variable influencing both the environmental characteristic and the behavioural outcome), selection processes (health-related behaviours determining where people live or owners of outlets coming to potential customers) and because associations may be in the opposite direction (physically active persons may get a larger social network as a consequence of their participation in physical activities). For the development of interventions and policy recommendations, it is important to further improve knowledge on the causality of relationships between environmental factors and physical activity and dietary intake. Although it is not possible to make a causal inference from observational studies, methodological improvements can help to get closer to enabling causal inferences. For this purpose, there is an increased interest in the use of propensity scores. A propensity score is based on a number of relevant covariates, and individuals with different exposures to environmental characteristics can be matched on these propensity scores.[53] As a result, 'similar' persons with and without environmental exposure can be observed, and this mimics a randomised study better than statistical adjustment in multivariate analyses.

Intervention research

We have described that most studies are cross-sectional with sometimes too little variance in exposure to environmental characteristics. Despite methodological advances, causal inferences from observational research will remain sub-optimal; experimental research is needed. Such experimentation may be possible for micro-level environmental factors, such as in cluster-randomised trials in schools or companies. Changing the larger, meso- or macro-level (physical) environment for purposes of evaluating the effects on health-related behaviours seems, however, unrealistic. There is, however, a possibility to evaluate changes in the environment that happen anyway, and such situations provide us with natural experiments. For example, Cummins *et al.* evaluated the introduction of a large-scale food retailing new supermarket in a deprived setting.[54] The quasi-experimental approach of this natural experiment did not find an intervention effect. Another study was able to demonstrate an increase in pedestrian activity after the introduction of a traffic calming scheme.[55] These studies illustrate the possibility (as well as the complexity) of evaluating natural experiments. There is a clear need to conduct more evaluations of these natural experiments.

At the same time, however, epidemiological modelling may be a tool to explore potential health consequences of changes in the environment, if enough valid information about environment–behaviour–obesity relationships is available. Such health impact assessments have been made for the assessment of the effects of interventions and policies,[56,57] but may also be valuable at the local level.

13.5.8 Taking the broader context into account

As mentioned, a majority of studies has linked *physical* environmental characteristics to physical activity. These studies are often conducted in the United States and in Australia. More than in many other fields of public health research, an intriguing question concerns the external validity of these results, because physical environments differ worldwide. The question is warranted to what extent results obtained from one study can be translated to other regions across the world. Currently, the issue of transferability of results from one country to another is most prominent for the local food environment. There is consistent evidence that the local food environment is related to dietary intake and obesity in the United States.[58–61] For example, the prevalence of obesity in the United States is lower in areas with supermarkets and higher in area with small grocery stores or fast food restaurants. In addition, it has been suggested that the local food environment may contribute to socio-economic disparities in dietary intake.[62] Such findings are, however, not, or poorly, replicated in studies in other parts of the world. In fact, in a small and heavily dense country as the Netherlands, no inequalities are found in the distance to supermarkets, and to the extent that there were differences, the density of supermarkets was higher in the less instead of the more affluent areas.[63]

These inconsistencies in findings have two major implications. Firstly, if there are differences in the association between environmental correlates of physical activity and diet between countries, there will be no consistency in evidence, and this needs to be taken into account in interpreting the results of review studies. Secondly, it highlights the need to go 'beyond' the measurement of the environment. It is crucially important to improve understanding of the 'drivers' that shape the local environment and that differ between countries.[64] In summarising and interpreting the results of research, there is a need to better take into account such drivers.

13.6   Concluding remark

In conclusion, there are good reasons to believe that environmental characteristics have contributed to the obesity epidemic. Research in environmental correlates of nutrition and physical activity has increased substantially in the past decade. The absence of a clear and coherent pattern of results yet must be seen as the outcome of a first generation of research. Given the major public health consequences of obesity, there is an urgent need to continue research along the lines discussed here.

References

1. Green, L., Kreuter, M. *Health Promotion Planning: An Educational and Ecological Approach*. 3rd Edition, Mountain View, CA, Mayfield, 1999.
2. Sallis, J.F., Owen, N. Ecological models of health behaviour. In: *Health Behavior and Health Education: Theory, Research, and Practice*. (Eds. Glanz, K., Lewis, F.M., Rimer, B.K.) 2nd Edition, San Francisco, CA, Jossey-Bass, 1996, 403–424.
3. Rice, N., Leyland, A. (1996) Multilevel models: application to health data. *Journal of Health Services Research and Policy*. 1:154–164.
4. Ajzen, I. (1991) The theory of planned behaviour. *Organisational Behaviour and Human Decision Processes*. 50:179–211.
5. Bandura, A. *Social Foundations of Thought and Action. A Social Cognitive Theory.*Eaglewoods Cliff, NJ, Erlbaum, 1986.
6. Armitage, C.J., Conner, M. (2001) Efficacy of the theory of planned behaviour: a meta-analytic review. *British Journal of Social Psychology*. 40(Pt 4):471–499.
7. Mackenbach, J.P., Stirbu, I., Roskam, A.J., Schaap, M.M., Menvielle, G., Leinsalu, M., Kunst, A. (2008) Socioeconomic inequalities in health in 22 European countries. *New England Journal of Medicine*. 358(23):2468–2481.
8. van Lenthe, F.J., Mackenbach, J.P. (2002) Neighbourhood deprivation and overweight: the GLOBE study. *International Journal of Obesity and Related Metabolic Disorders*. 26(2):234–240.
9. Frank, L.D., Engelke, P. (2001) The built environment and human activity patterns: exploring the impacts of urban form on public health. *Journal of Planning Literature*. 16: 202–218.
10. Humpel, N., Owen, N., Leslie, E. (2002) Environmental factors associated with adults' participation in physical activity: a review. *American Journal of Preventive Medicine*. 22(3):188–199.
11. Owen, N., Humpel, N., Leslie, E., Bauman, A., Sallis, J.F. (2004) Understanding environmental influences on walking; Review and research agenda. *American Journal of Preventive Medicine*. 27(1):67–76.
12. Trost, S.G., Owen, N., Bauman, A.E., Sallis, J.F., Brown, W. (2002) Correlates of adults' participation in physical activity: review and update. *Medicine and Science in Sports and Exercise*. 34(12):1996–2001.
13. Saelens, B.E., Sallis, J.F., Frank, L.D. (2003) Environmental correlates of walking and cycling: findings from the transportation, urban design, and planning literatures. *Annals of Behavioural Medicine*. 25(2):80–91.
14. Cunningham, G.O., Michael, Y.L. (2004) Concepts guiding the study of the impact of the built environment on physical activity for older adults: a review of the literature. *American Journal of Health Promotion*. 18(6):435–443.
15. Wendel-Vos, W., Droomers, M., Kremers, S., Brug, J., van Lenthe, F.J. (2007) Potential environmental determinants of physical activity in adults: a systematic review. *Obesity Reviews*. 8:425–440.

16. Swinburn, B., Egger, G., Raza, F. (1999) Dissecting obesogenic environments: the development and application of a framework for identifying and prioritizing environmental interventions for obesity. *Preventive Medicine.* 29:563–570.
17. Kaczynski, A.T., Henderson, K.A. (2008) Parks and recreation settings and active living: a review of associations with physical activity function and intensity. *Journal of Physical Activity and Health.* 5(4):619–632.
18. Committee on Physical Activity. *Transportation, and Land Use. Does the built environment influence physical activity? Examining the evidence.* Transportation Research Board, Institute of Medicine of the National Academies, 2005.
19. Panter, J.R., Jones, A.P., van Sluijs, E.M. (2008) Environmental determinants of active travel in youth: a review and framework for future research. *International Journal of Behavioural Nutrition and Physical Activity.* 5:34.
20. Saelens, B.E., Handy, S.L. (2008) Built environment correlates of walking: a review. *Medicine and Science in Sports and Exercise.* 40 (7 Suppl):S550–S566.
21. Ellaway, A., Macintyre, S. (1996) Does where you live predict health related behaviours?: a case study in Glasgow. *Health Bulletin (Edinb).* 54(6):443–446.
22. Giskes, K., Kamphuis, C.B., van Lenthe, F.J., Kremers, S., Droomers, M., Brug, J. (2007) A systematic review of associations between environmental factors, energy and fat intakes among adults: is there evidence for environments that encourage obesogenic dietary intakes? *Public Health Nutrition.* 10(10):1005–1017.
23. Kamphuis, C.B., Giskes, K., de Bruijn, G.J., Wendel-Vos, W., Brug, J., van Lenthe, F.J. (2006) Environmental determinants of fruit and vegetable consumption among adults: a systematic review. *British Journal of Nutrition.* 96(4):620–635.
24. van der Horst, K., Oenema, A., Ferreira, I., Wendel-Vos, W., Giskes, K., van Lenthe, F., Brug, J. (2007) A systematic review of environmental correlates of obesity-related dietary behaviors in youth. *Health Education Research,* 22:203–226.
25. Diez Roux, A.V. (2008) Next steps in understanding the multilevel determinants of health. *Journal of Epidemiology and Community Health.* 62(11):957–959.
26. Rosenheck, R. (2008) Fast food consumption and increased caloric intake: a systematic review of a trajectory towards weight gain and obesity risk. *Obesity Reviews.* 9(6):535–547.
27. Crawford, D.A., Timperio, A.F., Salmon, J.A., Baur, L., Giles-Corti, B., Roberts, R.J., Jackson, M.L., Andrianopoulos, N., Ball, K. (2008) Neighbourhood fast food outlets and obesity in children and adults: the CLAN Study. *International Journal of Pediatric Obesity.* 3(4):249–256.
28. van der Horst, K., Timperio, A., Crawford, D., Roberts, R., Brug, J., Oenema, A. (2008) The school food environment associations with adolescent soft drink and snack consumption. *American Journal of Preventive Medicine.* 35(3):217–223.
29. Zenk, S.N., Powell, L.M. (2008) US secondary schools and food outlets. *Health and Place.* 14(2):336–346.
30. Macintyre, S., McKay, L., Cummins, S., Burns, C. (2005) Out-of-home food outlets and area deprivation: case study in Glasgow, UK. *International Journal of Behavioral Nutrition and Physical Activity.* 2:16.
31. Powell, L.M., Chaloupka, F.J., Bao, Y. (2007) The availability of fast-food and full-service restaurants in the United States: associations with neighborhood characteristics. *American Journal of Preventive Medicine.* 33 (4 Suppl):S240–S245.
32. McLeroy, K.R., Bibeau, D., Steckler, A., Glanz, K. (1988) An ecological perspective on health promotion programs. *Health Education Quarterly.* 15:351–377.
33. Flay, B.R., Petraitis, J. (1994) The theory of triadic influence: a new theory of health behaviour with implications for preventive interventions. *Advances in Medical Sociology.* 4:19–44.
34. Kremers, S.P., de Bruijn, G.J., Visscher, T.L., van Mechelen, W., de Vries, N.K., Brug, J. (2006) Environmental influences on energy balance-related behaviors: A dual-process view. *International Journal of Behavioural Nutrition and Physical Activity.* 3:9.
35. Skogan, W. *Disorder and Decline: Crime and the Spiral of Decay in American Neighborhoods.* Berkely, University of Berkeley, 1990.

36. Pearce, J., Hiscock, R., Moon, G., Barnett, R. (2009) The neighbourhood effects of geographical access to tobacco retailers on individual smoking behaviour. *Journal of Epidemiology and Community Health*. 63(1):69–77.

37. Lindstrom, M., Moghaddassi, M., Merlo, J. (2003) Social capital and leisure time physical activity: a population based multilevel analysis in Malmo, Sweden. *Journal of Epidemiology and Community Health*. 57(1):23–28.

38. Christakis, N.A., Fowler, J.H. (2007) The spread of obesity in a large social network over 32 years. *New England Journal of Medicine*. 357(4):370–379.

39. Mackenbach, J.P., Roskam, A.J. Gewichtige verschillen: sociale stratificatie en overgewicht. In: *De Obesogene Samenleving*. (Eds. Dagevos, H., Munnichs, G.) Amsterdam, Amsterdam Univerisity Press, 2007 pp. 33–42.

40. Abel, T. (2008) Cultural capital and social inequality in health. *Journal of Epidemiology and Community Health*. 62(7):e13.

41. Veenstra, G. (2007) Social space, social class and Bourdieu: health inequalities in British Columbia, Canada. *Health and Place*. 13(1):14–31.

42. Drewnowski, A., Darmon, N. (2005) The economics of obesity: dietary energy density and energy cost. *American Journal of Clinical Nutrition*. 82 (1 Suppl):265S–273S.

43. Giskes, K., Van Lenthe, F.J., Brug, J., Mackenbach, J.P., Turrell, G. (2007) Socioeconomic inequalities in food purchasing: the contribution of respondent-perceived and actual (objectively measured) price and availability of foods. *Preventive Medicine*. 45(1): 41–48.

44. Giskes, K., van Lenthe, F.J., Kamphuis, C.B., Huisman, M., Brug, J., Mackenbach, J.P. (2009) Household and food shopping environments: do they play a role in socioeconomic inequalities in fruit and vegetable consumption? A multilevel study among Dutch adults. *Journal of Epidemiology and Community Health*. 63(2):113–120.

45. Day, K., Boarnet, M., Alfonzo, M., Forsyth, A. (2006) The Irvine-Minnesota inventory to measure built environments: development. *American Journal of Preventive Medicine*. 30(2):144–152.

46. van Lenthe, F.J., Huisman, M., Kamphuis, C.B., Giskes, K., Brug, J., Mackenbach, J.P. *Een Beoordelingsinstrument van Fysieke en Sociale Buurtkenmerken die Gezondheid Stimuleren dan wel Bevorderen*. Rotterdam, Department of Public Health, Erasmus Medical Center Rotterdam, 2006.

47. Giles-Corti, B., Timperio, A., Bull, F., Pikora, T. (2005) Understanding physical activity environmental correlates: increased specificity for ecological models. *Exercise Sport Science Review*. 33(4):175–181.

48. Kamphuis, C.B.M. Why do poor people perceive poor neighbourhoods. In: *Explaining Socioeconomic Inequalities in Health Behaviours: the Role of Environmental Factors*. (Ed. Kamphuis, C.B.M.) Rotterdam, Rotterdam Erasmus University (PhD-thesis), 2008 pp. 120–142.

49. Cerin, E., Mackinnon, D.P. (2008) A commentary on current practice in mediating variable analyses in behavioural nutrition and physical activity. *Public Health Nutrition*. 1–7.

50. Kremers, S.P., de Bruijn, G.J., Droomers, M., van Lenthe, F., Brug, J. (2006) Moderators of environmental intervention effects on diet and activity in youth. *American Journal of Preventive Medicine*. 32(2):163–172

51. Chaix, B., Merlo, J., Chauvin, P. (2005) Comparison of a spatial approach with the multilevel approach for investigating place effects on health: the example of healthcare utilisation in France. *Journal of Epidemiology and Community Health*. 59(6):517–526.

52. Chaix, B. (2009) Geographic life environments and coronary heart disease: a literature review, theoretical contributions, methodological updates, and a research agenda. *Annual Reviews Public Health*. 30:81–205

53. Boer, R., Zheng, Y., Overton, A., Ridgeway, G.K., Cohen, D.A. (2007) Neighborhood design and walking trips in ten U.S. metropolitan areas. *American Journal of Preventive Medicine*. 32(4):298–304.

54. Cummins, S., Petticrew, M., Higgins, C., Findlay, A., Sparks, L. (2005) Large scale food retailing as an intervention for diet and health: quasi-experimental evaluation of a natural experiment. *Journal of Epidemiology and Community Health*. 59(12):1035–1040.
55. Ogilvie, D., Mitchell, R., Mutrie, N., Petticrew, M., Platt, S. (2006) Evaluating health effects of transport interventions methodologic case study. *American Journal of Preventive Medicine*. 31(2):118–126.
56. Veerman, J.L., Barendregt, J.J., Mackenbach, J.P. (2006) The European Common Agricultural Policy on fruits and vegetables: exploring potential health gain from reform. *European Journal of Public Health*. 16(1):31–35.
57. Veerman, J.L., Barendregt, J.J., Mackenbach, J.P., Brug, J. (2006) Using epidemiological models to estimate the health effects of diet behaviour change: the example of tailored fruit and vegetable promotion. *Public Health Nutrition*. 9(4):415–420.
58. Morland, K., Diez Roux, A.V., Wing, S. (2006) Supermarkets, other food stores, and obesity: the atherosclerosis risk in communities study. *American Journal of Preventive Medicine*. 30(4):333–339.
59. Morland, K., Filomena, S. (2007) Disparities in the availability of fruits and vegetables between racially segregated urban neighbourhoods. *Public Health Nutrition*. 10(12):1481–1489.
60. Morland, K., Wing, S., Diez Roux, A., Poole, C. (2002) Neighborhood characteristics associated with the location of food stores and food service places. *American Journal of Preventive Medicine*. 22(1):23–29.
61. Morland, K.B., Evenson, K.R. (2009) Obesity prevalence and the local food environment. *Health and Place*. 15(2):491–495.
62. Morland, K., Wing, S., Diez Roux, A. (2002) The contextual effect of the local food environment on residents' diets: the atherosclerosis risk in communities study. *American Journal of Public Health*. 92(11):1761–1767.
63. Giskes, K., Van Lenthe, F.J., Brug, J., Mackenbach, J.P., Turrell, G. (2007) Socioeconomic inequalities in food purchasing: the contribution of respondent-perceived and actual (objectively measured) price and availability of foods. *Preventive Medicine*. 45(1):41–48.
64. Cummins, S., Macintyre, S. (2006) Food environments and obesity--neighbourhood or nation? *International Journal of Epidemiology*. 35(1):100–104.

14 Obesogenic Environments: Challenges and Opportunities

Seraphim Alvanides, Tim G. Townshend and Amelia A. Lake

14.1 Introduction

It is widely acknowledged that obesity is a social problem which has reached significant levels.[1] Interest in the relationship between the environment and obesity is not new,[2] but has gained recent momentum. However, evidence of this relationship is fragmentary and sometimes contradictory,[3] and as Chapter 13 has indicated, further progress is required, particularly in terms of developing theories and methods. UK rates of obesity are predicted to increase to half of the population by 2050.[4] Alongside this rise are associated increases in co-morbidities and health care costs.[5] While the Foresight report points to the 'normalisation' of overweight and obesity in our societies[4] the stakes are high if the rates of overweight and obesity are not reversed and this global obesity epidemic is not curbed.

It was proposed in Chapter 2 that a multifaceted approach to tackling obesity is needed and transdisciplinary working is urgently required. This edited volume has explored the influences that our surroundings have on factors such as food intake, physical activity and how people move within space and places. The chapters have discussed how our environment influences eating behaviours, physical activity levels and thereby energy balance, demonstrating that interdisciplinary working is crucial to this type of work. The book has illustrated that transdisciplinary working will become more common as health professionals work alongside planners, designers and policymakers to help design towns and cities which are healthy. In England, the cross-governmental strategy *Healthy Weights, Healthy Lives*[6] demonstrates how professionals and practitioners can work together in such a context to tackle the obesity epidemic. In this final chapter, we conclude the book focusing on three main strands that have been addressed: complexities, perceptions and objective measures, before suggesting future research and policy directions.

14.2 Complexities

Targets to address the obesity epidemic should be seen in the light of significant increases in obesity during the last two decades and overwhelming projections for the next four decades.[5] The complexity of obesity determinants have been illustrated in the Foresight systems map[7] and discussed in Chapters 1 and 2 of this volume. Many developed countries (and increasingly a number of developing countries) are now realising the size of the epidemic, its human impact and the economic cost on public health spending. There are promising developments, however. In England, for example, cross-government strategies and interventions are being developed, which take a more holistic perspective:

- *Life-course*: from children's early years to England's 'change4life' campaign[8]
- *Cross-sectional*: targeting different socio-economic groups
- *Geographical*: from local strategies within local authorities to the cross-government research and surveillance plan for England[6]

Such initiatives acknowledge the complexity of obesity and obesogenic environments and they are likely to result in policy interventions that shift from individual-level behaviours to population-level changes.[9] This collective volume has presented ample evidence on the complexity of obesogenic environments and suggested ways forward in addressing this complexity from a wide range of perspectives.

Starting with the complexities surrounding sedentary versus active lifestyles, Chapters 3, 4, 8 and 9 are in general agreement: there are strong links between availability (and accessibility) of environmental resources and increased physical activity levels. These supportive environments can be at the micro-scale of neighbourhood design (Chapter 3), at the broader scale, encouraging walking for recreation or physical activity (Chapters 4 and 9) or city scale and beyond, facilitating active travel within a broader mobility and transportation setting (Chapter 8). Measurement issues and constraints aside (discussed later in this chapter), there are problems with definitions of accessibility and provision both in terms of geographical distance (very local against city-wide and beyond) and in terms of availability of such resources (perceived against objective measures of access). Chapter 4 highlighted the limitations to how much our immediate or 'physical environment' can provide by way of opportunities for physical activity. While Chapter 3 illustrated that local environments can, and should, provide for physical activity. Chapter 3 also suggested ways forward in researching the contribution of urban design to tackling obesity. In addition, Chapter 8 made a compelling case for developing major policy initiatives and developing infrastructure that encourages active travel, such as walking and cycling, at the population level.

The environment appears to be a strong determinant for physical activity levels amongst children and youth on both sides of the Atlantic, as discussed in Chapters 6, 7 and 9. This influence takes place both indoors (home, school) and outdoors (from the immediate neighbourhood to the wider community, and the open space of nearby parks, recreation grounds, playing fields, town and city squares). With the progress in geospatial technologies such as Geographical Information Systems (GISs) and Geographical Positioning Systems (GPSs), the tools for collecting evidence, measuring and analysing such complex environments and environmental exposures are constantly evolving, as described in Chapters 5 and 6. However, children and young people are also constrained in their mobilities and influenced in their choices by parental preferences, fears and concerns, as demonstrated in Chapter 7. As definitions and measures of accessibility are better operationalised (Chapter 5) and geospatial technologies provide the means to collect such data (Chapter 6), there is further scope for implementing longitudinal studies to assess the quality, safety access and use of physical environment features and monitor their impact on physical activity and, potentially, obesity (Chapter 13).

The relationship between the food environment and obesity has been described as a relatively new field of research.[10] As highlighted by Chapter 11, while eating is a 'relatively simple act', why we eat what we eat is determined through a rather complex process. Our foodscape is constantly evolving and changing which is well illustrated by Pearce and Day's longitudinal perspective in Chapter 12. The complex association between neighbourhood food availability and deprivation has significant global differences (discussed also in Chapter 10). Regardless of the contradicting evidence, this evolving 'socio-spatial distribution' of food requires further investigation, particularly in relating individual intake of food to the foods available. Measuring the food environment, both at the macro- and micro-scale, and relating individual behaviours to the food environment require well-developed techniques and present methodological challenges. The importance of policy in determining what foods are available to purchase in our retail outlets is emphasised in Chapter 11.

14.3 Perceptions

The focus in this volume has been on environmental determinants of obesity. Chapters have explored social and physical environmental influences augmented by perceptions around availability, accessibility and affordability, in terms of food consumption and physical activity. Individuals' perceptions of their bodies have not been explicitly addressed in this volume, although it can be argued that social and cultural environments may also affect people's perceptions of themselves.[11] A number of chapters discussed how availability and affordability, alongside personal attributes such as income, gender and social background can influence the way in which we perceive our environments. Such perceptions play a major role in shaping what we consume and utilise, as food, services and recreation facilities. Ultimately, if individuals perceive the healthier goods and services as inaccessible, unavailable or unaffordable, they are more likely to opt for the non-healthy options. A number of chapters in this volume demonstrated that our social and physical environment can be a strong determinant in encouraging, supporting and sustaining healthy behaviours via induced perceptions.

Starting with the conceptual aspects surrounding perceptions, Chapter 4 explicitly addressed the distinction between availability and accessibility in relation to physical activity. Chapter 10 established how physical and economic environmental exposures influence perceptions of food environments and affect eating behaviours. The theoretical and conceptual models discussed in these chapters are supported by evidence from other contributions within two broad strands: physical activity and food environments. In terms of encouraging and increasing physical activity, Chapter 3 provided further evidence on the role of neighbourhood design and walkability, Chapter 8 discussed perceptions of the built environment in supporting active travel and Chapter 9 highlighted the role of greenspace (whether natural or 'designed') in encouraging healthy behaviour and improving quality of life. Chapter 7 complements the physical activity strand with evidence from the United States and suggestions for improving the environment for youth physical activity. Although Chapters 6 and 7 focus on children and young people, most of the environmental interventions can encourage active travel and physical activity for other sections of the population, as argued in Chapters 3, 8 and 9. Conversely, the perceived dangers of walking/cycling, limited access to greenspace and quality of public transport discourage many from leading active lifestyles, at all life stages.

Longitudinal evidence indicates that there is now increased opportunity to purchase food, compared with the past. Chapter 11 describes the increase in opportunities to purchase food over the last 20 years in England[12] and Pearce and Day (Chapter 12) illustrated similar increases in New Zealand between 1966 and 2005. In Chapter 10, Ball et al. question *which* environment should be measured, the subjective (perceived) or the objective. They use the example of Giskes et al.[13] whose study in Brisbane, Australia, found that perceived availability and prices of recommended foods in supermarkets were associated with the purchase of these foods. Conversely, objectively assessed availability and prices were not associated with purchases.

14.4 Objective measures

In order to fully comprehend the complexities of obesity,[7] researchers, practitioners and governing bodies need adequate evidence to facilitate policies, implement interventions and monitor their impact. It is important, however, to go beyond simplistic descriptions of variables and generic observation of trends. This can only be achieved by developing sophisticated instruments and measures that accurately reflect the environment and individual behaviours within this environment. The objective measures described in Chapters 3–6, 10 and 12 of this volume provide further evidence towards understanding the physical activity and food environments and their complexities.

Despite methodological progress with instrument definitions and technological advances in data collection tools (such as those illustrated in Chapters 4 and 6), there is still a conceptual gap between appropriate measures (e.g. perceived against objective) and broader methodological issues (e.g. cross-sectional against longitudinal designs). For example, many studies identify and measure either subjective or objective instances of the physical activity environment, but hardly any studies address them together, as discussed in Chapters 4, 6, 7 and 9. Similar limitations apply to food environments, where perceptions of access to food are usually examined in isolation to food availability and retailing opportunities, illustrated in Chapters 10 and 12. There is still some way in identifying which factors influence obesity and combining them effectively into objective measures that reflect accurately the food and physical activity environments.

Earlier in this volume, Chapter 3 made a compelling case by identifying limitations of current research approaches, study designs and suggesting ways for advancing the physical activity agenda. Taking this further, Chapter 13 revisited the limitations of research designs in addressing the complexity of obesogenic environments, and proposed innovative ways of researching nutrition and physical activity. These lines of thought are in accordance with the recommendations proposed by a work group convened to determine the future directions for measures of obesogenic environments.[14] In addition to developing standards and objective measures for the surveillance of obesity and its environmental determinants, the chapters of this volume are in agreement that we need to understand the relationships between perceived and objective measures. This can be achieved by conceptualising theoretical frameworks and aligning them with appropriate research designs, such as longitudinal studies and natural experiments.[14]

14.5 Future directions

A number of chapters in this volume demonstrated how the environments we inhabit can encourage sedentary lifestyles and unhealthy choices. Most chapters have suggested ways forward in understanding the complex nature of obesity and its determinants, our perceptions of the environment and the ways we can employ objective measures. In parallel with other global challenges (e.g. climate change), obesity can only be tackled by aligning the various agendas and seeking opportunities to tackle it at all levels. At the individual-level, the challenge is to effect changes on lifestyles and behaviours that can be sustained across the lifecourse. Such changes should tackle both sides of the obesity equation, by reducing the excess of energy intake and by increasing physical activity. The Foresight report highlighted that in Britain today, being overweight is the norm and that 'Britain is now becoming an obese society' (p. 20).[4] In order to prevent obesity and tackle this societal problem we need to make 'the default option the healthy choice', as argued by McKinnon *et al.* (p. 356).[9] Such a fundamental change will require coordinated policies and interventions, based on solid evidence, adequate measurement and continuous monitoring of obesity and its potential determinants.

The challenge of improving our environment to promote healthier choices presents the research community with an opportunity for transdisciplinary research. Exploring this complex issue from different research and policy perspectives, rather than approaching such a complex problem from disciplinary silos, has been discussed in Chapter 2. Tackling environmental influences on individual behaviours is an opportunity for government departments and international organisations to develop cross-government policies, beyond the current focus on the economic costs of obesity, and to facilitate the conditions in which healthy choices become the default option.[14]

References

1. Lake, A.A., Townshend, T. (2006) Obesogenic environments: exploring the built and food environments. *The Journal of the Royal Society for the Promotion of Health*. 126(6):262–267.
2. Jones, A., Bentham, G., Foster, C., Hillsdon, M., Panter, J. *Obesogenic Environments Evidence Review: Foresight Tackling Obesities: Future Choices Project*, London, Government Office for Science, 2007.
3. Townshend, T., Lake, A.A. (2009) Obesogenic urban form: theory, policy and practice. *Health & Place*. 15(4):909–916.
4. Foresight. *Tackling Obesities: Future Choices – Project Report*. 2nd Edition, London, Government Office for Science, 2007, available from http://www.foresight.gov.uk.
5. McPherson, K., Marsh, K., Brown, M. (2007) Modelling future trends in obesity and the impact on health. *Foresight Tackling Obesities: Future Choices*. 2nd Edition.
6. Department of Health. *Healthy Weight, Healthy Lives: A Cross-government Research and Surveillance Plan for England*. London, Department of Health, 2008.
7. Vandenbroeck, P., Goossens, J., Clemens, M. (2007) Foresight tackling obesities: future choices – building the obesity system map.
8. National Health Service (NHS). Change4Life, available from http://www.nhs.uk/change4life. Accessed February 2010
9. McKinnon, R.A., Orleans, C.T., Kumanyika, S.K., Haire-Joshu, D., Krebs-Smith, S.M., Finkelstein, E.A., Brownell, K.D., Thompson, J.W., Ballard-Barbash, R. (2009) Considerations for an obesity policy research agenda. *The American Journal of Preventive Medicine*. 36(4):351–357.
10. McKinnon, R.A., Reedy, J., Morrissette, M.A., Lytle, L.A., Yaroch, A.L. (2009) Measures of the food environment: a compilation of the literature, 1990–2007. *The American Journal of Preventive Medicine*. 36(4, Suppl.):S124–S133.
11. Hopkins, P.E. (2008) Critical geographies of body size. *Geography Compass*. 2(6): 2111–2126.
12. Burgoine, T., Lake, A.A., Stamp, E., Alvanides, S., Mathers, J.C., Adamson, A.J. (2009) Changing foodscapes 1980–2000, using the ASH30 study. *Appetite*. 53(2):157–165.
13. Giskes, K., Van Lenthe, F.J., Brug, J., Mackenbach, J.P., Turrell, G. (2007) Socioeconomic inequalities in food purchasing: the contribution of respondent-perceived and actual (objectively measured) price and availability of foods. *Preventive Medicine*. 45(1):41–48.
14. Story, M., Giles-Corti, B., Yaroch, A.L., Cummins, S., Frank, L.D., Huang, T.T.-K., Lewis, L.B. (2009) Work Group IV: future directions for measures of the food and physical activity environments. *The American Journal of Preventive Medicine*. 36(4, Suppl.):S182–S188.

Index